Childhood Brain & Spinal Cord Tumors

A Guide for Families, Friends & Caregivers

Second Edition

Tania Shiminski-Maher
Catherine Woodman
Nancy Keene

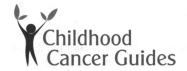

Childhood
Cancer Guides

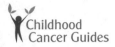
Childhood
Cancer Guides

Childhood Brain & Spinal Cord Tumors: A Guide for Families, Friends & Caregivers, Second Edition

by Tania Shiminski-Maher, Catherine Woodman, and Nancy Keene

Published by Childhood Cancer Guides, P.O. Box 31937, Bellingham, WA 98228.

Printed in the United States of America.

Printing History:
2001: First Edition

For information about special discounts for bulk purchases, please contact Independent Publishers Group Special Sales at specialmarkets@ipgbook.com.

ISBN 978-1-9410-8900-2

Library of Congress Control Number: 2014930516

 This book uses RepKover™, a durable and flexible lay-flat binding.

To our children—Abe, Alison, Emily, Ethan, Jake, Kathryn, Tucker

and

To all children with brain or spinal cord tumors—past, present, and future—and
those who love them

Table of Contents

Foreword

THE DIAGNOSIS OF a brain or spinal cord tumor in a child generates an extraordinary amount of pain, suffering, and turmoil in a family. The pain is compounded by the almost universal belief in the lay community that a child with a brain or spinal cord tumor has no hope of cure. Accordingly, the family is thrust into a torrent of emotion that makes it difficult to proceed in a calm and calculated fashion. Upon diagnosis, a family likely does not have the knowledge base required to address all of the different issues: how to cope with procedures and hospitalization, how to work in a positive fashion with the healthcare team, and how to deal with the intricacies of different treatment options.

This newly revised book fills an extraordinary void for parents whose child has been diagnosed with a brain or spinal cord tumor. Written in comprehensive and straightforward prose, it gives family members virtually everything they need to know in order to deal with this frightening diagnosis. It provides a framework for them to understand all of the issues they will face on the path from diagnosis through treatment and beyond.

A review of the table of contents in this book shows the remarkable breadth of information available to the reader. Parents are introduced to the kind of tumor their child might have and offered help with understanding procedures that can be frightening to the child and family members alike. They are taught how to work creatively with the healthcare team and, when necessary, to make a change. They are introduced to the major modalities used to treat a child with a brain or spinal cord tumor. Additionally, it covers equally critical issues that are rarely discussed with a family in a clinical setting and are poorly detailed in the literature, such as how to deal with schools; how to find additional support for the family; and how to deal with either the joy or fear at the end of treatment. It is also full of moving stories from children with brain tumors and their families.

This book is a gift and a welcome addition to the field of pediatric neuro-oncology. It will help countless families and healthcare providers learn all the ramifications of diagnosing a brain or spinal cord tumor in a child and the incredible turmoil that is subsequently experienced by the family. This book should be on the shelf of every healthcare professional who deals with children with brain and spinal cord tumors and should be made available to every family that has a child diagnosed with a brain or spinal cord tumor.

— Henry S. Friedman, MD
Deputy Director, The Preston Robert Tisch Brain Tumor Center
James B. Powell, Jr., Professor of Neuro-Oncology
Professor of Pediatrics
Duke University Medical Center
Durham, North Carolina

Introduction

We are all in the same boat, in a stormy sea,
and we owe each other a terrible loyalty.
— G. K. Chesterton

Tania Shiminski-Maher, a nurse practitioner, has worked for more than 30 years with children and teens who have brain and spinal cord tumors. Catherine Woodman's son Ethan is a long-term (12 years) survivor of medulloblastoma who is currently in college. She is also a psychiatrist who works at a major medical center. Nancy Keene's daughter, diagnosed at age 3 with high-risk acute lymphoblastic leukemia, is now a 25 year old out in the working world. We understand that nothing prepares a parent for the utter devastation of having a child diagnosed with cancer. We have walked the path from that life-changing moment through information gathering, treatment, rehabilitation, and management of late effects. We know that fear and worry are lessened by having accurate information and hearing the stories of other children and families who have walked the path before us. And we are honored to share with you what we and many other parents and healthcare providers have learned.

What this book offers

This book is not autobiographical. Instead, we wanted to blend basic technical information in easy-to-understand language with stories and advice from many parents and children. We wanted to provide the insights and experiences of parents who have all felt the hope, helplessness, anger, humor, longing, panic, ignorance, warmth, and anguish of their children's treatment for a brain or spinal cord tumor. We wanted parents to know how other children react to treatment, and we wanted to offer tips to make the experience easier.

Obtaining a basic understanding of topics such as medical terminology, common side effects of treatment, and how to interpret laboratory results can help improve quality of life for the whole family. Learning how to develop a partnership with your child's doctor can vastly increase your family's peace of mind. Hearing parents describe their own emotional ups and downs, how they coped, and how they molded their family life around hospitalizations is a tremendous comfort. And knowing there are other family members out there who hold their breath with each observation scan hoping for stable results can help you feel less alone. Our hope is that parents who read this book will find understandable medical information, obtain advice that eases their daily life, and feel empowered to be strong advocates for their children.

The parent stories and suggestions in this book are absolutely true, although some names have been changed to protect children's privacy. Every word has been spoken by the parent of a child with cancer, a sibling of a child with cancer, or a childhood cancer survivor. There are no composites, no editorializing, and no rewrites—just the actual words of people who wanted to share what they learned with families of children newly diagnosed with a brain or spinal cord tumor.

How this book is organized

We have organized the book sequentially in an attempt to parallel most families' journeys through treatment. We all start with diagnosis, then learn about the tumor and its treatment, try to cope with procedures, adjust to medical personnel, and deal with family and friends. We all seek out various methods of support and struggle with the strong feelings felt by of our child with a brain or spinal cord tumor, our other children, and ourselves. We try to work with our child's school to provide the richest and most appropriate education for our ill child. And, unfortunately, we sometimes must grieve, either for our child or for the child of a close friend we have made in our new community of families dealing with brain tumors.

Because it is tremendously hard to focus on learning new things when you are emotionally battered and extremely tired, we have tried to keep each chapter short. The first time we introduce a medical term, we define it in the text. Because both boys and girls get brain and spinal cord tumors, we did not adopt the common convention of using only masculine personal pronouns (e.g., he, him). We do not like using he/she, so we alternated personal pronouns (e.g., she, he) within chapters. This may seem awkward as you read, but it prevents half of the parents from feeling that the text does not apply to their child.

All the medical information contained in this second edition of *Childhood Brain & Spinal Cord Tumors* is current as of 2013. As treatment is constantly evolving and improving, there will inevitably be changes. For example, the technology that supports surgery and radiation treatments continues to improve. Scientists are currently studying some new medications and genetically determined responses to specific drugs that may dramatically improve treatments. You will learn in this book how to discover the newest and most appropriate treatments for your child. However, this book should not be used as a substitute for professional medical care.

We have included four appendices for reference: blood tests and what they mean; resource organizations; books and websites; and a cancer survivor's treatment record that should be filled out at the end of treatment. This personal summary of treatment can be used to educate all future healthcare providers about the types of treatment your child received and the follow-up schedule necessary to stay healthy.

How to use this book

While conducting research for this book, we were repeatedly told by parents to "write the truth." Because the "truth" varies for each person, more than 100 parents, children with brain or spinal cord tumors, and their siblings share portions of their experiences. This book is full of these snapshots in time, some of which may be hard to read, especially by families of newly diagnosed children. Here are our suggestions for a positive way to use the information contained in this book:

• Read the last chapter first. Many children survive and it helps to read their stories.

• Consider reading only the sections that apply to the present or the immediate future. Even if your child's prognosis indicates a high probability of cure, reading about recurrence or bereavement can be emotionally difficult.

• Realize that only a fraction of the problems that parents describe will affect your child. Every child is different; every child sails smoothly through some portions of treatment but encounters difficulties during others. The more you understand the variability of cancer experiences, the better you will be able to cope with your own situation, as well as be a good listener and helpful friend to other families you meet with differing diagnoses and circumstances.

• Take any concerns or questions that arise to your neuro-oncologist and/or nurse practitioner for answers. The more you learn, the better you can advocate for your child.

• Share this book with family and friends. Usually they desperately want to help and just don't know how. This book not only explains the disease and treatment but also offers dozens of concrete suggestions for family and friends.

If you want to delve into any topic in greater depth, Appendix C, *Books and Websites,* is a good place to start. It contains a list of reputable websites and an extensive list of books for parents and children of all ages. Reading tastes are very individual, so if something suggested in the appendix is not helpful or upsets you, put it down. You will probably find something else on the list that is more appropriate for you.

Best wishes for a smooth journey through treatment and a bright future for your entire family.

Acknowledgments

This book is truly a collaborative effort: without the help of many, it would simply not exist. We give heartfelt thanks to our families and friends who supported us along the way. Special thanks to our editor, Sarah Farmer, for her excellent editorial skills as well as humor, patience, tact, and honesty when needed. Thanks to Alison Leake, who used her eagle eye to copyedit the book, despite her busy work schedule. She did a great job! Special thanks to Susan Jarmolowski for making the interior design, layout, and cover gorgeous. We so appreciate the help of Gigi McMillan who updated Appendix B and Patty Feist who sent in lots of suggestions for books to add to Appendix C. Henry Friedman, MD, graciously took time from his busy schedule to update his Foreword. Thank you! Special thanks also to George Jallo, MD, for his help with the scans used for illustrations. We deeply appreciate all of you for helping make this a comprehensive, up-to-date resource for families of children with brain and spinal cord tumors and those who love them.

We send many thanks and much appreciation to two co-authors of the first edition of this book—Maria Sansalone and Patsy Cullen. Maria gathered stories from her friends in the brain tumor community that captured so many of the experiences and emotions of each member of their family. And Patsy drew from her 30 years of experience caring for children with brain tumors, conducting research to improve outcomes, and teaching the next generation of caregivers.

Both editions of this book are true collaborations between families of children with brain and spinal cord tumors and medical professionals. Many well-known and respected members of the pediatric oncology community, members of national organizations, and parents carved time out of their busy schedules to review chapters, make invaluable suggestions, and catch errors. We especially appreciate the patient and thoughtful responses to our many emails and phone calls. Thank you: Jeffrey C. Allen, MD; Diane Barounis, MSW, LCSW; Roberta Calhoun, ACSW; Deb Civello, RN, MA, CPON; Cass Cooney, MSN, PNP; Jillann Demes, MSW, LSW; Geri Jo Duda, RN; Fred Epstein, MD; Henry Friedman, MD; Russ Geyer, MD; Sharon Grandinette, MS, Ed; Deneen Hesser, RN, BS, OCN; George Jallo, MD; Larry Kun, MD; Laurie D. Leigh, MA; Mary Lovely, PhD, RN; Maureen McCarthy, BSCCS, Child Life Specialist; Tobey J. MacDonald, MD; Paul McKay; Gigi McMillan; Al Musella, DPM; Rosanna Ricafort, MD; Elizabeth A. Seay; Yvonne Soghomonian, RN; Nancy J. Tarbell, MD; Kathy Warren, MD; Sheri White; and Jeanne Young, BA.

More than words can express, we are deeply grateful to the parents, children with brain and spinal cord tumors, their siblings, and others who generously opened their hearts and relived their pain while sharing their experiences with us. To all of you whose words form the heart and soul of the book, thank you: Kathleen A. Barry; Cynthia Baumann-Retalic, mom of Kevin; Kathleen Bell; Kathy Bucher; Nancy Bullard, mother of three incredible young women; Tonya M. Burwell; Ricky Carroll; Angie M. Cheeks; Patricia V. Christiansen, mom to John V. Christiansen; Deb Civello; Lisa M. Clark, Christopher's mom; Mary Beth Collins; Maureen Colvin; Cheryl Coutts, proud mom of Morgan; Karen Covell, mother of two wonder boys, Christopher and Cameron; Grace Coville-McKenna; Aimee Dion Crisanti; Melissa and Andrew Croom; Renee Curkendall; Evan Darlington; Carol Dean, Mandy's mom; Lucindy M. DeLuca; Wade Demmert, proud dad of Mandy; Cynthia Diaz; Laura Duty, mother of Benjamin Duty; Sharon Eaton, Super "T's" mom; Sarah Farmer; Wes and Vicki Fleming; Tracy Flinders; Colette Gelman; Drew Head, father of Alissa; Cindy Herb and son Michael; Kellie Hicks; Shawn Honohan; Linda Horvat; Debbie Hoskin; Mary L. Hubbell; Margie Huhner, mom to Anna; George Hunter; Marcia Jacobs, angel Anjulie's mommy; Jenny Jardine; Darlene Behrend Jones; Larry Junck, MD; Susan Junghans, mother of angel David; Carolyn, mother of Paul Kazakos; Jan Klooster, mother of Dan Steven; Kathy Knight; C.J. Korenek; Louise and John Lamp, parents of Victoria; Missy Layfield; Debbie Lentini; Aidan Leslie; Melanie Logan and son, Darren Klawinski; Rachel Lourie; Christina McCarter; Maureen A. McCarthy; Danielle McCauley; Gillian McGovern; Alannah, Susan, and Paul McKay; Gigi McMillan; Susan Milliken; Katy Moffitt, proud mom of angel Jessica Ann Moffitt; Berendina Norton; Sandra M. Norton; Lauren Ott, RN; Josie and Kylie Pace; MaryJo Palermo-Kirsch, Kevin's momma; Stephanie Paul, proud mother of Derick Corey; Jane Peppler, mother of Ezra Farber; Diane Robinson Phillips; Robin and Emily Pierce; David Rank; Jim and Sally Reeves, parents of Jordan; Kris Riley, mom of Matt; Alison C. Roberto; Dona M. Ross; Ruth Sansalone; Carole-Lynn Saros; Kelly Saunders, mom to Hunter Goodon; Mindy Schwartz, Mikey's mom; Elizabeth A. Seay; Lee D. Smolen; Carol J. Sorsdahl; Anne Spurgeon; Loice Swisher, mother of Victoria Middleton; Trish Telcik; Bob Thomas and Megan Thomas; Terra Trevor; Denise Turek, mom to Jen; Sheri White; Catherine Woodman; Janie, Megan's Mom; Marcey, mom to Madison; Mark, father of Deli; Mark, loving husband of Janet; and those who wish to remain anonymous.

Thank you also to Nancy Keene and Honna Janes-Hodder for sharing their words. Some of the text for this book comes from their books for families of children with cancer: *Childhood Leukemia: A Guide for Family, Friends, and Caregivers, 4th edition* by Nancy Keene, and *Childhood Cancer: A Parent's Guide to Solid Tumor Cancers, 2nd edition* by Honna Janes-Hodder and Nancy Keene.

Despite the inspiration and contributions of so many, any errors, omissions, misstatements, or flaws in the book are entirely our own.

Chapter 1

Diagnosis

A journey of a thousand leagues begins with a single step.
— Lao-tzu

"WE HAVE THE RESULTS OF THE SCAN BACK; I'm afraid it's bad news. Your child has a tumor." For every parent who has heard those words, it is a moment frozen in time. In one shattering instant, life forever changes. Families are forced into a strange new world that feels like an emotional roller coaster ride in the dark. Strong emotions will batter every member of the family. However, with time and the knowledge that many children survive childhood brain and spinal cord tumors, hope will grow.

Signs and symptoms

The brain and spinal cord make up the central nervous system (CNS). These organs coordinate all of the functions necessary for life, including breathing, regulating heart rate, thinking, and moving. Tumors of the brain and spinal cord begin with the transformation of a single cell. This renegade cell reproduces, creating more abnormal cells. Eventually, this collection of abnormal cells forms a tumor in the brain or spinal cord. The location of the tumor (also called a mass), its rate of growth, and the associated swelling determine the signs and symptoms that develop in a child. Chapter 3, *Types of Tumors,* provides in-depth descriptions of the various types of brain and spinal cord tumors.

Parents are usually the first to notice that something is wrong with their child. Occasionally, a pediatrician notices a problem during a well-baby visit, or the tumor is discovered by chance on a scan or other test. Unfortunately, some of the signs and symptoms of brain and spinal cord tumors mimic common childhood illnesses, which can make diagnosis difficult.

The following are some of the signs and symptoms that may indicate the presence of a childhood brain tumor:

- Headaches (often with early morning vomiting)
- Dizziness

- Seizures (convulsions)
- Staring spells
- Loss of peripheral vision
- Double vision
- Nystagmus (jiggling of an eyeball from side to side)
- Inability to look up
- One eye turns inward or outward
- Weakness in hands on one or both sides of the body
- Unsteady gait
- Change in speech
- Trouble swallowing
- Drowsiness
- Facial drooping or asymmetry
- Nausea relieved by vomiting
- Hormonal or growth problems
- Hearing loss
- Changes in appetite or thirst
- Behavior changes
- Change in school performance

The following are signs and symptoms that may indicate the presence of a spinal cord tumor in a child:

- Back or neck pain, which may awaken the child from sleep
- Scoliosis (curvature of the spine, resulting in leaning of shoulders to one side or a noticeable hump in the back)
- Torticollis (tilting of the head and upper spine to one side)
- Weakness or sensory changes in arms or legs
- Changes in bowel and bladder control

These symptoms can be present for a long or short period of time, depending on the location and growth rate of the tumor. A child with a brain or spinal cord tumor usually has more than one symptom.

Most parents react to their concerns by taking their child to a doctor. Sometimes the symptoms are attributed to a normal childhood illness, and parents bring their child in for more visits before a brain tumor is suspected. This is easier to understand when you consider that, in their entire careers, most pediatricians see only one or two children with brain or spinal cord tumors. Ultimately, the doctor orders a scan or refers the child to a specialist, such as a pediatric neurologist, for further tests (see Chapter 6, *Coping with Procedures.*)

> *Alannah was 4 years old when she was diagnosed with a brainstem glioblastoma. On December 23, my daughter's school called my wife to have her pick up Alannah because she had vomited, although she appeared fine afterward.*
>
> *On Christmas Eve, Alannah woke up, and after playing for awhile, began complaining of a headache. We assumed she had picked up some sort of virus at her school. Later that day, we went to my parents' house for a traditional Christmas Eve gathering. Alannah began having trouble walking, and appeared to be looking at everything with her eyes shifted to the left. We laid her down in the guest room and a few minutes later, she threw up again. We still figured that we were dealing with a "bug," so we cleaned her up and went home. The following morning, she seemed fine except that her eyes were still fixed to the left. Later in the day, she started to have trouble with her balance and walking again. We took her to our local urgent care, still expecting to be told that she had a virus.*
>
> *First, she was examined by a nurse practitioner. After checking Alannah's eyes, she quickly called in the doctor on duty. After a brief examination, he told me that he wanted to send her to the hospital by ambulance for a CT [computed tomography] scan. He said that while it might be a virus affecting her brain, he wanted the scan done to be sure that nothing else was wrong. Once we arrived at the hospital, several doctors examined Alannah. After waiting for about 2 hours, the CT scan was performed. Shortly thereafter, the physician called my wife and I out of the room and showed us the scan. She showed us what she called a "mass" on Alannah's brainstem, and told us that she would admit Alannah to the hospital and order an MRI. After another couple of hours in the ER we were transferred to a room on the fifth floor, in shock and disbelief, waiting for them to discover their mistake, and send us home.*

The diagnosis of a brain or spinal cord tumor is sometimes not as quick as Alannah's:

> *The first signs were so subtle: the slight but constant inward turn of our son's left eye became apparent to us within the first few months of life. By the time he was 7 months old, we were concerned enough to bring it to our pediatrician's attention. He felt it was just normal uncoordinated eye movement. Every well-baby visit we brought the same problem to his attention. When our son was a year old, we were finally referred to an eye specialist—a pediatric ophthalmologist. Another year of visits began: the specialist insisted his eye was fine. We were just as certain the*

eye wasn't right, and we thought we could now see the eyeball jiggling. Then the ophthalmologist referred us to a pediatric orthoptist at a local Lions' Club clinic. She listened to our concerns, examined our son's eyes, and wrote a letter for our pediatrician verifying the abnormalities. Based on her report, our pediatrician agreed to schedule an MRI. Our son was 2 years and 2 months old by the time he was diagnosed with a moderately large optic glioma.

Where should your child receive treatment?

After tentatively diagnosing a brain or spinal cord tumor, most physicians refer the child to the closest major medical center with expertise in treating children with brain and spinal cord tumors. It is very important that your child is treated at a facility that has a full complement of specialists who are experienced in treating children with cancer, who know the latest treatment and research advances, and who work together as a team on behalf of your child. An effective treatment team will include pediatric oncologists, neurosurgeons, radiation oncologists, pathologists, pediatric nurse practitioners, child life specialists, rehabilitation specialists, education specialists, psychologists, and social workers. Institutions that specialize in treating children with brain and spinal cord tumors will provide state-of-the-art treatment, offering your child the best chance for cure.

> *Just after surgery, a number of doctors came by and introduced themselves as members of our team. At first, I was startled to learn that a radiation oncologist had been assigned to us, because radiation was not part of our son's current treatment plan. But then she explained that each member of the team would see us whenever we came to the children's hospital pediatric brain tumor clinic. I feel better knowing our child isn't an unknown quantity to these specialists, in case we ever do need them.*

Physical responses

Many parents become physically ill in the weeks following diagnosis. This is not surprising, given that most parents stop eating or grab only fast food, have trouble sleeping, and are exposed to all sorts of illness while staying in the hospital. Every waking moment is filled with excruciating emotional stress, which makes the physical stress much more potent.

> *Our daughter had many strong seizures while in the hospital, and my stomach would churn. I'd have to leave the bedside when the nurse would come to help. I had almost uncontrollable diarrhea. Every new stressful event just dissolved my gut; I could feel it happening.*

To try to prevent illness, it is helpful to try to eat nutritious meals, get a break from your child's bedside to take a walk outdoors, and find time to sleep. Care needs to be taken not to overuse drugs or alcohol in an attempt to control anxiety or cope with grief. Although physical illnesses usually end or improve after a period of adjustment, emotional stress often continues throughout treatment.

Emotional responses

The shock of diagnosis results in an overwhelming number of intense emotions. Cultural background, individual coping styles, basic temperament, and family dynamics all affect an individual's emotional response to stress. There are no set stages of response, and parents frequently find themselves vacillating from one emotional extreme to another. Many of these emotions reappear at different times during the child's treatment. All of the emotions described below are normal responses to a diagnosis of cancer in a child.

Children's and teens' emotional responses to diagnosis are discussed in Chapter 17, *Communication and Behavior.*

Confusion and numbness

In their anguish, most parents remember only bits and pieces of the doctor's early explanations of their child's disease. This dreamlike state is an almost universal response to shock. The brain provides protective layers of numbness and confusion to prevent emotional overload. This allows parents to examine information in smaller, less-threatening pieces. Pediatric neurosurgeons and oncologists understand this phenomenon and are usually quite willing to repeat information as often as necessary. Many centers have nurse practitioners, physician assistants, and nurses who translate medical information into understandable language and answer questions. Do not be embarrassed to say you do not understand or that you forgot something you were told. It is sometimes helpful to write down instructions and explanations, record them on a small tape recorder or smartphone, or ask a friend or family member to help keep track of all the new and complex information.

> When I left the doctor's office, I was a mass of hysteria. I couldn't breathe and felt as if I was suffocating. Tears were flowing nonstop. I had lost total control of myself and had no idea of how to stop my world from turning upside down.
>
> • • • • •
>
> For a brief moment I stared at the doctor's face and felt totally confused by what he was explaining to me. In an instant that internal chaos was joined with a scream of terror that came from some place inside me that, up until that point, I never knew existed.

Denial

Denial is when parents cannot acknowledge what is happening to their child. Psychologically, they are unable to accept it. Parents simply cannot believe that their child has a life-threatening illness. Denial helps parents survive the first few days after diagnosis, but gradual acceptance must occur so the family can begin to make the necessary adjustments to treatment. Life has dramatically changed. When parents accept what has happened, understand their fears, and begin to hope, they will be better able to advocate for their child and their family.

> I walked into the empty hospital playroom and saw my wife clutching Matthew's teddy bear. Her eyes were red and swollen from crying. I had no idea what had happened. A minute later the doctor came into the room with several residents (doctors who are receiving specialized training after they completed medical school). He told me that Matthew had a tumor and that he was very sick. I remember thinking that there had to have been a mistake. Maybe he was reading the wrong chart? My initial reaction was that it was physically impossible for one of my children to have a tumor. Tumors only grow in the elderly. Kids don't get tumors!

Guilt

Guilt is a common and normal reaction to a diagnosis of a brain or spinal cord tumor. Parents sometimes feel they have failed to protect their child, and they blame themselves. It is especially difficult because the cause of their child's tumor, in most instances, cannot be explained. There are questions: How could we have prevented this? What did we do wrong? How did we miss the signs? Why didn't we bring her to the doctor sooner? Why didn't we insist that the doctor do a scan? Did he inherit this from me? Why didn't we live in a safer place? Was it because of the fumes from painting the house? Why? Why? Why? Nancy Roach describes some of these feelings in her booklet *The Last Day of April*:

> Almost as soon as Erin's illness was diagnosed, our self-recrimination began. What had we done to cause this illness? Was I careful enough during pregnancy? We knew radiation was a possible contributor; where had we taken Erin that she might have been exposed? I wondered about the toxic glue used in my advertising work or the silk screen ink used in my artwork. Bob questioned the fumes from some wood preservatives used in a project. We analyzed everything—food, fumes, and TV. Fortunately, most of the guilt feelings were relieved by knowledge and by meeting other parents whose children had been exposed to an entirely different environment.

It may be difficult to accept, but parents need to understand that they did nothing to cause their child's illness. Years of research have revealed little about what causes childhood brain and spinal cord tumors or what can be done to prevent them.

Fear and helplessness

Fear and helplessness are two faces of the same coin. Nearly everything about this new situation is unknown, and the only thing parents really do know—that their child has a life-threatening illness—is too terrifying to contemplate. Each new revelation about the situation raises new questions and fears: Can I really flush a catheter or administer all these drugs? What if I mess something up? Will my boss fire me if I miss too much work? Who will take care of my other children? How do I tell my child not to be afraid when he can see I am scared to death? How will we pay for this? The demands on parents' time, talents, energy, courage, and strength are daunting.

> I stood at the elevator bank in the basement of Children's Hospital waiting for the elevator, saying to all those around me: "I can't even say those words out loud! Come on everybody say it with me: My daughter has a brain tumor! A brain tumor! A b-r-a-i-n t-u-m-o-r! Now that we know how to spell it, let's say it over and over ... braintumorbraintumorbraintumorbraintumorbraintumor!" Needless to say, I'm sure all the docs, nurses, and patients who were standing there with me just chalked it up to my temporary insanity, shock, denial, and complete flip-out that I was going through.

A child's diagnosis instantaneously strips parents of control over many aspects of their lives and can change their entire world view. All the predictable and comforting routines are gone, and the family is thrust into a new world that is populated by an ever-changing cast of characters (interns, residents, fellows, pediatric oncologists, IV teams, nurses, and social workers); a new language (medical terminology); and seemingly endless hospitalizations, procedures, and drugs. This transition is especially hard on parents who are used to a measure of power and authority in their home or workplace.

> My husband had a difficult time after our son was diagnosed. We have a traditional marriage, and he was used to his role as provider and protector for the family. It was hard for him to deal with the fact that he couldn't fix everything.

Until adjustment begins, parents sometimes feel utterly helpless. Physicians they have never met are presenting treatment options for their child. Even if parents are comfortable in a hospital environment, feelings of helplessness may develop because there is simply not enough time in the day to care for a very sick child, deal with their own changing emotions, educate themselves about the disease, notify friends and family, make job decisions, and restructure the family schedule to deal with the crisis. The sense of helplessness often diminishes as parents gain a better understanding of the new environment and accept it as their new reality.

> It's not a nice way to have to live. What's waiting around the next corner? That's a scary question. One of my biggest fears is the uncertainty of the future. All that we can do is the best we can and hope that it's enough.

• • • • •

Sometimes I would feel incredible waves of absolute terror wash over me. The kind of fear that causes your breathing to become difficult and your heart to beat faster. While I would be consciously aware of what was happening, there was nothing I could do to stop it. It's happening sometimes very late at night, when I'm lying in bed, staring off into the darkness. It's so intense that for a brief moment, I try to comfort myself by thinking that it can't be real, because it's just too horrible. During those moments, these thoughts only offer a second or two of comfort. Then I become aware of just how wide my eyes are opened in the darkness.

Many parents explain that helplessness begins to disappear when a sense of reality returns. They begin to make decisions, study their options, learn about the disease, and become comfortable with the hospital and staff. As their knowledge grows, so does their ability to participate constructively as members of the treatment team. For further information, see Chapter 7, *Forming a Partnership with the Treatment Team.*

However, do not be surprised if feelings of fear, panic, and anxiety erupt unexpectedly throughout your child's treatment.

Anger

Anger is a common response to the diagnosis of a life-threatening illness. It is nobody's fault that children are stricken with brain and spinal cord tumors. Because parents cannot direct their anger at the cancer, they may target doctors, nurses, spouses, siblings, or even their ill child. Because anger directed at other people can be very destructive, it is necessary to find ways to express and manage the anger.

Life isn't fair, but yet the sun still comes up each morning. To be angry because your child has a brain tumor is normal. The question is where to direct that anger. Sometimes I feel as if I'm angry at the entire world. In my heart, though, my outrage is directed solely at each and every tumor cell feeding on my child.

Expressing anger is normal and can be cathartic. Trying to suppress this powerful emotion is usually not helpful. Some suggestions from parents for managing anger follow.

Anger at healthcare team:

- Try to improve communication with the doctors

- Discuss your feelings with one of the nurses or nurse practitioners

- Discuss your feelings with social workers

- Ask to meet with members of the various medical teams who are caring for your child to address or clarify communication issues

- Talk with parents of other ill children, either locally or by joining an online support group

Anger at family:

- Exercise a little every day
- Do yoga or relaxation exercises
- Keep a journal or tape-record your feelings
- Cry in the shower or pound a pillow
- Listen to music
- Read other people's stories about brain or spinal cord tumors
- Talk with friends
- Talk with parents of other ill children
- Join or start a support group
- Improve communication within the family
- Try individual or family counseling
- Live one moment at a time

Anger at God:

- Share your feelings with your spouse, partner, or close friends
- Discuss your feelings with clergy or church, synagogue, or mosque members
- Re-examine your faith
- Know that anger at God is normal
- Pray
- Give yourself time to heal

It is important to remember that angry feelings are normal and expected. Discovering healthy ways to cope with anger is vital for all parents.

Sadness and grief

No one is prepared to cope with the news that their child might die. Intense feelings of sorrow, loss, and grief are common, even when the prognosis is good. Parents often describe feeling engulfed by sadness. They fear they may simply not be able to deal with the enormity of the problems facing their family. Parents grieve the loss of normalcy and realize life will never be the same. They grieve the loss of their dreams and aspirations for their child. They may feel sorry for themselves and may feel ashamed and embarrassed by these feelings.

> *I have an overwhelming sadness and, unfortunately for me, that means feelings of helplessness. I wish I could muster up a fighting spirit, but I just can't right now.*

· · · · ·

> *While I have moments of deep sadness and despair, I try not to let them turn into hours and certainly not days. I am too aware of the fact that I may have the rest of my life to grieve.*

Parents also grieve the loss of the child they knew. Children who achieve remission or cure from a brain or spinal cord tumor often have permanent late effects from treatment. The loss of the child as he once was can be very difficult for all members of the family.

Parents travel a tumultuous emotional path where overwhelming emotions subside, only to resurface later. All of these are normal, common responses to a catastrophic event. For many parents, these strong emotions begin to become more manageable as hope grows.

Hope

After being buffeted by illness, anger, fear, sadness, grief, and guilt, most parents welcome the growth of hope. Hope is the belief in a better tomorrow. Hope sustains the will to live and gives the strength to endure each trial. Hope is not a way around, it is a way through. There is reason for hope.

Thirty-five years ago, very few children with brain or spinal cord tumors were cured. Technological advances, including computer-assisted surgical planning, advanced imaging techniques, newer chemotherapy drugs, and focused radiation therapies, have changed that. Additional research continues to develop new treatments using gene therapy and individual tumor targeted therapies. Over the last 4 decades, because of these advances, as well as research and participation in clinical trials (see Chapter 5, *Choosing a Treatment*), many children are now long-term survivors.

Families often discover a renewed sense of both the fragility and beauty of life after the diagnosis. Outpourings of love and support from family and friends provide comfort and sustenance. Many parents speak of a renewed appreciation for life and consider each day with their child as a precious gift.

> *When we were given the diagnosis of glioblastoma multiforme (GBM), it took time and layers of understanding before we could come to grips with everything. This whole concept of brain disease is so frightening and so surreal; it can't possibly be*

grasped in a few weeks. We realized that the adjustment wouldn't be made in a single step, but that we'd reach plateaus of "new normal" along the way. In other words, don't be surprised if you feel like you have a pretty good grip on things and then suddenly lose it one day. As with life as usual, some days will be better than others. If you feel deeply sad or completely overwhelmed one day, remind yourself that it's a mood like all the others in your repertoire, and there is an excellent reason for it, but in time you will feel better able to cope.

A Japanese proverb says: "Daylight will peep through a very small hole."

The immediate future

You are not alone. Many have traveled this path before you and they will share their wisdom and support with you. The next several chapters will help you understand your new reality and make the decisions you will face at each stage of your journey. In their own words, parents will explain the choices they made and how they adjusted, learned, and became active participants in their child's treatment. Sharing experiences with parents and survivors of childhood brain and spinal cord tumors may help your family develop its own unique strategy for coping with the challenges ahead.

A Mother's View

Memory is a funny thing. I'd be hard-pressed to remember what I had for dinner last night, but like many people, the day of the Challenger explosion and, even further back, the day of John Kennedy's death are etched in my mind to the smallest detail.

And like a smaller group of people, the day of my child's diagnosis is a strong and vivid memory, even seven years later. Most of the time, I don't dwell on that series of images. It was, after all, a chapter in our lives, and one that is now blessedly behind us. But early each autumn, when I get a whiff of the crisp smell of leaves in the air, it brings back that dark day when our lives changed forever.

Many of the memories are painful and, like my daughter's scars, they fade a little more each year, but will never completely disappear. While dealing with the medical and physical aspects of the disease, my husband and I also made many emotional discoveries. We sometimes encountered ignorance and narrow-mindedness, which made me more sad than angry. Mistakes were made, tempers were short, and family relations were strained. But we saw the other side, too. Somehow, our sense of humor held on throughout the ordeal, and when that kicked in, we had some of the best laughs of our lives. There was compassion and understanding when we needed it most. And people were there for us like never before.

I remember two young fathers on our street, torn by the news, who wanted to help but felt helpless. My husband came home from the hospital late one night to find that our lawn had been mowed and our leaves had been raked by them. They had found a way to make a small difference that day.

Another time, a neighbor came to our house bearing a bakery box full of pastries and the message that his family was praying for our daughter nightly around their supper table. The image of this man, his wife, and his eight children joining in prayer for us will never leave me.

A close friend entered the hospital during that first terrible week we were there, to give birth to her son. I held her baby, she held me, and we laughed and cried together.

Sometimes, when I look back at that time, I feel as though everything that is wrong with the world and everything that is right are somehow distilled in one small child's battle to live. We learned so very much about people and about life.

Surely people who haven't experienced a crisis of this magnitude would believe that we would want to put that time behind us and forget as much of it as possible. But the fact is, we grew a little through our pain, like it or not. We see through new eyes. Not all of it is good or happy, but it is profound.

I treasure good friends like never before. I view life as much more fragile and precious than I used to. I think of myself as a tougher person than I was, but I cry more easily now. And sure, I still yell at my kids and eagerly await each September when they will be out of my hair for a few hours each day. But I hold them with more tenderness when they hop off the school bus into my arms. And I like to think that some of the people around us, who saw how suddenly and drastically a family's life can change, hold their children a little dearer as well.

Do I want to forget those terrible days and nights seven years ago? Not on your life. And I hope the smell of autumn leaves will still bring the memories back when I'm a grandmother, even if I can't remember what I had for dinner last night.

— Kathy Tucker
CURE Childhood Cancer Newsletter
Rochester, NY

Chapter 2

The Brain and Spinal Cord

The world breaks everyone and afterward
many are strong at the broken places.

— Ernest Hemingway
A Farewell to Arms

IF YOUR CHILD HAS A BRAIN OR SPINAL CORD TUMOR, it's helpful to understand the basics of brain and spinal cord anatomy. Learning about the structure and function of the brain and spinal cord makes it easier to understand doctors' explanations about types of tumors and treatment plans.

This chapter provides an overview of brain and spinal cord anatomy, with several figures to help you visualize the different parts of the brain. It then discusses symptoms associated with tumors in various locations in the brain and spinal cord. The chapter also includes a table summarizing all the tumor locations and associated symptoms.

The brain

The brain, cushioned by watery fluid on all sides, resides inside the skull. It resembles a fleshy, shelled walnut in shape. Like a walnut, it has two distinct but connected halves. These are called the left and right cerebral hemispheres. Although the hemispheres appear to be mirror images of each other, the similar-looking parts of each do different things.

Like a walnut's exterior, the brain's surface folds in and out. These wrinkles increase the surface area of the brain. Its surface is divided by especially deep grooves, called fissures or sulci. The brain contains major nerves—such as the optic nerves, which connect it to the eyes. There are also nerves that control movement of arms and legs, the ability to maintain a heart rate, and level of awareness. Blood vessels carry oxygen and nutrients to all parts of the brain and spinal cord, and channels called aqueducts allow the watery fluid (called cerebrospinal fluid [CSF]) to move throughout the brain and spinal cord (central nervous system or CNS).

The brain has several protective coverings that prevent injury. The bones of the skull and the spine provide the outermost protection. Inside the skull are three thin membranes called the meninges, which surround the brain and spinal cord. The outer meninge is called the dura mater, the inner meninge is the pia mater, and the middle meninge, which carries the blood vessels, is called the arachnoid (see Figure 2-1). The brain and spinal cord are also protected by the CSF that flows between the layers of meninges.

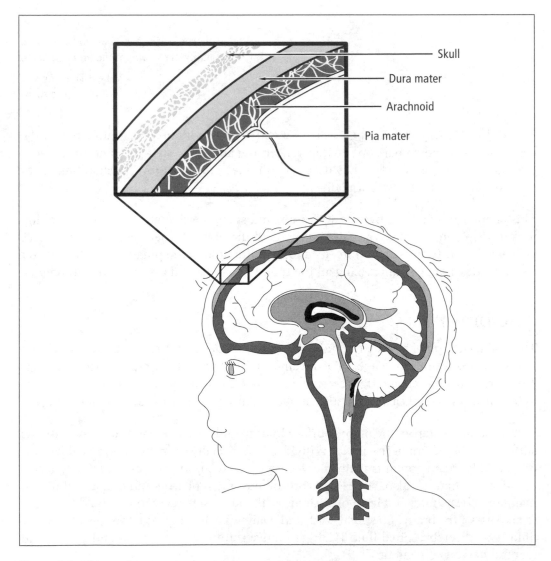

Figure 2-1: The meninges

Cerebrum

The largest region in the brain is the cerebrum (also called the supratentorial region). It is made up of two cerebral hemispheres (left and right). The two hemispheres are separated by a large groove, called the cerebral fissure. Deep within the cerebral fissure is a bundle of nerve fibers called the corpus callosum, which transmits information between the two sides of the cerebrum.

The cerebrum interprets sensory input from all parts of the body and also controls body movements. It is the part of the brain responsible for thinking, reasoning, learning, controlling movement, and processing emotions and memories.

The cerebrum is divided into four areas (called lobes) on each side of the brain: the frontal, temporal, parietal, and occipital lobes. The corpus callosum connects the two parts of each lobe on both sides of the brain. Structures on one side of the brain control the opposite side of the body. For example, any movement of the arms and legs on the right side of the body is controlled by the left cerebral hemisphere.

Your child's doctors will attempt to determine which side of your child's brain is dominant. Dominance is important for tumors that are near the hearing or speech and language processing areas. It may be difficult for the surgeon to remove all of the tumor on a dominant side in these areas without damaging speech or hearing. Pre-operative testing (functional MRI scans) and intraoperative monitoring (mapping) are vital when dealing with tumors in the dominant hemisphere. These tools, discussed in Chapter 6, *Coping with Procedures,* and Chapter 10, *Surgery,* allow the surgeon to remove as much tumor as possible while preserving function. The parts of the cerebrum are shown in Figure 2-2.

Frontal lobes

The frontal lobes, located directly behind your forehead, are your brain's main planning and personality centers. They process and store information that helps you think ahead, use strategy, and respond to events based on past experiences and other knowledge. A small part of the frontal lobe is involved in articulating speech. Another small strip of the frontal lobe helps control movement. Malfunctions in the frontal lobe may lead to poor planning, impulsiveness, and certain types of speech problems. Symptoms are more pronounced if the tumor crosses the corpus callosum and affects both frontal lobes. Symptoms of frontal lobe tumors include:

- Seizures

- Changes in ability to concentrate

- Poor school performance

- Changes in social behavior and personality

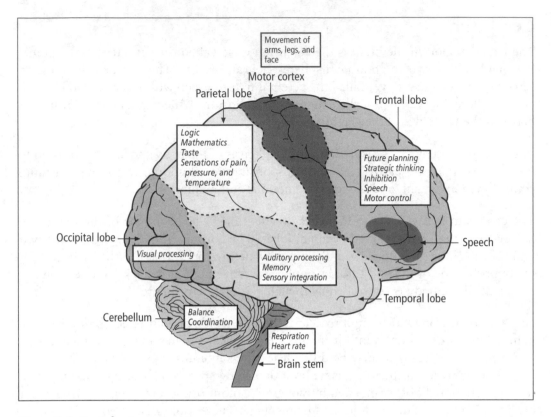

Figure 2-2: Basic brain anatomy

Toward the back section of the frontal lobe is the motor cortex, the part of the brain that controls movement of the head and body parts on the opposite side of the body. Because the location of motor nerves varies a little in each person, mapping of the motor cortex using a functional MRI, and using this information while monitoring during surgery, helps surgeons know the exact location of these nerves so as not to injure them during tumor removal. For more information, see the "MRI" section of Chapter 6, *Coping with Procedures,* and the "Intraoperative monitoring" section of Chapter 10, *Surgery.*

Temporal lobes

The temporal lobes are located at the sides of the brain. Hearing, memory, and speech and language processing are managed by the temporal lobes. They are the places where information taken in from the various senses is integrated, permitting complex thoughts, movements, and sensations to be formulated and acted upon. Within the temporal lobes is the amygdala, which controls social behavior, aggression, and excitement. The hippo-campus, located in the temporal lobes, is involved in storing memories of recent events. Depth perception and sense of time are also controlled by the temporal lobes.

Tumors in the temporal lobes can cause seizures and changes in behavior. When a tumor grows in the temporal lobes, the brain has a hard time filtering out extra information, and sensory information and memories may start to blend together in unfamiliar ways. Sounds may be perceived as having colors, for example, or your child may have an unsettling feeling of déjà vu.

> *Our son is now 6 years old, and he's had his brain tumor since he was a baby, so he's lived with it for quite a while. He has partial complex seizures that cycle from one a week to two or three times a day for a couple days a week. This has been going on regardless of what medication we've used, so far.*
>
> *They start with a blank stare, then he says, "Um, um" or "Mom, Dad" a few times, or sometimes, if it's at night, he may be more disoriented and cry out. Then he flushes pink, sometimes he smacks his lips or picks at his clothes with his fingers. At one point, you can tell he can't hear or even see, but then he becomes more aware, and he'll take a breath when we ask. Then he usually spits up and wants to nap.*
>
> *And the medications can cause their own side effects, like dull affect, behavior changes, and light sensitivity. Our neurologist's office had a poster up about an epilepsy support group in the area, so I've been going to those.*

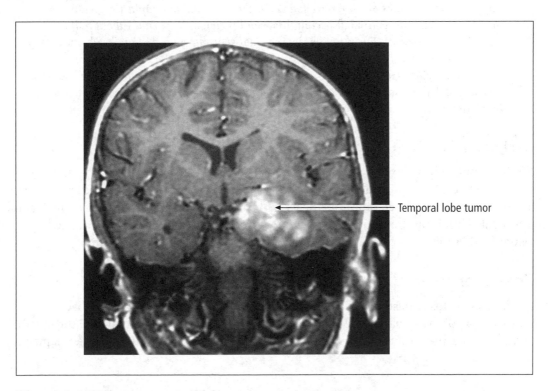

Figure 2-3: MRI showing temporal lobe tumor

Parietal lobes

Directly behind the frontal lobes and above the temporal lobes are the parietal lobes. In some people, the motor cortex, which controls arm and leg movement, extends into the parietal lobes. The parietal lobes process all sorts of sensory information coming in from the body, including data about temperature, pain, and taste. The parietal lobes also control language and the ability to do arithmetic. When the parietal lobes are not functioning properly, sensory information is not processed correctly, and your child may have a hard time making sense of her environment.

The rear of each parietal lobe, next to the temporal lobe, has an area important in processing the auditory and visual information needed for language. When children have tumors in these lobes, they do not understand what is being said when someone speaks to them.

Abnormal movements or weakness in the arms and legs, memory problems, language problems, and seizures are associated with tumors in the parietal lobes. During a seizure affecting these areas, strange physical sensations may be felt, such as a crushing pressure or a tingling feeling in part of the body.

> Megan was 20 months old when we found out that she had an anaplastic ependymoma occupying the entire left occipital-parietal region of her brain (about half the size of her little head). For 6 to 8 weeks, she had sporadic vomiting and crabbiness in the morning. By the time we'd arrive at the doctor's office, she would be fine. Then she developed a right-sided tremor that was so strong it shook her whole body when she tried to use her right arm. The pediatrician ordered an MRI and found the brain tumor.

Occipital lobes

The occipital lobes serve as the visual centers of the brain. They are responsible for making sense of the information that comes to the brain from the eyes through the optic nerves. The left occipital lobe deals with input from the right eye, and the right lobe deals with input from the left eye. Tumors in the occipital lobes are associated with visual field cut (loss of central or peripheral vision) on one side or the other.

Posterior fossa

The posterior fossa (also called the infratentorium) is located at the very back of the brain, on top of the spinal cord. It includes the cerebellum, the brainstem, and the fourth ventricle (see the "Ventricular system" section and Figure 2-6 later in the chapter).

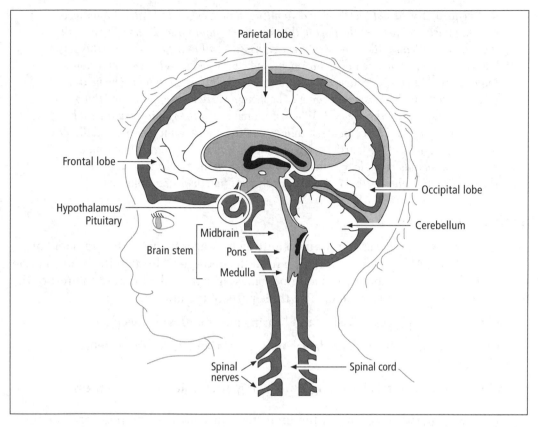

Frontal lobe

Hypothalamus/
Pituitary

Brain stem

Midbrain

Pons

Medulla

Parietal lobe

Occipital lobe

Cerebellum

Spinal
nerves

Spinal cord

Figure 2-4: Side view of the brain

Sixty percent of all childhood brain tumors originate in the posterior fossa. Symptoms of tumors in this area of the brain include:

- Signs of increased intracranial pressure (headache, vomiting, unsteady gait, double vision, sleepiness, or lethargy)

- Weakness of cranial nerves (visual or hearing problems, weakness or drooping on one side of the face, eye movement problems, difficulty swallowing, difficulty breathing)

- Unsteady gait (ataxia)

Cerebellum

The cerebellum is about one-eighth the size of the cerebrum. Tumors growing in the cerebellum can cause coordination and balance problems. The child may have an uneven walking pattern or may continually fall to one side. Difficulty judging distances or reaching for and grabbing an object are symptoms of a tumor in this area.

Red-headed, 2-year-old Matthew had vomiting almost every day. After 3 months of running back and forth to the doctor, the babysitter and I noticed some "tipsy walking," as we called Matt's ever-so-subtle dizziness. A call to the doctor with this report led us to the office of a neurologist. A neurological exam and a little observation found us with an order to have an MRI to rule out a brainstem tumor. The neurologist was sure the diagnosis was going to be benign vertigo of infancy, something usually outgrown by the age of 3. Whew, 1 more year of the vomiting and we'd be done. Wrong again. The neurologist told us our son had a brain tumor (medulloblastoma, on the floor of the fourth ventricle), that it was malignant, and he would need surgery as soon as possible. His tumor was located in the cerebellum, at the base of the brainstem, right where the circuits for all vital functions are connected.

Brainstem

The brainstem is the relay center for transmitting messages between the brain and other parts of the body. All sensory information from the body goes through the brainstem on its way to the rest of the brain, and all motor messages from the brain to the rest of the body travel through the brainstem. The three parts of the brainstem are:

- Midbrain, which processes vision and hearing and coordinates sleep and wake cycles
- Pons, which controls eye and facial movements and links the cerebellum to the cerebrum
- Medulla, which controls breathing, swallowing, heart rate, and blood pressure

The 12 cranial nerves originate in the brainstem, primarily in the pons and medulla. They control eye and facial movements, vision, taste, hearing, swallowing, and movement of the neck and shoulders.

Symptoms of tumors in the brainstem include:

- Abnormal eye movements or a droopy eyelid
- Drooping of the face or facial asymmetry
- Difficulty swallowing or breathing
- An uneven walking pattern
- Weakness on one or both sides of the body, often seen first in an arm and/or a leg

Ayla's eyes were "off" from each other. Her right eye would look at you and the left eye would go off. Our pediatrician thought it could be cross-eye, and suggested waiting it out, but in another week, her eye was completely turned in and you couldn't even see the pupil. The eye doctor we saw said there was no reason that he could see for her eyes to cross, so we went to a neurologist, who did a neurological exam, and said Ayla showed no neuro problems. But, he ordered a scan just in case, not expecting to find anything. He thought it could possibly be a virus. The scan found a 5x5 cm tumor in the posterior fossa, cerebellopontine angle, fourth ventricle, and arising from the brainstem.

Diencephalon

Near the center of the brain is the diencephalon, which is made up of several tiny but extraordinarily important structures: the thalamus, the hypothalamus, the pituitary gland, and the pineal gland.

All sensory information passes through the thalamus before being sent to the forebrain for more advanced interpretation—except for information gathered via the sense of smell, which takes a different route. The hypothalamus is small, but it has a big role in managing everything from hunger to digestion to muscle contractions. It has direct control over the pituitary gland, which produces hormones and similar chemicals. The pineal gland helps to govern the body's sense of time and rhythm, including regulation of the reproductive cycle.

Tumors that grow in the diencephalon cause:

- Disruption of hormone production
- Abnormal growth (usually delayed growth)
- Excessive thirst and frequent urination
- Drowsiness or changes in level of consciousness
- Difficulty with vision
- Memory problems
- Weakness of one or both sides of the body

> *Florence has recovered from a germinoma, a malignant tumor of the pituitary gland. She was ill from ages 11 to 15, and the diagnosis took 2 years. This tumor seems to be very rare. Prior to diagnosis, there was a long period of weight loss, incessant thirst, and teachers and doctors who kept saying this was all psychological. Florence would get up in the morning, go to the kitchen, and start the awful drinking, glass after glass. One time I really lost it. I shouted at her, "Why are you doing this? Do you know what you are doing? You are going to make yourself very ill. Do you know what manipulative behavior is?" I shouted and shouted; she didn't argue or cry. She just stood there and smiled at me sadly. She said, "I just can't help it." I thought, "That is it. This is a real illness." By then she was thin and she hadn't grown for months.*

A young doctor gave her an injection of vasopressin. The effect was miraculous; she ran along the corridor, skipped up and down, she felt marvelous. The young doctor came back, very excited. He said, "We have a very good result." I stared at him. He said, "Well, perhaps a bad result from your point of view. Florence has diabetes insipidus. This is a permanent condition, the hormone which governs her kidneys is not being produced, and she has been drinking to stop herself from dying of dehydration." After more searching, I finally found a consultant, and when he heard the symptoms, he said he knew what the cause could be. It was a germinoma—a rare tumor whose symptoms often begin with diabetes insipidus.

Optic nerves

The optic nerves carry information from the eyes to the occipital lobes. The nerve from the right eye goes to the left occipital lobe, and the nerve from the left eye goes to the right occipital lobe. These two nerves cross at a place called the optic chiasm, near the hypothalamus. Tumors that affect the optic nerves cause changes in visual acuity (the ability to see) or visual fields (peripheral vision).

After they discovered the optic tract tumor on the MRI, they sent us to vision specialists at the eye clinic. There Jamie saw an ophthalmologist who checked for optic nerve swelling, an orthoptist who checked acuity, and a visual function specialist, who found a complete loss of left-sided peripheral vision. The field cut is especially noticeable when he's in new environments, and he bumps into things on the left, although mostly he remembers to make the extra effort to turn his head to check out things on that side.

Spinal cord

At the base of the brain (in the back), the brain becomes the spinal cord—a long, tough bundle of nerve fibers that runs down the back and is protected from harm by the vertebrae of the spine. The spinal cord is the pathway for nerve impulses that travel to and from the brain to all parts of the body. Tumors can grow inside or outside the spinal cord or, in some cases, twine around the cord. Symptoms of tumors in the spinal cord include:

- Back or leg pain that awakens the child from sleep
- Curvature of the spine
- Weakness in arms or legs
- Changes in sensation (tingling, numbness) in the back, arms, or legs
- Changes in bowel and bladder function

Danny (age 8) began having infrequent bouts of headaches and vomiting at odd times, not always in the morning. He also told me that he was having strange half-second blackouts. After a couple visits to the pediatrician, we found he had swelling of the optic discs, papilledema. Other than that, he passed all neurological tests. Finally, a CT scan showed hydrocephalus. Just before a shunt was placed, an MRI of the head showed multiple lesions all over the brain. Our doctors recommended a spinal MRI to check if the brain lesions were spread from the spine. The MRI of the spine showed the same pattern of unusual lesions. It was like a sugar coating all along the meningeal lining of the spine without any hard central mass.

Figure 2-5 shows an MRI scan of a tumor causing the spine to curve.

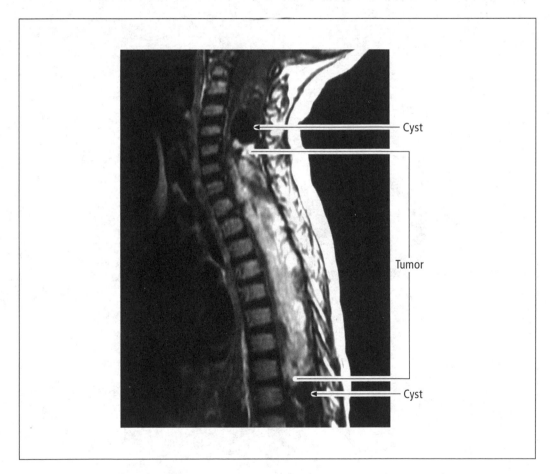

Figure 2-5: A spinal cord tumor

Ventricular system

The ventricular system, shown in Figure 2-6, is made up of four fluid-filled chambers in the brain, called ventricles. These areas in the brain circulate CSF that bathes the brain and spinal cord. Under normal conditions, the brain produces approximately 1 pint of CSF a day. Healthy bodies absorb the amount produced each day. Disruptions in the balance between the amount of CSF produced and reabsorbed can result in too much CSF, which increases the pressure in the brain. This fluid buildup, called hydrocephalus, occurs in two ways:

- A tumor grows in or pushes into a ventricle, blocking the normal flow of CSF

- Blood, tumor cells, a scar, or dead tissue obstructs the subarachnoid space and prevents the absorption of CSF

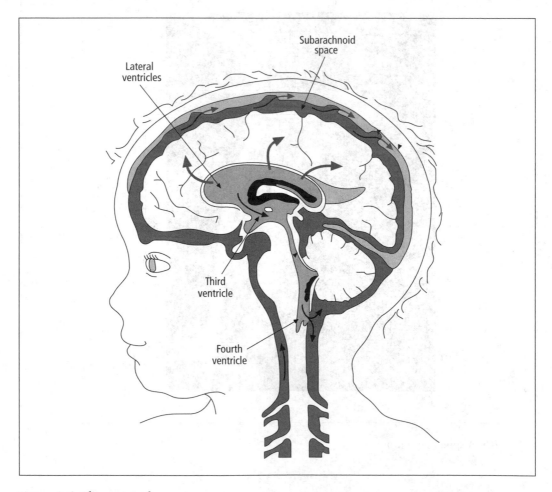

Figure 2-6: The ventricular system

My son Paul had multiple admissions for pneumonia and a collapsed lung as a baby. The doctors were sure he had cystic fibrosis. After many tests, they decided maybe they were wrong. Summer started and everything was going well. In August he again started getting sick. Over the next 2 months, Paul's balance deteriorated. By October he could no longer walk. Our family doctor sent us to see a neurologist. On the day of our appointment, we went to the neurologist and were told we didn't have an appointment, that we would have to reschedule. The nurse had forgotten to write us in the book. I insisted we be seen and we sat in the office until the doctor saw us. The doctor thought Paul might have muscular dystrophy. She wanted to do a baseline MRI. We took the films back to her office to view after the MRI. She told us Paul had hydrocephalus. She was showing us the films and explaining, when she said, "Oh my God, he has a tumor. I'm so sorry." They started preparing to admit him to pediatric intensive care unit. His hydrocephalus was life-threatening and he was in surgery 3 hours later to place a VP shunt. Paul had his tumor completely removed; he was 21 months old. His tumor was in the posterior fossa and was determined to be an ependymoma.

Table of symptoms based on tumor location

The table below summarizes the symptoms associated with tumors in various parts of the brain.

Part of the Brain	Symptoms
Frontal lobes	• Seizures • Changes in ability to concentrate • Poor school performance • Changes in social behaviors and personality
Temporal lobes	• Partial complex seizures (staring spells) • Behavior problems (aggressive, impulsive)
Parietal lobes	• Seizures often involving shaking of an arm or leg on the side that is opposite of the tumor • Difficulty processing information • Language and memory problems • Weakness of arm or leg on side opposite of tumor
Occipital lobes	• Loss of central or peripheral vision
Cerebellum	• Problems with balance • Uncoordinated gait • Difficulty judging distances

Part of the Brain	Symptoms
Brainstem	• Abnormal eye movements or a droopy eyelid • Drooping of the face or facial asymmetry • Difficulty swallowing or breathing • An uneven walking pattern • Weakness on one or both sides of the body, often seen first in an arm and/or a leg
Diencephalon	• Disruption of hormone production • Abnormal growth • Excessive thirst and frequent urination • Drowsiness • Difficulty with vision • Memory problems • Weakness of one or both sides of the body
Optic nerves	• Visual changes (loss of peripheral vision, decrease in visual acuity)
Spinal cord	• Back or leg pain that awakens the child from sleep • Curvature of the spine • Weakness in arms or legs • Changes in sensation (tingling, numbness) in the back, arms, or legs • Changes in bowel and bladder function
Ventricular system	• Hydrocephalus • Lethargy • Headache • Vomiting

Increased intracranial pressure

A general term for symptoms that result from the mass of the tumor occupying space within the brain is "increased intracranial pressure." As the mass grows it compresses the brain, causing pressure. Pressure also increases if the tumor obstructs the normal fluid pathways, causing hydrocephalus. Symptoms of increased intracranial pressure include:

• Double vision or other visual changes

• Pressure on the optic discs (called papilledema), seen by a physician when looking into eyes with an ophthalmoscope

• Headaches (which awaken the child from sleep)

• Vomiting (typically in the morning, which often temporarily relieves the nausea and headache)

• Unsteady gait

- Sleepiness or lethargy
- Memory problems

> *In July, Jennifer had her second appointment with a doctor in 1 weeks' time because her headaches were so severe. The primary physician sent Jennifer to the hospital for a CT scan. I figured it would be in a couple of weeks due to the holiday weekend. He said within 2 hours. The nurse was drawing Jennifer's blood, when another nurse came in and said that the hospital wants Jennifer down there as soon as possible. They were holding the radiologist there, waiting on Jennifer. We left the primary physician's office around 11 a.m., and at noon, I was informed that Jennifer had an abnormality found on the brain. We were told to go to lunch and then report to the MRI department around 1 p.m. We reported to the MRI department and were told that Jennifer would be admitted to the hospital as soon as the MRI was done. I asked, "Would someone like to tell me what is going on?" I saw a telephone and called Jennifer's primary physician. This was the first time that I did not have to speak to a nurse; he got right on the phone. He said, "I am so sorry, I was waiting on the results of the MRI and was going to talk to you and Jennifer. The CT scan revealed a huge mass on the left side of the brain."*

From the CNS to the body

The brain and spinal cord, which make up the CNS, communicate with the rest of the body via nerves. Nerves are thin strings of tough fiber that extend throughout the body. The brainstem and spinal cord branch off into many nerves that carry information to and from every part of the body. Together, these nerves are known as the peripheral nervous system.

The peripheral nervous system carries commands from the CNS to various body parts and returns information gathered from your senses. For example, nerves close to the skin's surface are sensitive to touch and tell the brain if they notice a crawling sensation. In response, your brain may trigger commands that cause you to absentmindedly brush a hand over the affected area or scratch it.

Other nerves transmit information to and from the body's internal organs, including the heart, stomach, and intestines. These nerves and the parts of the spinal cord and brain that control them are called the visceral or autonomic nervous system.

Most of the time, the workings of the peripheral, autonomic, and central nervous systems go completely unnoticed. The majority of their interconnected activities concern basic physical functions: breathing, digesting food, producing hormones, pumping blood, and the like. Although it's possible to stop and purposefully make yourself aware of some of these processes, most people pay no attention as long as everything is working well. Brain and spinal cord tumors disrupt the normal, smooth functioning of these nervous systems.

At the hospital a tall dark-haired man met us in his office with a firm handshake. His kind brown eyes looked into mine. They held compassion and looked straight into me. They were willing eyes that held the horizon of the unknown. He was to be our neurosurgeon.

He showed us the scans from the MRI. It was like looking at a large negative. It is a picture of a slice from the body—as if you put a potato or an egg in a slicer and pulled out one slice to examine it. A foreign, alien feeling gripped me. From nothing wrong to brain tumor. This should not be happening. This was not normal. This is something that happens in someone else's life. Slow down. I wanted to say. Show me. Point with your finger to where it is. Tell me what is supposed to be in this picture and what is not?

That lemon-sized spot. That's not supposed to be there? Well, what is it? He explained that the best procedure would be to perform a craniotomy and surgically remove the tumor, find out what kind it was, and proceed from there. In just a few hours we went from suntanned vacationers to scared parents giving permission for someone to surgically explore our child's brain.

I wanted to slip away. I wanted to hold the picture in my hands and study it. I wanted to zoom in on the unwanted mass and understand why it was there. The mass, what does it mean? She's that sick. She's sitting in my lap. She can walk. She can smile. She looks normal. Can an intruder hide that well? The scans are removed. I didn't hold them. She's in my lap. I'm supposed to be strong.

We left the office and went to Admitting. It takes a long time to process the papers. Another opinion, yes, another opinion would be good. Yes, we probably should ask for a second opinion. We were at the best facility, weren't we? We were with the best doctors. It was Friday night. Who would give us a second opinion tonight? She was being admitted. Should we wait? Could we wait? We risked a stroke, death, physical impairment.

I have learned since that the damage done in a rush surgery or by inexperienced hands results in handicaps that might have been prevented. I was lucky not to know this.

At 4:30 p.m. a nurse called the waiting room. She was out of surgery and the neurosurgeon would be coming to talk with us. The man with the silent eyes approached. I rose. Knowing that what he said would change me. If she had survived the surgery, what would her life be like? If she had not survived, how would I?

He approached the waiting room with a lightness in his step. Coming straight to the point he said, "Your daughter had an astrocytoma. Her surgery was longer than normal because the tumor was embedded in her brainstem. There is the possibility that some small part of the tumor is still remaining. This will be followed by future CT scans and MRIs."

I was seized by an incredible urgency to see her face. I needed to see her. To prove to myself that all of this had been real. And to prove she was still here. She was in recovery. I stood over her and reached for her hand. Her head was turned to one side and I tried to find her eyes. The room was cold and silent except for the beeps of the monitors. She looked small in the huge bed. There was a bandage around her head. It smelled like cold. It felt like cold. It was a place you would run from if you could. I stood there knowing she might not be okay. She might not ever run or laugh or play. This is the moment for prayers. And you hope.

She opened her eyes as if she came from heaven. Her eyes lighting a cathedral with a single candle.

Chapter 3

Types of Tumors

Fresh activity is the only means of overcoming adversity.
— Johann Wolfgang von Goethe

TUMORS IN THE BRAIN OR SPINAL CORD (also called central nervous system tumors) account for 25 percent of all childhood cancers and are the second most common cancer in children. Symptoms vary depending on the location of the primary tumor. Tumors in the brain and spinal cord may exist for long periods with no growth, or they can dramatically increase in size in just a few days. Recent advances in diagnosis and treatment have improved the long-term survival rates for many children with brain or spinal cord tumors.

This chapter begins with a discussion of the causes of brain tumors. It then describes the many types of brain and spinal cord tumors, including their typical location, rate of growth, and treatment. It ends with a brief overview of the most commonly used treatments for brain and spinal cord tumors.

Who gets central nervous system tumors?

More than 4,000 children younger than age 20 are diagnosed with brain or spinal cord tumors in the United States each year. Because there are many different kinds of brain and spinal cord tumors, the number of children diagnosed with each particular type is small. The incidence of childhood brain and spinal cord tumors is higher in males than females, and higher among white children than any other racial/ethnic group.

Genetic factors

Most brain and spinal cord tumors occur randomly and have no apparent cause. They are, however, associated with several inherited syndromes such as Von Recklinghausen neurofibromatosis, tuberous sclerosis, Turcot syndrome, Li-Fraumeni syndrome, and von Hippel-Lindau syndrome. Children with these genetic conditions have a greatly increased risk for developing brain tumors. Together, however, they account for less than 5 percent of childhood brain and spinal cord tumors. Because of their high risk for tumors, children with these conditions get periodic MRI scans and other evaluations to check for tumors.

Environmental factors

Very little is known about environmental causes of brain or spinal cord tumors. The best-documented cause of brain tumors is previous radiation to the brain. The risk of a second brain tumor increases with the dose of radiation received.

Other environmental factors, such as electromagnetic radiation and pesticide exposure, have not been confirmed as causes of brain and spinal cord tumors. Many research studies have evaluated possible environmental causes, but no conclusive results have yet been found.

Types of brain and spinal cord tumors

Tumors of the brain and spinal cord are classified based on the cell from which they originate and by their rate of growth. Slow-growing tumors are sometimes present for months or years. Symptoms of slow-growing tumors are subtle and these tumors are sometimes found incidentally. Symptoms that develop over a short period of time usually indicate the presence of a fast-growing tumor.

To identify the type of tumor, a sample of the tumor is obtained during surgery (biopsy or tumor removal). Then, a pathologist (a doctor who specializes in examining body tissues) looks at one or more pieces of the tumor under a microscope. Unfortunately, it can be difficult to classify some brain tumors. Different pathologists may look at the same tumor sample and give it a different name. Sometimes it is necessary to have several neuropathologists examine the tumor samples before a diagnosis can be reached. This process can be very frustrating and confusing for parents.

In this chapter, the most common types of tumors found in the brain and spinal cord are described and alternative names for the same tumors are provided. The most common types of childhood brain and spinal cord tumors are:

- Astrocytomas
- Atypical teratoid/rhabdoid tumors (AT/RT)
- Brainstem gliomas
- Choroid plexus tumors
- Craniopharyngiomas
- Ependymomas

- Germ cell tumors

- Medulloblastomas

- Optic pathway and hypothalamic gliomas

- Primitive neuroectodermal tumors (PNET)

Malignant or benign tumor?

The terms malignant and benign are confusing when applied to many brain and spinal cord tumors. All fast-growing tumors are considered malignant. Even if entirely removed with surgery, these tumors will usually grow back unless a child undergoes further treatment such as radiation and/or chemotherapy. Thus, the terms "malignant," "fast-growing," or "cancer" usually mean the same thing when used to describe fast-growing brain and spinal cord tumors.

Slow-growing tumors (also called low-grade tumors) are technically classified as benign. If these tumors are totally removed with surgery, they rarely regrow. Many slow-growing tumors, however, are found deep within the brain or brainstem, where aggressive surgery is not possible. In these cases, other treatments (like chemotherapy and/or radiation) are used in an attempt to shrink or halt further tumor growth. Therefore, even if a tumor deep in the brain is slow-growing, it may require the same treatments as malignant brain tumors—and these treatments can cause the same long-term side effects. Some healthcare providers call benign tumors that are deep in the brain "malignant by location."

In this book, tumors are referred to as fast-growing or slow-growing. However, one must also consider the location of the tumor to understand the symptoms, likelihood of successful treatment, and possibility of late effects.

A discussion of the specific tumor types (in alphabetical order) follows.

Astrocytomas

Astrocytomas (also called gliomas) are the most common type of brain and spinal cord tumor in children. They develop from brain cells called astrocytes. They can be slow-growing or very fast-growing and can arise anywhere in the brain or spinal cord. About 80 percent of astrocytomas are slow-growing.

Common names of slow-growing astrocytomas or gliomas include:

- Juvenile pilocytic astrocytoma

- Oligodendroglioma

- Mixed glioma

- Ganglioglioma

- Subependymal giant cell astrocytoma (SEGA)

- Pleomorphic xanthoastrocytoma (PXA)

Slow-growing astrocytomas in the brain: Slow-growing astrocytomas in the brain usually arise in the cerebral hemispheres, the cerebellum, or in the thalamus and hypothalamus. If a slow-growing astrocytoma is in an accessible location, surgery is the primary treatment. Surgery is possible in many areas of the cerebrum and is always possible in the cerebellum. Multiple surgical procedures may be needed if the neurosurgeon is unable to remove the entire tumor during the first surgery. Chemotherapy and radiation are used for slow-growing tumors that are deep within the brain (hypothalamic or optic pathway glioma) where surgery is not possible, or when only part of the tumor is removed.

Slow-growing astrocytomas in the spine: Slow-growing astrocytomas account for 75 percent of all spinal cord tumors in children. Surgery is the primary treatment, but it is usually not possible to remove all of the tumor. Multiple surgical procedures are generally needed if the tumor regrows. Radiation therapy is used for tumors that grow despite multiple surgeries. Chemotherapy is not usually given to children with slow-growing spinal cord tumors, so its effectiveness is unknown.

Fast-growing astrocytomas in the brain: Some astrocytoma tumors (20 percent) grow rapidly. They usually grow in the cerebrum or brainstem, and are rarely found in the spinal cord. The three types of fast-growing astrocytomas are:

- High-grade anaplastic astrocytoma

- Glioblastoma multiforme

- Gliomatosis cerebri

Fast-growing astrocytomas are difficult to cure even with the most aggressive treatments. Surgery, followed by aggressive multi-drug chemotherapy and radiation therapy, is used to treat these tumors. High-dose chemotherapy followed by an autologous stem cell transplant is also sometimes used to treat fast-growing astrocytomas that do not respond to chemotherapy (see Chapter 14, *Peripheral Blood Stem Cell Transplantation*).

Atypical teratoid/rhabdoid tumor

Atypical teratoid/rhabdoid tumors (AT/RTs) are fast-growing and occur most often in children younger than age 2. They account for less than 2 percent of all childhood brain tumors. They can be found anywhere in the brain, and they can quickly spread throughout the brain and spinal cord.

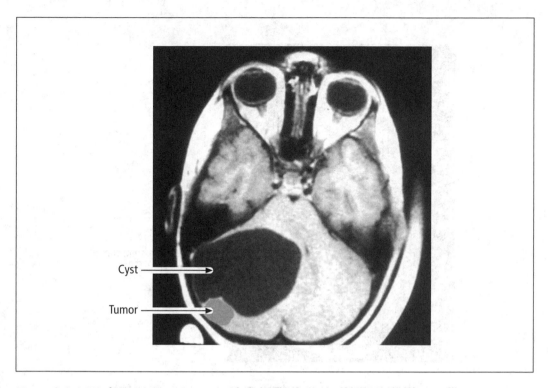

Figure 3-1: MRI showing astrocytoma with associated cyst in the cerebellum

Treatment generally involves surgical removal of the tumor and then cycles of high-dose chemotherapy, each followed by a stem cell transplant (called tandem transplants). Radiation therapy may also be used.

Brainstem gliomas

Astrocytomas that grow in the brainstem are called brainstem gliomas. They make up 10 to 15 percent of all pediatric brain tumors. Ninety percent of these tumors are fast-growing and cause rapidly developing symptoms. They usually involve the pons (also known as pontine gliomas) and have a diffuse appearance on the MRI scan. Radiation therapy, sometimes with chemotherapy, is the treatment for brainstem gliomas. Surgery is not a treatment option because aggressive surgery in the brainstem is life-threatening and results in severe neurological impairment.

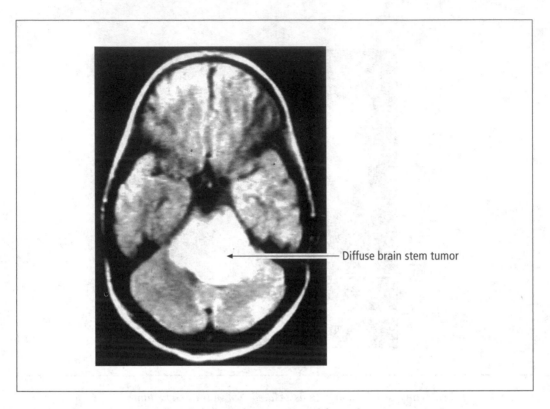

Diffuse brain stem tumor

Figure 3-2: MRI showing diffuse brain stem tumor viewed from above

About 10 percent of brainstem tumors are slow-growing brainstem gliomas. They usually are located in the medulla, and symptoms develop over a long period of time. Treatment generally involves radiation and observation. Surgery is not typically an option.

Choroid plexus tumors

Choroid plexus papillomas (slow-growing) and choroid plexus carcinomas (fast-growing) arise from the choroid plexus, which is the part of the brain that produces cerebrospinal fluid. These tumors account for 1 to 3 percent of all childhood brain tumors and most often occur in infants. The tumor is usually diagnosed at the same time as hydrocephalus (excess fluid in the brain). For choroid plexus papillomas, surgery is the treatment. For choroid plexus carcinomas, surgery followed by chemotherapy and/ or radiation is the treatment. More than one surgery is sometimes needed for both types of choroid plexus tumors.

Craniopharyngiomas

Craniopharyngiomas grow in the area of the brain that contains the hypothalamus, pituitary, and optic chiasm (called the suprasellar region). They account for approximately 5 to 10 percent of all childhood brain tumors. Treatment is controversial because aggressive surgery often cures the child, but can cause life-long memory, visual, behavioral, and hormonal problems. To lessen long-term side effects, a common treatment option is the removal of part of the tumor followed by radiation therapy. Proton beam radiation is sometimes used to treat these tumors. If the tumor has a large cyst associated with it, treatment may include directly injecting chemotherapy into the cyst to reduce its size.

Ependymomas

Ependymomas make up 8 to 10 percent of childhood brain tumors. They develop in the cells that line the ventricles of the brain. About 70 percent of ependymomas occur in the posterior fossa, usually in the fourth ventricle. Ependymomas can also occur in the cerebral hemispheres and in the spinal cord.

Surgery is the first treatment for ependymomas. It can be difficult, however, to totally remove an ependymoma in the fourth ventricle because it is so close to the brainstem. Treatment of ependymomas after surgery has historically been controversial. Following surgery, some neuro-oncologists recommend only observation if there is no evidence of residual disease. Other neuro-oncologists recommend local radiation therapy even if there is no evidence of residual disease. If there is residual tumor after surgery, then radiation therapy with or without chemotherapy is given.

Germ cell tumors

These tumors arise from various types of germ cells that produce hormones. Part of determining the specific type of germ cell tumor a child has involves sampling the blood and cerebrospinal fluid for the presence of these hormones. Different types of germ cells give rise to different types of tumors, including germinomas, nongerminomas, and teratomas.

These tumors grow in the center of the brain—usually in the suprasellar or pineal regions. Germ cell tumors can spread to other areas of the brain and spinal cord. Treatment varies depending on the cell type and the location of the tumor.

Medulloblastomas

Medulloblastomas account for about 20 percent of all brain and spinal cord tumors in children younger than 15. The majority of diagnoses are in children between ages 5 to 10. The most important factors associated with this type of tumor are location and whether the tumor has spread to other areas of the brain and spinal cord. Medulloblastomas normally grow in the posterior fossa, starting in the cerebellum. As medulloblastomas grow, they sometimes extend into the cerebellar hemispheres, fourth ventricle, or brainstem. Because they can interfere with the normal flow of cerebrospinal fluid, hydrocephalus (excess fluid in the brain) is often present at diagnosis.

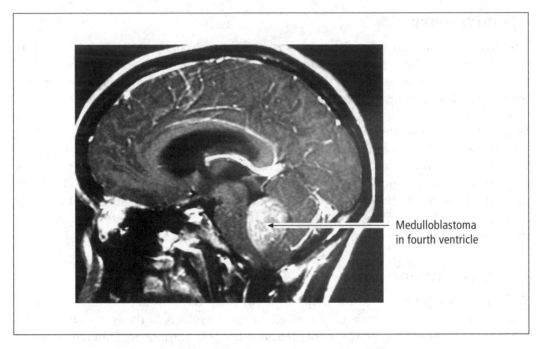

Medulloblastoma in fourth ventricle

Figure 3-3: MRI showing medulloblastoma growing in the fourth ventricle

Unlike most other brain and spinal cord tumors, medulloblastoma cells can spread throughout the brain and the spinal cord. For this reason children have an MRI scan of the entire brain and spine at diagnosis to determine if the tumor has spread. The diagnosing physician will also do an analysis of the cerebrospinal fluid by lumbar puncture to check for the presence of tumor cells.

Treatment plans vary depending on the child's age at diagnosis, the amount of tumor removed, and the extent of tumor spread. Surgery (in one or several operations) is the first treatment for medulloblastoma. Total removal is sometimes difficult if the tumor has spread to the brainstem or the floor of the fourth ventricle. Following surgery, treatment usually begins with radiation, followed by chemotherapy.

Over the past 2 decades, new prognostic categories have been developed by the World Health Organization based on the location of the medulloblastoma tumor and the presence or absence of specific biomarkers that help predict outcome. These categories are classic, desmoplastic, large cell, anaplastic, medullomyoblastoma, and melanocytic medulloblastoma. The ability to subtype medulloblastomas allows the treatment team to tailor the amount of radiation and chemotherapy used to treat the tumor. The subtypes that are associated with a more favorable outcome require less treatment than subtypes that are more aggressive.

Medulloblastoma tumors are grouped into two broad treatment categories: standard-risk and high-risk. Standard risk is defined as medulloblastomas that:

- Occur in a child older than age 3, and

- Have been completely removed by surgery, and

- Have not spread to other areas of the brain and spinal cord.

Children with standard-risk medulloblastoma receive craniospinal radiation and chemotherapy after surgery. Proton radiation treatment is sometimes used to treat standard risk medulloblastoma. A medulloblastoma tumor is considered high-risk if:

- Some tumor remains after surgery, or

- The tumor has spread to other areas of the brain and spinal cord, or

- The child is younger than age 3, regardless of the amount of tumor removed.

High-risk medulloblastoma treatment plans include surgery, craniospinal radiation, aggressive chemotherapy, and, in some cases, peripheral blood stem cell transplantation. Radiation therapy is usually delayed until children are at least 3 years old.

Optic pathway/hypothalamic gliomas

Approximately 5 percent of pediatric brain tumors are gliomas that grow around the optic nerves or hypothalamus. These slow-growing tumors sometimes are diagnosed in children with neurofibromatosis 1 (NF1 or Von Recklinghausen). Optic pathway/hypothalamic tumors may lie dormant for extended periods of time. Observation with careful clinical examination and serial MRI scans is the treatment of choice.

More aggressive treatment is necessary if an MRI shows tumor growth or if the child develops symptoms (usually visual or hormonal). Surgery, chemotherapy, and radiation are all treatment options for optic pathway/hypothalamic tumors. The precise combination of therapies depends on the age of the child, severity of symptoms, and the location of the tumor.

Primitive neuroectodermal tumors (PNET)

PNET and medulloblastoma were once considered the same type of tumor that arose in different locations in the brain. Historically, medulloblastoma was the name given to this tumor when it grew in the posterior fossa. PNET was the term used when a tumor grew outside of the posterior fossa in the cerebral hemispheres. Recent research has shown that the two tumors are biologically distinct, but, despite these differences, the treatment for PNET and high-risk medulloblastoma is the same—surgery, craniospinal radiation, and chemotherapy.

The four subtypes of PNET are central nervous system (CNS) neuroblastomas, ganglioneuroblastomas, medulloepitheliomas, and ependymoblastomas. In addition, three biological subtypes have been identified, but enough is not known yet about them to tailor treatment based on any of the subtypes.

Table of types of tumors, usual location, and treatment

Type of Tumor	Usual Location	Usual Treatment
Astrocytoma (glioma)—slow-growing	Cerebral hemispheres and cerebellum	Total surgical removal, if necessary in stages
	Hypothalamus or optic pathway	Chemotherapy and radiation
	Spine	Surgery and sometimes radiation
Astrocytoma (glioma)—fast-growing	Cerebral hemispheres and brainstem	Surgery, chemotherapy, radiation, and sometimes peripheral stem cell transplant
Atypical teratoid/rhabdoid tumor (AT/RT)	Anywhere in the brain	Surgery, chemotherapy, radiation, and sometimes peripheral stem cell transplant
Brainstem glioma—fast-growing	Brainstem (pons)	Radiation alone or with chemotherapy
Brainstem glioma—slow-growing	Brainstem (medulla)	Observation, radiation
Choroid plexus papilloma—slow-growing	Choroid plexus	Surgery
Choroid plexus carcinoma—fast-growing	Choroid plexus in the ventricles	Surgery, chemotherapy, and radiation

Type of Tumor	Usual Location	Usual Treatment
Craniopharyngioma	Suprasellar region (hypothalamus, pituitary, and optic chiasm)	• Surgery alone if total removal, followed by observation • If partial removal, followed with radiation • If a cyst, chemotherapy may be injected into it
Ependymoma	Ventricular system, most commonly the fourth ventricle; rarely, in cerebral hemispheres or spinal cord	Surgery, observation, radiation, and sometimes chemotherapy
Germ cell tumor	Pineal region or suprasellar region	Varies depending on cell type and location. Can be surgery, radiation, chemotherapy, and sometimes peripheral stem cell transplant
Medulloblastoma	Posterior fossa	Surgery, craniospinal radiation, chemotherapy, and sometimes peripheral stem cell transplant
Optic pathway/hypothalamic glioma	Hypothalamus, optic nerves	Observation, then chemotherapy if tumor grows. Surgery and radiation are sometimes used.
Primitive neuroectodermal tumor (PNET)	Usually the cerebrum, but can be anywhere in the brain or brain stem	Surgery, chemotherapy, and radiation

Treatment

At diagnosis, most parents do not know how to find the best doctors and treatments for their child. State-of-the-art care is available from physicians who participate in the Children's Oncology Group (COG), sponsored by the National Cancer Institute (NCI). COG's members—pediatric surgeons and oncologists, neurologists, radiation oncologists, researchers, and nurses—develop the standard of care for patients worldwide and conduct new studies to discover better therapies and supportive care for children with all types of cancer. The NCI also sponsors a consortium called the Pediatric Brain Tumor Consortium (PBTC) that consists of 11 institutions in the United States (all of which are members of COG). For further information about COG and PBTC, read Chapter 5, *Choosing a Treatment*.

Treatment of brain and spinal cord tumors includes one or more of the following:

• Surgery

• Chemotherapy

• Radiation

- Stem cell transplantation
- Observation
- Biologic modifiers and targeted therapies

Research continues to evaluate new types of treatment. At the present time, areas of exploration include reduced radiation dose, new methods of delivering radiation, new chemotherapy drugs, targeted therapies, and biological modifiers. The goal of these new treatments is to increase cure rates and lessen the likelihood of late effects from treatment.

The following sections provide a very brief overview of treatments. For more detailed information, refer to the chapters on surgery, chemotherapy, radiation, and stem cell transplantation.

Surgery

Surgery is the primary treatment for most brain and spinal cord tumors. It is used to establish the diagnosis and to remove as much of the tumor as possible. For detailed information, see Chapter 10, *Surgery.*

> *The surgery to remove the tumor took about 4 hours, and there were no major complications. Scott spent 3 hours in the recovery room before being ready to go to the ICU. His first words after waking were, "I love you, Mom," which obviously touched Karen. While in the recovery room, we realized that Scott's stuffed Yoshi toy, who also went to the operating room, returned with a head bandage identical to Scott's. Someone had a sense of humor!*

· · · · ·

> *Kirsten's tumor had shrunk enough after four cycles of chemotherapy for a near total resection. However, the tumor was still considered active, and after surgery she went on to receive three more cycles of chemotherapy.*

Chemotherapy

Chemotherapy is a term that refers to drugs that kill cancer cells. It is used to treat all fast-growing brain and spinal cord tumors and many slow-growing tumors. Response rates are considerably improved when more than one chemotherapy drug is given at a time. Some commonly used chemotherapy drugs include vincristine, cisplatin, carboplatin, etoposide, temazolomide, irinotecan, and cyclophosphamide. For detailed information, see Chapter 11, *Chemotherapy.*

Chemotherapy is sometimes given at the same time as radiation therapy in an attempt to increase radiation's effectiveness. In this case, the chemotherapy is referred to as a radio-sensitizer.

> Luke (2 years old) had side effects from his chemo protocol that were relatively minor compared to what other children experience. He did have nausea, but it usually consisted of one to three vomiting episodes over 1 or 2 days and was over quickly. Over the entire eight course cycle he did have numerous neutropenic bouts (low blood counts), with several visits to the emergency room for night-onset fevers resulting in short-term hospitalizations to get IV antibiotics. He did get two or three infections in his catheter, which also required hospitalizations for antibiotics. However, he only needed one blood and one platelet transfusion during the entire protocol. He ate incredibly well all during his protocol and even gained steadily in weight and height.

Generally, treatment with chemotherapy is mapped out in a protocol which includes a list of the medications to be used and how they are administered, the recommended dosages, and a schedule for when the medications will be given over the course of treatment. Protocols are explained in detail in Chapter 5, *Choosing a Treatment*.

Radiation therapy

Radiation therapy, also called irradiation or radiotherapy, is the use of high-energy x-rays to kill cancer cells. Many brain and spinal cord tumors are sensitive to radiation.

The primary role of radiation is to destroy tumor cells. Radiation is given locally to the area of the tumor and is given to the entire brain and spine if the tumor has spread or is likely to spread to other areas of the brain and spinal cord. For detailed information, see Chapter 13, *Radiation Therapy*.

> Radiation was tough but it was also short. Ethan was still mute after surgery and pretty uncooperative, so we had no idea what he wanted to know. We opted to tell him everything: that he had cancer, that he needed radiation to treat the cancer, that they would be putting him to sleep everyday to do the radiation, and that he would lose all his hair, but through it all we would be with him.

> The radiation to the head and spine lasted 13 days and was the hardest part. Ethan was nauseated (despite ondansetron). He stopped eating completely at one point, and had odd cravings at others. We met with the pediatric oncology dietician and when we asked what we should do if Ethan would only eat French fries. Her response was to take him to McDonalds three times a day. While we were shocked at the time, it really helped us readjust our expectations and priorities. Calories became king. Brownies for breakfast? So be it. We were so proud when he ate two instead of just one. These priorities continued into the year of chemotherapy and have served us well.

Stem cell transplantation

In the last decade, peripheral blood stem cell transplantation (PBSCT) has been used to treat children with difficult-to-treat malignant or relapsed brain and spinal cord tumors. In this procedure, high-dose chemotherapy is given; this kills bone marrow as well as tumor cells. Normal stem cells are then infused into the child's veins. The stem cells migrate to the cavities inside the bones, where new, healthy blood cells are then produced. For some tumors, the current treatment is a series of two or three PBSCTs (referred to as tandem stem cell transplants). For more information about these types of transplants, see Chapter 14, *Peripheral Blood Stem Cell Transplantation*.

> Sean (18 months old) has now had two rounds of high-dose chemo with stem cell transplants. The first went off without a hitch, the second was a bit of a nightmare. He got an infection, colitis, and then a staph infection in his line. He was in the hospital for about 10 days after the stem cell transplant. With Sean's diagnosis of atypical teratoid/rhabdoid tumor (AT/RT), we know that our time with him may be limited and we want to make sure we are focused on giving him the best shot at survival and, as important, the best shot at a joyful, loving life, however long.

Observation

Unlike many other cancers, brain tumors (especially slow-growing tumors) may have periods of little or no growth. For this reason, the physician may decide to check the tumor with MRI scans at designated intervals. Observation may be recommended if the tumor is quite small and causes no symptoms. A period of observation usually occurs after partial removal of a deep, slow-growing tumor (especially in a young child). Observation always occurs after completion of treatment for a fast-growing brain or spinal cord tumor.

> Brendon was diagnosed with a slow-growing tumor of the brainstem when he was 7 years old, after 2 years of confusing symptoms and dozens of doctor appointments. The first children's hospital told us, "We can't do chemo and we can't radiate it. It's too deep for surgery. Take him home; he has less than 6 months to live." We saw an article in a magazine about a famous pediatric neurosurgeon, and called him. He called us right back and 2 days later he operated and took out about 90 percent of the tumor. The treatment was just observation then. We had MRIs every few months. When Brendon was 10 he started getting symptoms again—trouble swallowing, breathing problems, growing paralysis. The tumor was growing inward so surgery wasn't an option. So, we did chemo and it relieved many of the symptoms. Then we observed again. This has been the pattern for the last decade—treat, observe, treat, observe. Brendon is now 16.

Biological modifier therapy and targeted therapies

Many researchers devote their lives to unlocking the mystery of what causes brain tumors to form and how to change or stop tumor growth. Over the past 2 decades, slow but steady progress has been made. Two newer approaches in treating children with brain and spinal cord tumors are biological modifier therapy and targeted therapies.

Biological modifier therapy uses living cells, substances derived from living cells, or synthetic versions of cells to treat tumors. Some types of biological modifier therapy use the immune system to identify and kill tumor cells, and other types target tumor cells directly. For example, one biological therapy, called immunotherapy, uses synthetic copies of proteins (antibodies) to attack foreign cells like cancer. Another biological therapy uses cytokines (proteins that act as hormone regulators) to stop tumor growth or interrupt cell movement.

Targeted cancer therapies use drugs or other substances that block either the growth or spread of cancer by interfering with the molecules involved in tumor growth. Targeted therapies interfere with cancer cell division in different ways. Some therapies focus on the proteins that are involved in cell signaling pathways, which form a communication system that governs basic cellular functions and activities such as cell division, cell movement, and cell death. By blocking signals that tell cancer cells to grow and divide uncontrollably, targeted cancer therapies can help stop cancer progression and may cause cancer cells to die. Other targeted therapies can indirectly cause cancer cell death by stimulating the immune system to recognize and destroy cancer cells and/or by delivering toxic substances directly to the cancer cells.

New biological and targeted therapies are being tested for brain and spinal cord tumors. To learn more about the newest targeted and biological therapies, go to *www.cancer.gov*. You can search the website for information about new therapies and for a list of clinical trials available for your child's brain or spinal cord tumor. An additional source of information is CancerNet, which you can reach by calling 888-273-3508 or online at *http://cancernet.gov.*

Our daughter Morgan was diagnosed with medulloblastoma in the cerebellum when she was 2 years old. We researched, took her to one of the top pediatric neurosurgeons in the country, and he totally resected it. We did more research on treatment options, since radiation at her age would be devastating. But, we also wanted to kill the cancer. We decided on a clinical trial that involved very high dose chemotherapy with stem cell rescue [transplantation]. Those treatments were incredibly difficult.

Two years later, the tumor grew again at the same place, but we caught it early. It was again totally removed, and we again began a research effort on options for treatment. We chose a new type of radiation. We, like many other families of kids with brain tumors, had to use many different treatment methods over time. We are so grateful that new, and more effective, treatments had been developed to help our daughter.

Morgan is now 18 years old. She is a senior in high school and is currently looking at colleges. Does she have learning disabilities? Yes. Are they stopping her from pursuing her dreams? No.

Chapter 4

Telling Your Child and Others

To name things is to tame them.
— Tim O'Brien
Tomcat in Love

YOU HAVE JUST LEARNED your child is gravely ill. There is so much to take in, so much to do, and all you really want to do is wake up and end this nightmare; but you are the only one who knows this news. What will you tell your sick child? And what can you say to your other children, or your parents? Should you tell your friends and neighbors? What can you possibly say?

Telling your child

It is important to defy any urge you have to shield your child from the truth, because honesty is one of the most important gifts you can give him. Your child needs to know what is happening now and what is to come. Because you are coping with a bewildering array of emotions yourself, sharing information and providing reassurance and hope may be difficult. In the past, shielding children from the painful reality of cancer was the norm. Most experts now agree that children feel less anxiety and cope with treatments better if they have a clear understanding of their illness. It is important to provide age-appropriate information soon after diagnosis and to create a supportive climate so children feel comfortable asking questions of both parents and the medical team. Sharing strengthens the family, allowing all members to face the crisis together.

> *Before Alissa's first surgery for spinal astrocytoma when she was 6 years old, I took a little chalkboard, drew a stick figure with circles for vertebrae. I pointed to her back, and explained what the spinal cord does. I told her, "You have something growing in there that needs to be removed. The doctors need to cut your back and remove it." We didn't use any baby talk. We told her and her brother Nicholas exactly what was going on.*

When to tell your child

You should tell your child as soon as possible after diagnosis. Sick children know they are sick, and all children know when their parents are upset, frightened, and withholding information. In the absence of the truth, children imagine—and believe—scenarios far more frightening than the reality. With no warning, they have found themselves in strange surroundings; all of their normal activities stop occurring; total strangers are performing scary and painful procedures on them; their parents are upset; and everywhere they look, they see sick or disabled children. They may not be talking about their fears, often in an effort to protect their parents, but they know something is very wrong.

> We immediately told Ethan that he had a brain tumor. His father and I were crying and he knew something was wrong, so we felt this was the best approach. He was 6 years old at the time, and we told him he had something growing in his head that should not be there and he needed surgery to take it out. He knew about cancer before he had it, and he knew that it was a bad thing to have, but he has handled the knowledge that he had it very well. Now that he is older, when he looks back on those early days he says that he was glad that we told him what was going on and that he was never frightened. I wish that I could say the same, but I am grateful that we were able to make him feel comfortable about what he was facing.

The most loving thing a parent can do is to tell the truth before the child is overwhelmed by the fear of what she has imagined. Staying silent has another side effect: it undermines the credibility of the parent with the child. This will be a very long and frightening journey, and your child must believe you are in this together and that she can always count on you to support her and tell her the truth.

> We felt we had to tell Jessica the truth from the very beginning. She needed to know that she could trust us. Talking about it helped her understand why the treatments were necessary. We told her that her hair would fall out, but that it didn't matter. She would still be beautiful to us, with or without hair. We told her when something would hurt and when it wouldn't. We told her we were all in this together and that we would discuss everything every step of the way.

Who should tell your child

Who tells your child about his illness is a personal decision, influenced by the age and temperament of the child, religious beliefs, and sometimes physician recommendation. Children ages 1 to 3 usually fear separation from parents, so the presence of strangers in an already unfamiliar situation may increase their anxiety. Many parents tell their small child in private, while others prefer to have a family physician, oncologist, social worker, member of the clergy, or other family members present. Many children's hospitals have child life specialists who can help explain the diagnosis and treatment to children in an age-appropriate manner. They can help you develop a strategy to speak with your child about the diagnosis. Often, they have age-appropriate materials (books, pictures, dolls) to help with the conversation.

> *When we first found out that the MRI showed a moderately large tumor, we didn't tell Billy, who was 2 years old, until a few days later. I think we needed to be clear for ourselves what the plan was going to be. Over the next few days, we started to tell him that the MRI pictures showed that he had a boo-boo in his head, and soon we would take a trip to a hospital with Grammie where the boo-boo would be fixed. When the day came for surgery, Grammie was with us when we told him again about the boo-boo inside his head, that this was the day for it to be fixed, and that he would take a nap while the doctors fixed the boo-boo. He asked if we would be with him, and we each reassured him that we all would be there when he woke up. I had decided not to mention any pain or about bandages near his eyes, but I think now that we know a little better, we might have said something about that, too.*

Children ages 4 to 12 sometimes benefit from having the treatment team (neuro-oncologist, nurse, social worker, child life specialist, or psychologist) present. It provides an opportunity to promote the sense that everyone is united in their efforts to help your child get well. Staff members can answer the child's questions and provide comfort for the entire family. Children in this age group frequently feel guilty and responsible for their illness. They may harbor fears that the cancer is a punishment for something they did wrong. Parents, social workers, psychologists, child life specialists, and nurses can help explore unspoken questions and provide reassurance.

> *My 6-year-old son Brian was sitting next to me when the doctor called to tell me that he had cancer. I whispered into the phone, "What should I tell him?" The doctor said to tell him that he was sick and needed to go to a special children's hospital for help. As we were getting ready to go to the hospital, Brian asked if he was going to die, and what were they going to do to him. We didn't know how to answer all the questions, but told him that we would find out at the hospital. My husband told him that he was a strong boy and we would all fight this thing together. I was at a loss for words.*
>
> *At the hospital, they were wonderful. What impressed me the most was that they always talked to Brian first, and answered all his questions before talking to us. When Zack (Brian's 8-year-old brother) came to the hospital 2 days later, the doctors took him in the hall and talked to him for a long time, explaining and answering his questions.*
>
> *I was glad that we were all so honest, because Brian later confided to me that he had first thought he got cancer because he hadn't been drinking enough milk.*

Adolescents have a powerful need for control and autonomy that should be respected. At a time when teens' developmental tasks include becoming independent from their families, teens with cancer are suddenly totally dependent on medical personnel to save their lives and on parents to provide emotional support. Teenagers sometimes feel more comfortable discussing the diagnosis with their physician in private. In some families, a diagnosis of cancer can create an unwelcome dependence on parents and can add new stress to the already turbulent teen years. Other families report that the illness helped forge closer bonds between teenagers and their parents.

> Just when I had expected her to become a rebellious teenager, Florence (15 years old) became even closer to me than before. She knew that I had believed her when she started having symptoms from the pituitary tumor and sometimes she said I'd saved her life.

Children and teens react to the diagnosis of cancer with a wide range of emotions, as do their parents. They may lapse into denial, feel tremendous anger or rage, or be extremely optimistic. As treatment progresses, both children and parents often experience a variety of unexpected emotions.

> We've really marveled as we watched Joseph go through the stages of coping with all of this just as an adult might. First of all, after he was diagnosed in April, he was terrified. Then in for 2 months he was alternately angry and depressed. When we talked to him seriously during that time about the need to work with the doctors and nurses against the cancer no matter how scary the things were that they asked him to do, he looked us right in the eye and screamed, "I'm on the cancer's side!" Then over the course of a few weeks he seemed to calm down and made the decision to fight it, to cooperate with all the caregivers as well as he possibly could and to live as normal a life as he could. It's hard to believe that someone could do that at 4 years old, but he did it. By his 5th birthday on July 26th, he'd made the transition to where he is now: hopeful and committed to "killing the cancer."

What to tell your child

Children need to be told that they have a tumor in their head or spine and what that means, using words and concepts appropriate for their age and level of emotional development. The sooner they are comfortable with the word *tumor*, the less mysterious it will seem and the more powerful they will feel in dealing with the disease. Very young children might be satisfied to hear, "A tumor is growing in your head and it should not be there. We are going to the hospital so the doctors can take it out." Older children may benefit from reading books, alone or together with a parent; surfing reliable Internet sites; or asking members of the treatment team questions to get the information that matters most to them.

Key concepts to convey to your child include:

- The disease is called a brain (or spinal cord) tumor and this is what it means (supply age-appropriate description).

- No one knows what causes brain tumors, and it is not the child's fault she got sick.

- Some things about brain tumors are scary—for the child and the parents—and it is okay to feel afraid, confused, angry, or sad.

- It may be necessary to spend a lot of time in the hospital.

- There might be some unpleasant side effects, such as hair loss and nausea, but most of them are temporary.

- The parents, the child, and the healthcare team all have jobs to do to help the child get well, and everyone will work together to make that happen.

- Questions or worries are normal, and the child should feel free to ask a parent or someone on the healthcare team any questions she wants to ask.

- There are many things you as parents cannot control, but you will never lie to him and will always try to make sure there are no surprises.

- School-age children might not be able to go to school for a few months, but there are ways they can keep in touch with their classmates while they are out of school.

- Cancer is not contagious; friends and family cannot catch it.

> My 4-year-old daughter told me very sadly one day, "I wish that I hadn't fallen down and broken inside. That's how the cancer started." We had explained many times that nothing she did, or we did, caused the tumor, but she persisted in thinking that falling down did it. She also worried that if she went to her friend Krista's house to play that Krista would catch cancer.

Children will have many questions throughout their treatment. Parents must assure the child that this is normal and that they will always answer the child's questions honestly. Gentle and honest communication is essential for the child to feel loved, supported, and encouraged.

> Our daughter was diagnosed as a preschooler. The older she gets, the more she asks: where's my tumor, why do I have it, what are all the medications for. She wants more of the details, and she needed to know the brain tumor wasn't her fault. We were talking about it recently, and she asked, "Why do I have it, Mommy, was I bad?"

When your child asks a question, take a moment to be sure you heard and understood it correctly and to formulate a thoughtful answer that your child will understand. Parents are under tremendous stress and have many things on their minds. In this distracted state, it is easy to toss off an easy answer or answer a question the child did not ask; but doing this can increase the child's confusion and undermine their trust in the parent as a source of information. Barbara Sourkes, PhD, explains the importance of understanding the child's question before responding:

> Coping with the trauma of illness can be facilitated by a cognitive understanding of the disease and its treatment. For this reason, the presentation of accurate information in developmentally meaningful terms is crucial. A general guideline is to follow the child's lead: he or she questions facts or implications only when ready, and that readiness must be respected. It is the adult's responsibility to clarify the precise intent of any question and then to proceed with a step-by-step response, thereby granting the child options at each juncture. He or she may choose to continue listening, to ask for clarification, or to terminate the discussion. Offering less information with the explicit invitation to ask for more affords a safety gauge of control for the child. When these guidelines are not followed, serious miscommunications may ensue. For example, an adult who hears "What is going to happen to me?" and does not clarify the intent of the query may launch into a long statement of plans or elaborate reassurances. The child may respond with irritation, "I only wanted to know what tests I am going to have tomorrow."

Telling the siblings

The diagnosis of a brain or spinal cord tumor is traumatic for siblings. Family life is disrupted, time with parents decreases, and a large amount of attention is paid to the ill child. Brothers and sisters need as much knowledge about what is going on as their sick sibling does. Information provided should be age appropriate, and all questions should be answered honestly. Healthcare providers (physicians, physician assistants, nurse practitioners, child life specialists, and social workers) can help parents educate the well siblings. Siblings can be extremely cooperative if they understand the changes that will occur in the family and their role in helping the family cope. Maintaining open communication and respecting their feelings helps siblings feel loved and secure.

> We always, always explained everything that was happening to Brian's older brother Zack (8 years old). He never asked questions, but always listened intently. He would say, "Okay. I understand. Everything's all right." We tried to get him to talk about it, but through all these years, he just never has. So we just kept explaining things at a level that he could understand, and he has done very well through the whole ordeal. The times that he seemed sad, we would take him out of school and let him stay at the Ronald McDonald House for a few days, and that seemed to help him.

We have tried to spend one-on-one time with each of the other kids. These are some other things that have been good for us:

- *The kids have been going to the hospital with Ethan one at a time, and getting a sense that this is no picnic, what he is going through.*

- *If one of us is out of town and Ethan is in the hospital, I have hired a babysitter to be with him in the evening and have done something special with the other kids for one of the nights. This works great if you live close enough to the hospital where your child is being treated.*

- *My husband and I have each taken the older kids on the traditional summer trips. This has been hard on Ethan, but none of this is perfect.*

- *My husband and I have each taken one school subject for the kids and have really spent time with them on it. I did reading with Tucker (I read everything he does and we talk about it), French with Abe, and Spanish with Jake. My husband has different topics, and we do something every day. We were too dysfunctional to be able to do more than one subject, so we decided to focus, and it has been a lot of fun for us.*

We talk about lots of things as a family and help the kids as needed, but these are "special" things. This has been a long year for us, but I think these things helped.

Even with good communication and support, parents may see siblings experiencing difficult emotions, such as anger, guilt, jealousy, and sadness, and changes in behavior, such as regression, school problems, and symptoms of illness to gain attention. These result from the stress of living with a brother or sister diagnosed with cancer. Chapter 15, *Siblings*, explores sibling issues in detail and contains many suggestions from both parents and siblings who have gone through this experience.

Notifying the family

Notifying relatives is one of the first painful jobs for the parents of a child newly diagnosed with cancer. Depending on the family dynamic, the family may be a refuge or a source of additional stress.

I called my mother and asked her to tell everyone on my side of the family. My husband called his sister and asked her to tell everyone. We asked that they not call us for a few days because we needed a little time to feel less fragile and didn't want to cry in front of Catherine too much.

• • • • •

We approached each grandmother differently and got totally unexpected responses. We thought the first grandmother, who knew the most about the symptoms we were investigating, could take the news over the phone, but it was too much for her. The other grandmom had heart problems, and we sent my brother to her house to tell her. When he got there, she wanted to know why we didn't call right away. She said, "Don't worry about me, just worry about this little one."

Family members often react in surprising ways, with unexpected help coming from some people and a disappointing lack of support from others. Parents must be prepared for these unexpected responses and try not to take them personally. Usually, the other person is struggling to process this difficult news in his or her own way and may be trying to spare the parent from more stress by not asking too many questions.

My dad had always been my rock, but when I told him about my son's illness, he basically didn't say anything and he never came to the hospital. I was furious with him. It took me a long time to realize that he needed me to be strong for him, too. He was just devastated by the thought that his only grandchild might be taken from him and there was nothing he could do to stop it.

Notifying friends and neighbors

The easiest way to notify friends and neighbors is to delegate one person to do the job. Calling only one neighbor or close friend prevents you from having numerous tearful conversations. Most parents are at their child's bedside and want to avoid more emotional upheaval, especially in front of their child. Parents need to recognize that friends' emotions will mirror their own: shock, fear, worry, helplessness. Because most friends want to help but don't know what to do or say, they will welcome any suggestions you can give about what might be helpful.

Tell a trusted friend exactly what information you want him or her to pass on and, most importantly, whether you would welcome visits, phone calls, or cards. The more clarity you can provide, the less stress you will experience and the better your friends can support you. If you want visitors, for example, let people know when visiting hours are and whether there are any restrictions set by the hospital (or by you or your child) about who can come and for how long.

There were many days I wanted to hide in bed and pull the covers over my head. I know everyone was well meaning and genuinely cared, but the constant stream of people through the house and phone ringing added to the stress we were already under. We already had a home care nurse coming 5 days a week, a physical therapist coming 3 days a week, in addition to constant phone calls to follow up on blood work and tests, appointments to schedule, and family members to keep track of. Bubba, our dog, loved all the commotion, but the rest of us tired quickly.

Not everyone you know will want or need the same level of detailed information. You may wish to encourage visits from close acquaintances but ask others to wait for phone or email updates. However, think twice before leaving anyone off the notification list. Many parents report that individuals they barely knew ended up being some of their most helpful and supportive resources.

Many families set up phone trees to provide ongoing updates—the parent calls one person, who calls a designated group of people, who then call others. More information about this topic is available in Chapter 16, *Family and Friends*.

Notifying your child's school

You should notify the principal as soon as possible about your child's diagnosis. It is a good idea to do this in writing (either by email or letter), in part because it is a less emotional way to convey the news, but also because it enables you to be certain you pass along all the relevant information. In the first contact, it is helpful to include the following information (see Chapter 18, *School*, for a sample letter):

- The diagnosis and a brief description in layman's terms of what it means
- A very brief outline of what is expected to happen next and how that will impact your child's ability to attend school
- The address, email address, and phone number where you can be reached
- A brief description of the educational resources available at the hospital or any other educational information you have been given by the hospital social worker or child life specialist and their contact information
- How your child's teacher or classmates can reach your child, especially when your child is in the hospital

You can also express your hope that you, the school, and the hospital will work together to ensure that your child's education sustains as few interruptions as possible. You can ask the principal to share your letter with the teacher (or teachers) or you can send them separate emails or notes.

When notifying students at the school, the wishes of your child (especially if a teenager) about notification of school and friends should be respected. If you and your child want to ask the teachers and students to stay in touch, inform them that she may sometimes feel too tired to answer right away. Personal visits may not be feasible or welcome, at least at first, but cards, letters, pictures, classroom videos, or other updates will make your child feel less isolated and will remind her that there are people who care for her outside of her immediate family and the hospital staff. In some schools it may be possible to attend school virtually—when it is feasible and the technology is available. More information is available in Chapter 18, *School*.

Using technology to communicate

After the initial contacts have been made, the people in your life will be eager for updates. During those first few weeks of treatment, parents have very little time to chat and often lack the energy to carry on lengthy or meaningful conversations. The nights can be long, however, and nighttime provides an excellent opportunity to use technology to keep people informed about what is happening and how you are feeling.

Many hospitals now have free wireless Internet access (Wi-Fi) in the room, in the parents' lounge, or in a communal room. Some Internet service providers offer their own Wi-Fi adapters that can be plugged into a laptop to provide access anywhere there is cell phone service. Smartphones and other personal data devices also all have Internet access.

Once connected to the Internet, many options exist for keeping in touch, including Facebook®, Twitter®, and blogs. Some parents establish an email group and send regular updates to the list. One easy way to communicate with your friends and family is to use CaringBridge (*www.caringbridge.org*), which provides free websites to families and friends of critically ill individuals. Its templates make it easy to set up an attractive site, and the software allows you to add text and photos. Parents, siblings, or the sick child can create journal entries that track the progress of treatment and discuss fears, inspirations, hopes, or needs. There is a guest book where well-wishers can post words of love and encouragement. Finally, you can make the site as public or private as you wish and link your site to other places, such as a blog or Facebook® page. The CaringBridge websites do not have annoying pop-ups or advertisements of any kind.

I was diagnosed at the age of 16 with a low-grade astrocytoma. I've had seven surgeries, including shunt revisions, and radiation. I have a large family, and I have a lot of little cousins. When I was diagnosed, I explained everything to them, and they seemed to take it pretty well. Kids can deal with issues like this, better than most adults. My youngest cousin was 5 years old. She has really grown up learning about brain tumors and knowing that her cousin has a brain tumor. She has coped with it, and understands what I have to do to fight this monster. She tells her friends that I'm her favorite cousin and she wants to be just like me! It has drawn us much closer since I was diagnosed, and I believe it is because we did not hide anything from her. We answered the questions she had, and tried to explain everything to her. She knows almost everything that we know about brain tumors, and explains to others the importance of having your brain checked. The way she deals with it makes me laugh a lot of times, and that is what I need.

Chapter 5

Choosing a Treatment

The challenge in pediatric oncology remains clear: to strive for the cure and health of all children through the development of more effective yet less damaging treatment for our young patients.

— Daniel M. Green, MD and Giulio J. D'Angio, MD
Late Effects of Treatment for Childhood Cancer

THE FIRST FEW weeks after diagnosis are utterly overwhelming. In the midst of confusion, fear, and fatigue, you might need to make an important and sometimes difficult decision: whether to choose the best-known treatment (standard treatment) or enroll your child in an experimental treatment (clinical trial). This chapter explains helpful things to know before deciding on a treatment for your child, including the difference between standard treatment and clinical trials. It also covers questions to ask about proposed treatments, informed consent, the pros and cons of selecting a clinical trial, and stories from parents about the decisions they made.

Treatment basics

To receive the best-available treatment, it is essential that the child with a brain or spinal cord tumor be treated at a pediatric medical center by board-certified pediatric oncologists or neuro-oncologists with extensive experience treating these types of tumors. For most children, treatment begins within days of diagnosis and requires aggressive supportive care. The goal of treatment is to achieve complete remission by obliterating all cancer cells as quickly as possible.

Treatment of childhood brain and spinal cord tumors includes one or more of the following:

- Surgery (see Chapter 10)

- Chemotherapy (see Chapter 11)

- Radiation Therapy (see Chapter 13)

- Peripheral Blood Stem Cell Transplantation (see Chapter 14)

Standard treatment

The standard treatment (or standard of care) for each type and stage of tumor is the treatment that has worked best for the most children up to that point in time. The current standards of care are the result of decades of clinical research studies. As researchers analyze the results from ongoing or completed clinical trials, they accumulate knowledge and make changes in standard treatments. In the 1990s, for example, most children with medulloblastoma received high doses of whole-brain radiation as standard care. Carefully controlled clinical trials later demonstrated that many children with medulloblastoma can be given a much lower dose than was used in the 1990s. Thus, the standard of care was changed.

To learn about the standard of care for your child's type and stage of tumor, contact the National Cancer Institute's (NCI) Physician's Data Query (PDQ) by calling (800) 422-6237 (800-4-CANCER) or by going to the pediatric section of its website at *www.cancer.gov/cancertopics/pdq/pediatrictreatment*. PDQ provides information about pediatric brain and spinal cord tumors, state-of-the-art treatments, and ongoing clinical trials. Two versions are available online: one for patients and their families that uses simple language and contains no statistics, and one for professionals that is technical, thorough, and includes citations to the scientific literature.

> *The study that our institution was participating in at the time of my daughter's diagnosis was attempting to lessen the treatment to reduce neurotoxicity yet still cure the disease. My family began a massive research effort on the issue, and we had several family friends who were physicians discuss the case with the heads of pediatric oncology at their institutions. The consensus was that since my daughter was at the high end of the high-risk description, it was advisable to choose the standard treatment, which was more aggressive than the proposed clinical trial.*

The protocol

If your child receives standard treatment, you will be given a written copy of the treatment plan, called a protocol. Just like a recipe for baking a cake, a protocol has a list of ingredients, the amounts to use, and the order to use them in so the protocol has the best chance for success. The protocol lists the treatments, drugs, dosages, and tests for each segment of treatment and follow-up. If your child is enrolled in a clinical trial, you will receive a copy of the short protocol but can obtain the entire protocol document by asking for it (see later section called "The entire clinical trial document").

The portion of the protocol devoted to the schedule for treatments and tests may be longer than 20 pages. The family may also be given an abbreviated version (one to two pages) for quick and easy reference on a daily basis. This abbreviated part of the protocol is frequently called the "roadmap." Parents and teenage patients should review these documents carefully with the treatment team to be certain they understand them.

> *It took me a long time to get over my hang-up that things needed to go exactly as per protocol. Any deviations on dose or days were a major stress for me. It took talking to many parents, as well as doctors and nurses, to realize and feel comfortable with the fact that no one ever goes along perfectly and that the protocol is meant as the broad guideline. There will always be times when your child will be off drugs or on half dose because of illness or low counts or whatever. It took a long time to realize that this is not going to ruin the effectiveness, that the child gets what she can handle without causing undue harm.*

Clinical trials

If a clinical trial is open for your child's particular type and stage of tumor, you will be asked to consider enrolling your child in it within days of diagnosis. You then must choose between the standard treatment and the clinical trial.

Clinical trials are carefully controlled research experiments that use human volunteers to develop better ways to prevent or cure diseases. Pediatric clinical trials attempt to improve upon existing treatments. A clinical trial can involve a totally new approach that is thought to be promising, or it may entail fine-tuning existing treatments, reducing the toxicity of known treatments, or developing new ways to assess responses to treatments. Many children are needed in each clinical trial for the results to be statistically meaningful.

In some cases, such as with average-risk medulloblastoma, the standard treatment has a high likelihood of resulting in complete and lasting remission. For other types of tumors, the prognosis is poor on the standard treatment, and parents may be more motivated to choose a clinical trial. Occasionally, parents choose to enroll their child in a clinical trial because they want to contribute to better treatments in the future. Other parents may be wary of participating in an experimental program and may opt for standard treatment. There is no "right" choice. Obtain all the information you can, weigh the pros and cons, and make a decision based on your values and comfort with the choice.

Your treatment team may tell you about studies that are sponsored by pharmaceutical companies, especially those designed to support patients through the effects of treatment. Such supportive care trials evaluate antibiotics, anti-nausea drugs, and new agents to raise blood counts, minimize pain, or control other symptoms. The oversight and control of these trials involves an entirely different mechanism than the oncology treatment studies discussed in this chapter. Ask your doctor or nurse to discuss these studies with you if your child is invited to participate in one.

You also may be asked for permission to allow biological studies of your child's tumor. These studies involve performing specific tests on pieces of your child's tumor to better understand how the cancer works with the hope that knowledge will lead to the development of better treatments. The neurosurgeon or pediatric oncologist may ask your permission to send any tumor left over after diagnosis to a tumor bank for research. Because brain tumors can have subtle differences (called subtypes), biological studies help researchers better identify and understand the subtypes. The categorization of different types of medulloblastoma has come from this type of research. Scientists are also using banked tumor cells to test response to new medications and immunotherapy.

Types of clinical trials

There are three main types of clinical trials offered to children with brain or spinal cord tumors.

Phase I. Drug studies begin in laboratories, where the drugs are evaluated using chemical or biological models, tissue samples, and other methods to see if there is a chance the drug might be effective at treating disease. If laboratory evidence suggests a drug may work in humans, it is first tested in a Phase I study. These studies examine how the body processes (metabolizes) the drug, establish the highest dose that can safely be given to a patient (the maximum tolerated dose, or MTD), and evaluate the side effects.

In pediatric Phase I trials, the dose of a new drug is gradually increased in small groups of children until it becomes too toxic; essentially, one small group of children gets a low dose, the next small group gets a slightly higher dose, and so on, until an unacceptable number of children experience unacceptable toxicities. Phase I studies are true experiments and their purpose is not to cure the participants. The true beneficiaries of Phase I studies are future patients. In most cases, parents are not asked to enroll their child in a Phase I study unless all other treatment options have failed. Parents often enroll their children in these trials in the hope that a new and untried drug will be effective against their child's disease, but they need to recognize that the chances of achieving remission are low. Because they require careful monitoring, Phase I studies are only conducted in a select few hospitals.

Phase II. Phase II trials refine the safety parameters and evaluate new drugs' effects on specific tumors. This is the stage at which many drugs fail—meaning they are not as effective as originally predicted or they have unexpected or serious side effects in many patients. Sometimes patients are enrolled when their tumors have regrown after treatment. Occasionally, Phase II trials are designed to test an exceptionally promising agent against a tumor for which other effective therapies exist.

Phase III trials. These clinical trials determine if a new treatment is better than the usual or standard therapy. Some Phase III trials are designed solely to improve survival; others try to maintain survival rates while lowering toxicity of treatment. In pediatric Phase III studies, some children will receive the standard therapy, while others receive some modification, such as higher or lower doses of medication or radiation, different combinations of drugs, or shorter or longer treatments. Some children will derive direct benefit if a new treatment proves superior to standard therapy. Others will receive the same therapy they would have received if not enrolled on the study (the standard arm). To ensure the results are accurate, Phase III studies require thousands of participants and several years to complete.

The NCI offers several resources to help parents understand the clinical trial process. You can call the NCI at (800) 422-6237 or visit its clinical trials website at *www.cancer. gov/clinical_trials*.

The information in the rest of this chapter pertains to Phase III trials that are reviewed and funded by the NCI. Issues for enrolling in Phase I and Phase II trials are very different, as are concerns when enrolling in trials sponsored by private companies.

Design of clinical trials

In 2000, four pediatric cancer research groups merged to form a single pediatric cancer research organization called the Children's Oncology Group (COG), which is supported by the NCI (*www.childrensoncologygroup.org*). Approximately 200 institutions that treat children with cancer are members of COG. The NCI also sponsors a consortium called The Pediatric Brain Tumor Consortium (PBTC) that consists of 11 institutions in the United States (all of which are members of COG):

- Children's Hospital Los Angeles (California)
- Children's National Medical Center (Washington, DC)
- Children's Memorial Hospital (Chicago, Illinois)
- Cincinnati Children's Hospital Medical Center (Ohio)
- The Brain Tumor Center at Duke (Durham, North Carolina)
- Lucile Packard Children's Hospital (Palo Alto, California)
- Memorial Sloan Kettering Cancer Center (New York)

- National Cancer Institute (Bethesda, Maryland)
- St. Jude Children's Research Hospital (Memphis, Tennessee)
- Texas Children's Cancer Center (Houston)
- University of Pittsburgh (Pennsylvania)

The purpose of the PBTC is to test new agents and therapies for pediatric brain tumors and to evaluate cutting-edge diagnostic technology (Phase 1 and Phase II trials). All members of PBTC have well-established, multidisciplinary brain tumor programs and are capable of performing technically challenging studies. You can learn more about this group at its website *www.pbtc.org*.

Study arms

Phase III studies have multiple arms, which means participants are sorted into different groups (called arms) that receive different treatments. Every Phase III trial has one arm that is the current standard of care. Each of the other arms contains one or more experimental components, such as:

- New drugs
- Old drugs used in a new way (e.g., different dose or new combinations of old drugs)
- Duration of treatment that is shorter or longer than standard care
- The addition, deletion, or change in dose of certain treatments (such as radiation therapy)
- The use of new supportive care interventions, such as preventative antibiotics or new drugs to control nausea

When the trial is completed and all the data is analyzed, the effectiveness of each experimental arm is compared to the "standard of care" arm. When designing pediatric clinical trials, the first priority is to protect the children from harm. Researchers are ethically bound to offer treatments they think will be at least as safe and effective as the standard of care.

> *Sean missed the deadline for enrolling in a clinical trial when he was diagnosed. However, when his tumor regrew we did enroll him on a trial. The particular trial he was in was a randomized computer trial that decided if he was getting one or two chemotherapy agents. We felt if we enrolled him in the trial, maybe the results would help other children.*

Randomization

Phase III trials require a process called randomization, meaning that after parents agree to enroll their child in a clinical trial, a computer randomly assigns the child to one arm of the study. The parents will not know which treatment their child will receive until the computer assigns one. The purpose of computer assignment is to ensure patients are evenly assigned to each treatment plan without bias from physicians or families. One group of children (the control group) always receives the standard treatment to provide a basis for comparison to the experimental arms. At the time the clinical trial is designed, there is no conclusive evidence to indicate which arm is superior. Thus, it is impossible to predict whether your child will benefit from participating in the study.

> We had a hard time deciding whether to go with the standard treatment or to partici-
> pate in the study. The "B" arm of the study seemed, on intuition, to be too harsh for
> her because she was so weak at the time. We finally did opt for the study, hoping we
> wouldn't be randomized to "B." We chose the study basically so that the computer
> could choose and we wouldn't ever have to think "we should have gone with the
> study." As it turned out, we were randomized to the standard arm, so we got what
> we wanted while still participating in the study.

Researchers closely monitor ongoing studies and modify the study if one arm is clearly identified as superior during the course of the trial or if an arm has unacceptable side effects.

Supervision of clinical trials

The ethical and legal codes ruling medical practice also apply to clinical trials. In addition, most research is federally funded or regulated (all COG trials are), with rules that protect patients. COG and PBCT also have review boards that meet at prearranged dates for the duration of a clinical trial to ensure the risks of all parts of the trial are acceptable relative to the benefits.

The treating institution is required to report all adverse side effects to COG, which reports them to the U.S. Food and Drug Administration. If concerns are raised, the study may be temporarily halted while an independent Data Safety and Monitoring Board and the study committee review the situation. If one arm of the trial is causing unexpected or unacceptable side effects, that portion is stopped, and the children enrolled are given the better treatment.

All institutions that conduct clinical trials also have an Institutional Review Board (IRB) that reviews and approves all research taking place there. The purpose of such boards and committees—made up of scientists, doctors, nurses, and citizens from the community—is to protect patients. Funding agencies (e.g., NCI) review and approve trials before children are enrolled.

Questions to ask about clinical trials

To fully understand the clinical trial that has been proposed, here are some important questions to ask the oncologist:

- What is the purpose of the study?

- Who is sponsoring the study? Who reviews it? How often is it reviewed? Who monitors patient safety?

- What tests and treatments will be done during the study? How do these differ from standard treatment?

- Why is it thought that the treatment being studied may be better than standard treatment?

- What are the possible benefits?

- What are all possible disadvantages?

- What are the possible side effects or risks of the study? What are the side effects of the study compared to those of standard treatment?

- How will the study affect my child's daily life?

- What are the possible long-term impacts of the study compared with the standard treatment?

- How long will the study last? Is this shorter or longer than standard treatment?

- Will the study require more hospitalization than standard treatment?

- Does the study include long-term follow-up care?

- What happens if my child is harmed as a result of the research?

- Will you compare for me the study versus standard treatment in terms of possible outcomes, side effects, time involved, costs, and quality of life?

- Have insurers been reimbursing for care on this protocol?

After discussing the clinical trial with the oncologist, you will need a copy of the information to review later. Many parents record the conversation or bring a friend to take notes; others write down all the doctor's answers for later reference.

> *Our 18-year-old daughter Morgan was diagnosed with a medulloblastoma in her cerebellum when she was 2 years old. A clinical trial involving very high-dose chemotherapy followed by stem cell transplant was proposed. We asked numerous*

questions, and I wrote down all the answers in my notebook. The two primary questions were: How many kids die during and after this treatment? Are her chances of long-term survival worth the pain we were going to put her through? We struggled with the concept of hurting her if it wasn't going to do any good. We also asked about the specific drugs, their side effects, and what to expect from each treatment. It was a very difficult process and decision.

Pros and cons of clinical trials

Making the decision whether to have your child participate in a clinical trial is often difficult. The following list of reasons why some families chose whether or not to enroll may help clarify your feelings about this important decision.

Why some families choose to enroll:

- Children receive either state-of-the-art investigational therapy or the best standard therapy available.

- Clinical trials can provide an opportunity to benefit from a new therapy before it is generally available.

- Children enrolled in clinical trials may be monitored more frequently throughout treatment.

- Review boards of scientists oversee the operation of clinical trials.

- Participating in a clinical trial often makes parents feel they did everything medically possible for their child.

- Information gained from clinical trials will benefit children with cancer in the future.

Reasons why families choose not to enroll:

- The experimental arm may not provide treatment as effective as the standard, or it may generate additional side effects or risks.

- Some families do not like the feeling of not having control over choosing the child's treatment.

- Some clinical trials require more hospitalizations, treatments, clinic visits, or tests that may be more painful than the standard treatment.

- Some families feel additional stress about which arm is the best treatment for their child.

- Insurance may not cover investigational studies. Parents need to carefully explore this issue prior to signing the consent form.

When my son was diagnosed with an optic glioma, we were told we had two options: a clinical trial or standard treatment. We decided to get a second opinion before making our decision. Our pediatrician, my husband, and I met in the doctor's office for a telephone conference with a pediatric oncologist from a major brain tumor center. We each presented our concerns, including our pediatrician, who thought of some issues we hadn't considered. I think we all came away better informed of our options.

Informed consent

True informed consent is a process—not merely an explanation and signing of documents. Informed consent requires that:

- All treatments available to the child have been explained—not just the treatment available at your hospital or through your doctor, but all the treatments that could be beneficial, wherever they are given.

- The parents and, to the extent possible, the child, have discussed these options and decided they want to consider one of them.

- The option selected is thoroughly discussed, with all its benefits and risks clearly explained.

- Those aspects of the study that are considered experimental and those that are standard are clearly described.

A fully informed medical decision is one that weighs the relative merits of a therapy after full disclosure of benefits, risks, and alternatives. During the discussions between the doctor(s) and family, all questions should be answered in language that is clearly understood by the parents and child, and there should be no pressure on parents to enroll their child in a study. The objective of the informed consent process is that all family members are comfortable with their choice and can comply with it. Studies show that the more questions parents ask during the informed consent process, the better they understand what they are agreeing to.

We had many discussions with the staff prior to signing the informed consent to participate in the clinical trial. We asked innumerable questions, all of which were answered in a frank and honest manner. We felt that participating gave our child the best chance for a cure, and we felt good about increasing the knowledge that would help other children later.

Informed consent is a process that occurs over several meetings during which the physician provides information and the parents ask questions (and get answers). Sometimes the informed consent process does not work as it should because of several factors, including the state of mind of the parents, the communication style of the doctor, and the system (if any) in place to discuss treatment options. Usually, this situation is the result of miscommunication arising from some combination of the following:

- No formal meeting times were established in advance to discuss treatment options, so parents do not understand the importance of the discussion they are having with the doctor and the treatment team.

- Parents, who are tired, confused, and mentally numb, may appear to understand things they are barely hearing.

- The doctor does not recognize that the parents are not following what he is saying and that they need more guidance and time to absorb the choices.

- The doctor is unconsciously promoting the choice she believes is the best one and she interprets the lack of questions as agreement.

- There is no one in the room except the doctor and the parents; therefore, there is no one to intervene if communication breaks down.

It is a good idea to ask the treatment team immediately after diagnosis when and how the treatment decision will be made and to ask for specific meeting dates and times to discuss treatment, even if it means a slight delay before starting treatment. Parents may also want to invite a trusted friend or their child's pediatrician to attend this meeting to ensure they understand their options.

Studies have shown that when treatment team members who are not doctors are present during the informed consent meetings, parents have a better understanding of their choices. You may want to ask that a nurse or a social worker be present for the meetings.

> *Two days after my child was diagnosed, the oncologist told me it was time to begin treatment. I do remember him talking a lot, but I swear it actually sounded like "Wah, wah, wah, protocol, wah, wah, wah, very successful, wah, wah, wah, sign here." And I did. It was several days before it sank in that I had authorized an experimental treatment protocol and not the standard of care. The irony is that I worked in clinical research. I knew how this was supposed to go. But I was alone and tired and frightened and went along like a sheep. Did he railroad me? Maybe; but I don't think he meant to and in the end it was my responsibility to hold it together and ask what needed to be asked. But it just wasn't in me at the time. Later, I told the doctor this and he was astonished to learn that I hadn't heard a word he said. My child is doing well now, so I am happy, but if I had it to do again, I might not have made the choice I did.*

The clinical trial consent form

The form parents sign will have language similar to the following: "The study described above has been explained to me, and I voluntarily agree to have my child participate in this study. I have had all of my questions answered, and understand that all future questions that I have about this research will be answered by the investigators listed above."

By the time a study is published in the literature, doctors on the cutting edge of treatment are 2 to 4 years into improving that treatment or learning of its shortcomings. For this reason, it is best to make decisions in partnership with knowledgeable medical caregivers, rather than on your own.

No matter how comfortable you are with your child's treating oncologist, it may be helpful to have another medical caregiver help sort out your options. Often, that person will be the family's pediatrician or family doctor. Second opinions can be obtained from physicians at other COG institutions or one of the members of PBTC. They will arrange to review the information (e.g., scans, pathology, biological and molecular tumor cell characteristics) and then will provide a second opinion. It is most useful to get a second opinion from a center that treats significant numbers of patients with your child's diagnosis. Most pediatric oncologists are willing to facilitate this process for you.

Assent

Assent means that children and adolescents are involved in decisions about their treatment. Children younger than age 18 do not have the right to refuse standard treatment for their cancer. They do, however, have the right to accept or reject experimental treatments. All clinical trials are considered to be experimental treatments. Regardless of whether children will receive the standard treatment or an experimental treatment, they have rights to have the disease, treatment, and procedures explained to them at an age-appropriate level.

Doctors and parents are required to allow children to provide input to the extent of the child's abilities. According to the American Academy of Pediatrics (AAP), assent means that the child:

• Is aware of the nature of his or her disease

• Understands what to expect from tests and treatments

• Has had his or her understanding assessed

• Has had an opportunity to accept or reject the proposed treatment

Parents can read or download a copy of the AAP policy statement ("Informed Consent, Parental Permission, and Assent in Pediatric Practice") at *http://pediatrics. aappublications.org/content/95/2/314.full.pdf+html.* This policy was reaffirmed by the AAP in 2011. In part, the policy states, "In situations in which the patient will have to receive medical care despite his or her objection, the patient should be told that fact and should not be deceived." This policy applies to standard treatment.

Clinical trials, however, are research. An added layer of protection is added for research trials, and IRBs decide whether assent of the child is needed. If parents and the child disagree, usually several discussions are held with mediators (for example, a social worker or pediatric psychologist) to try to reach an agreement. If parents and their child still disagree, an advocate for the child is appointed and a decision about treatment is made by the hospital ethics committee.

In short, parents can legally make decisions about standard care, but both parents and children have decision-making rights about whether or not to participate in research.

Saying no to a clinical trial

Parents, older children, and teens have the legal right to decide whether or not to participate in a clinical trial. If the family chooses for the child not to participate in the proposed clinical trial, the child is given the best-known treatment (standard treatment) for his type of tumor.

> We just were not comfortable with the concept of a clinical trial. It seemed like gambling to us. We also felt totally overwhelmed about making decisions on important subjects that we didn't understand. Even though we asked many, many questions, we just couldn't come to grips with the whole idea in the 2 days after our daughter was diagnosed. So, we declined the trial and had the best-known treatment. We were happy with our decision.

The entire clinical trial document

If your child is enrolled in a clinical trial, the roadmap described earlier is actually a very small portion of a lengthy document describing all aspects of the study. The entire document usually exceeds 100 pages and covers the following topics: study hypothesis, experimental design, scientific background and rationale with relevant references from the scientific literature, patient eligibility and randomization, therapy for each arm of the study, required observations, pathology guidelines, radiation therapy guidelines (if applicable), supportive care guidelines, specific information about each drug, relapse therapy guidelines, statistical considerations, study committee members, record-keeping requirements, reporting of adverse drug reactions, and a consent form.

The full protocol is intended for use by specialists in oncology medicine and nursing and is not written in lay language. It is highly technical and can be confusing or overwhelming for parents.

However, some parents are medical professionals or people who want to better understand their child's illness and treatment. These parents may want to have a copy of the study document for several reasons. First, it provides a description of some of the clinical trials that preceded the present one and explains the reasons the investigators designed this particular study. Second, it provides detailed descriptions of drug reactions, which comfort many parents who worry that their child is the only one exhibiting extreme responses to some drugs. Third, motivated parents who have only one protocol to keep track of occasionally prevent errors in treatment. Finally, for parents who are adrift in the world of cancer treatment, it can return to them a bit of control over their child's life.

> Since knowledge is comfort for me, I really wanted to have the entire clinical trial document, despite its technical language. Whereas the brief protocol that I had listed day, drug, and dose, the expanded version listed the potential side effects for each drug, and what actions should be taken should any occur. I learned the parameters.

Other parents find that reading hundreds of pages of technical information is overwhelming or just not helpful. As with almost every topic discussed in this book, families need to make individual choices based on what works best for their unique needs.

If your child is enrolled in a clinical trial and you would like a copy of the entire document, ask your child's neuro-oncologist for one. If the neuro-oncologist will not provide it, call COG (626-447-0064) and ask for a copy. Informed consent documents for COG trials specifically state that families will receive a copy of the full protocol upon request. After reading the protocol, it may be helpful to schedule an appointment with your physician, nurse practitioner, or research nurse to discuss any questions or concerns.

The protocol is not for general distribution, because it is unethical to use these protocols outside a controlled research setting. Parents who obtain a copy should not circulate it.

Removing a child from a clinical trial

Parents have the legal right to withdraw their child from a clinical trial at any time, for any reason. But before doing so, it's a good idea to discuss questions or concerns with your child's doctor. The decision to withdraw from a trial should not be held against the parent, and the child will still receive the best available care for her type of cancer. On the consent form signed by the parent, there will be language similar to this: "You are free not to have your child participate in this research or to withdraw your child at any time without penalty or jeopardizing future care."

*Jesse was enrolled in a clinical trial to assess long-term neuropsychological conse-
quences of cranial radiation. The testing was free, and we were glad to participate.
Unfortunately, the billing department of the hospital continually billed us in error.
We tried to correct the problem, but it became such a hassle that we withdrew from
the study.*

Making a decision

As soon as possible after diagnosis, parents sit down with the medical team to discuss
treatment options. If your child is being treated at a research hospital, the first discussion is usually about standard treatment and a clinical trial, if a trial is open and your
child qualifies. Parents are often very conflicted about choosing a treatment.

*We did a study and my son received 1.8 Gy, with a boost to the entire posterior fossa.
I have struggled with lots of guilt over the decision. We were thrown into such a
whirlwind and decisions had to be made so quickly. My husband and I debated and
debated, prayed and prayed, and then when we decided to go ahead with the study,
we both agreed to no regrets. But, it did feel as if we were playing Russian roulette
with our child.*

The choice to opt for standard treatment or a clinical trial is a strictly personal one, but
parents should only make it after they are certain they understand the implications of
each path. The doctor is legally and ethically bound to alert parents to the full range of
medically appropriate treatment options available to their child and to help the parents
understand what each option entails before asking them for written consent (and older
children and teens to provide assent) to begin a particular treatment plan. The doctor
may recommend a particular treatment option that he believes to be in the best interest
of the child, but he may not coerce or deceive the parents into approving a treatment.
Once the parents have consented to standard treatment or a clinical trial, the doctor is
obligated to abide by their decision.

Protocol changes

Many parents express anguish when their child's doses or schedules for chemotherapy
change during treatment. It is very common for doses to be lowered or treatment to be
delayed while a child recovers from low blood counts, infection, or toxic reactions to
the treatment. In fact, almost every child has dose reduction(s) or delays in treatment.
The protocol is a guideline that will be modified, depending on your child's response
to treatment.

I didn't know what a protocol was when my son was diagnosed, and I understood from the doctors that this was the "exact" regime that must be followed to cure him. It frightened me whenever changes were made in the protocol. With time, I came to view the protocol as merely a guideline that is individualized for each patient according to his tolerance and reaction to the drugs. We ended up deleting whole sections of the protocol due to extreme side effects. He has been off therapy for 15 years now and is doing great.

When we were struggling with the decision of whether to join the study, I asked the oncologist how would we ever know if we made the right decision. He said something very wise. "You will never know and you should never second guess yourself, no matter how the study turns out. Statistics are about large groups of kids, not your child. Your child might respond no matter which arm she is on or she might show no benefit from a treatment arm where most other kids do well. Statistics for you will be either 100 percent or 0 because your child will either live or die. I can't tell you which will be the better treatment, that is why we are conducting the study. But no matter what, we will be doing absolutely the best we can."

Chapter 6

Coping with Procedures

Mommy, I didn't cry but my eyes got bright.
— A 4-year-old with cancer

THE PURPOSE OF THIS CHAPTER IS TO PREPARE both child and parent for several common procedures by providing detailed descriptions of each. Because almost all procedures are repeated frequently during the long treatment for childhood brain and spinal cord tumors, it is important to establish a routine that is comfortable for you and your child. The procedure itself may cause discomfort, but a well-prepared, calm child fares far better than an unprepared and frightened one.

Planning for procedures

Procedures are needed to make diagnoses, check for spread of disease, give treatments, and monitor responses to treatment. Some procedures are pain-free and easy to tolerate once both the parent and child know what to expect. Other procedures can cause both physical and psychological distress in the child, which can be amplified if the child sees that the parent is also traumatized. The best way to prepare the child is for parents to prepare themselves, intellectually and emotionally, to provide the support and comfort their child will need to endure the upcoming procedures. In most cases, although the procedure itself is non-negotiable, options are available to lessen the pain or stress. Parents need to know what these choices are to be effective advocates for their children.

A family-centered approach works best when planning and implementing procedures. The procedures are often as frightening, or more so, for parents than for children. Because memories of the procedures can be long lasting, children, parents, and staff should work together to plan for and cope with procedures.

Many hospitals have a child life program. These programs exist to minimize psychological trauma and maintain, as much as possible, normal living patterns for hospitalized children. The American Academy of Pediatrics considers child life programs the standard of care for hospitalized children. As soon as possible after admission, find out whether your hospital has a child life program or an equivalent support team.

> Matthew was in sixth grade when he was diagnosed, and he was worried about the surgery for implanting the port. He didn't know what the scar would look like and he was concerned about AIDS, because it had been in the news a lot that year. The child life worker came in and really helped. She showed him what a port looked like; then they explored the pre-op area, the actual surgery room, and post-op. She showed him on a cloth doll exactly where the incision would be and how the scar would look. Then she introduced him to "Fred," the IV pump. She said that Fred would be going places with him, and that Fred would keep him from getting so many pokes. She told Matthew that he could bring something from home to hang on Fred. Of course, he brought in a really ugly stuffed animal. Throughout treatment, she really helped his fears and my feelings about losing control over my child's daily life.

Child life specialists or other team members may accompany children to, and provide support during, procedures. They establish relationships with children based on warmth, respect, empathy, and understanding of developmental stages. They also communicate with the other members of the treatment team about the psychosocial needs of children and their families.

One way to help child life specialists do their job is to communicate openly with them from the beginning. In particular, it is helpful to share insights about your child's temperament and history to help the specialist understand how to approach your child. Discuss with the child life professional or social worker when and how to prepare for upcoming procedures. Usually, parents need to experiment with how much advance notice to give younger children about procedures. Some children do better with several days to prepare, while others worry themselves sick if they are informed too far in advance. Sometimes, needs change over the years of treatment, so good communication and flexibility are essential.

> I started giving my 4-year-old daughter 2 days' notice before procedures. But she began to wake up every day worried that "something bad was going to happen soon." So we talked it over and decided to look at the calendar together every Sunday to review what would happen that week. We put stickers on "procedure days" so she knew what to expect. She was a much happier child after that.

Although it may not always be possible, try to schedule procedures so the same person does the same procedure each time. Call ahead to check for unexpected changes to prevent any surprises for your child. Repetition can provide comfort and reassurance to children. Ritual can also be important. A child may prefer a precise sequence of steps or the use of certain cue words to signal the start of a procedure. If the staff knows the child and complies with her wishes, the child is usually calmer and more compliant.

Parents can ask for the medical professional with the most experience to perform procedures. The most-experienced person is not always the senior one. Nurses, for example, are often better than doctors at drawing blood. In the case of procedures that must be performed by a doctor, the nurses or technicians usually know which one is best at which procedure. Don't hesitate to ask.

Parents should have a choice whether or not to be present during a medical procedure. If your child does better when you are not in the room, ask the child life specialist or another member of the treatment team to be present solely to comfort your child. Teens often want to handle the procedure on their own and it is normally best to respect their wishes.

During procedures, a parent's role is to be supportive and loving. In most cases, the best place to position yourself is at your child's head, at eye level. Speak calmly and positively to your child. You can tell stories, sing songs, or read a favorite book. It helps to praise your child for good behavior, but don't reprimand or demean your child if problems occur.

> We decided from the very beginning that, even though it's no fun to have a bone marrow aspiration or a spinal tap, we were going to make something positive out of it. So we made it a party. We'd bring pizza, popcorn, or ice cream to the hospital. We helped Kristin think of the nurses as her friends. We'd celebrate after a procedure by going out to eat at one of the neat little restaurants near the hospital.

Giving children some control over what happens helps tremendously, but only give choices when they truly exist.

> Katy and I wrote down her requests for each procedure that first week in the hospital. For example, during spinal taps she wanted me (not a nurse) to hold her in position; she wanted xylocaine to be given with a needle, not with the pneumatic gun; and she had a rigid sequence of songs that I sang.

Oncology clinics usually have a special box full of toys or a selection of rewards for children who have had a procedure. It sometimes helps for the child to have a treat to look forward to afterward. Some parents bring a special gift to sneak into the box for their child to find.

Pain management

The goal of pediatric pain management should be to minimize discomfort during procedures. The two methods to achieve this goal are psychological (using the mind) and pharmacological (using prescription drugs). These two methods can be used together to provide an integrated approach.

Psychological methods

It is essential to prepare for every procedure. Unexpected stress is more difficult to cope with than anticipated stress. If parents and children understand what is going to happen, where it will happen, who will be there, and what it will feel like, they will be less anxious and better able to cope. Here are some ways to prepare your child:

- Verbally explain each step in the procedure
- Meet the person who will perform the procedure, if possible
- Tour the room where the procedure will take place
- Let small children use dolls to play-act the procedure
- Let older children observe a demonstration on a doll
- Have adolescents watch a video that demonstrates the procedure
- Encourage discussion and answer all questions

> Ever since I was diagnosed with my brain tumor when I was 16, I have been doing research. When I go in for tests, I try and learn as much as possible about what this test will show, and how it is done. I think the research that I have done since I was diagnosed has greatly helped me. I feel like the things that are being done will one day help another person in my shoes. Because I am learning new information, it keeps the testing from getting too boring.

Hypnosis, imagery, and distraction are three techniques widely used to help children cope with painful procedures. Following are descriptions of each.

Hypnosis is a well-documented method for reducing discomfort during painful procedures. When performed by a qualified healthcare professional (e.g., psychologist, physician, nurse, social worker, or child life specialist), hypnosis can help your child control painful sensations, release anxiety, and diminish pain. The professional guides the child into an altered state of consciousness that helps to focus or narrow attention. To locate a qualified practitioner, visit the American Society of Clinical Hypnosis' website at *www.asch.net* or call (630) 980-4740.

Imagery is a way to create a mental image of pleasurable sights, sounds, tastes, smells, and feelings. It is an active process that helps people feel as if they are actually entering the imagined place. Focusing on pleasant images allows the child to shift attention from the pain. The child can actually alter the experience of pain, which simultaneously gives the child control while diminishing pain. Ask if the hospital has someone who can teach your child this very effective technique.

The following description of using imagery was written by Jennifer Rohloff when she was 17 years old and is reprinted with permission from the *Free to Be Yourself* newsletter of Cancer Services of Allen County, Indiana.

My Special Place

Many people had a special place when they were young—a special place that they still remember. This place could be an area that has a special meaning for them, or a place where they used to go when they wanted to be alone. My special place location is over the rainbow.

I discovered this place when I was 12 years old, during a relaxation session. These sessions were designed to reduce pain and stress brought on by chemotherapy. This was a place that I could visualize in my mind so that I could go there anytime that I wanted to—not only for pain, but when I was happy, mad, or sad.

It is surrounded by sand and tall, fanning palm trees everywhere. The blue sky is always clear, and the bright sun shines every day. It is usually quiet because I am alone, but often I can hear the sounds of birds flying by.

Every time I come to this place I like to lie down in the sand. As I lie there, I can feel the gritty sand beneath me. Once in a while I get up and go looking for seashells. I usually find some different shapes and sizes. The ones I like the best are the ones that you can hear the sound of the ocean in. After a while I get up and start to walk around. As I walk, I can feel the breeze going right through me, and I can smell the salt water. It reminds me of being at a beach in Florida. Whenever I start to feel sad or alone or if I am in pain, I usually go jump in the water because it is a soothing place for me. I like to float around in the water because it gives me a refreshing feeling that nobody can hurt me here. I could stay in this place all day because I do not worry about anything while I am here.

To me this place is like a home away from home. It is like heaven because you can do anything you want to do here. Even though this place may seem imaginary or like a fantasy world to some people, it is not to me. I think it is real because it is a place where I can go and be myself.

Distraction can be used successfully with all age groups, but it should never be used as a substitute for preparation. Babies can be distracted by colorful, moving objects. Parents can help distract preschoolers by showing them picture books or videos, telling stories, singing songs, or blowing bubbles. Many youngsters are comforted and distracted from pain by hugging a favorite stuffed animal. School-aged children can watch videos or TV, or listen to music, and several institutions use interactive video games to help distract older children or teens.

> *My daughter went through her therapy prior to the days when kids were given any pain medications for procedures. She and I would make up a schedule of songs for me to sing during the spinal tap or bone marrow. I would stroke her skin and sing softly to her. She visibly relaxed, and the staff found it soothing, as well. I'll never forget the time that the oncologist, nurse, and I were all quietly singing "Somewhere Over the Rainbow" during a spinal tap.*

Relaxation, biofeedback, massage, acupuncture, Reiki (Japanese energy healing), and accupressure are all also used successfully to manage pain. Ask the hospital's child life specialist, psychologist, or nurse to discuss and practice different methods of pain management with you and your child.

Pharmacological method

Most pediatric oncology clinics sedate or anesthetize children for procedures that are painful or that require them to lie completely still. If your clinic does not offer this option, strongly advocate for it. Sedation and anesthesia have the advantage of calming children, reducing pain, and, in many cases, obliterating all memory of the procedure. Four classes of drugs are used for this purpose:

- **Sedatives,** which depress the central nervous system and result in relaxation. The child or teen may fall asleep, but will remain conscious.

- **General anesthetics,** which induce a loss of consciousness to prevent the child or teen from experiencing pain or remembering a procedure.

- **Local anesthetics,** which temporarily interrupt nerve transmission at a specific site on the body to lessen pain.

- **Analgesics,** which relieve pain. Narcotics are a subclass of analgesics that induce sleep and are potent pain relievers. Many commonly prescribed pain relievers combine narcotic and non-narcotic drugs to achieve greater pain relief with less drowsiness and a lowered risk of addiction.

Sedatives and general anesthetics are given intravenously. Some facilities take the child into the operating room (OR) for the procedure; others use a preoperating area or clinic sedation room and allow the parent to be present the entire time. Certain drugs must be administered by an anesthesiologist (a doctor specializing in anesthesia) in a hospital setting. Drugs commonly used during procedures include:

- **Valium® or Versed®, plus morphine or fentanyl.** Valium® and Versed® are sedatives that are used with pain relievers such as morphine or fentanyl. These drugs can be given in the clinic, but the possibility of slowed breathing requires expert monitoring and the availability of emergency equipment. The combination of a sedative and a pain reliever will result in your child being awake but sedated. Your child may move or cry, but he will not remember the procedure. Often, EMLA® or lidocaine are also used to ensure the procedure is pain-free.

> *My son was treated from ages 14 to 17. During his spinal taps he would get Versed® once he was positioned on the table. I would always sit at his head and keep his shoulders forward while his head rested on my arm. (Kind of a hug.) As the Versed® took effect, he would look up at me with huge eyes and give me a grin a mile wide, then he would say something off the wall. He had to spend an hour flat after the spinal tap. He'd be groggy the whole time, constantly asking me what time it was and how soon we could leave. He'd forget he asked and ask me again 5 minutes later. This continued for the whole hour. Later, we'd laugh about it. He never remembered anything from the LPs.*

- **Propofol.** Propofol is a general anesthetic and will cause your child to lose consciousness. It must be administered in a hospital by an anesthesiologist. It is given intravenously and has the benefit of acting almost immediately with little recovery time. At low doses, propofol prevents memory of the procedure but may not relieve all the pain; thus, it is often used with EMLA® or lidocaine.

> *Patrick (12 years old) hates the lack of control involved when having a procedure and getting propofol. He attempts to regain some control by verbally explaining to the doctors just exactly how he wants it done each time. He has his own little routine—tells them jokes, sings "I Want to Be Sedated" (you know, the Ramones song), etc. Patrick's biggest problem is the taste from the propofol. We have tried so many different things when he wakes up to mask the taste—Skittles®, gum, Gatorade®. We now have a supply of Atomic Fireballs®. I give him one as soon as they bring him out, and he says that really helps cover the taste.*

There are many types of drugs and several methods used to administer them, from very temporary (10 minutes) mild sedation to full general anesthesia in the OR. Discuss with your oncologist and anesthesiologist which method will work best for your child.

> *Let's face it, kids don't care about lab work or protocols, they just want to know if they are going to be hurt again. I think that one of our most important jobs is to advocate, strongly if necessary, for adequate pain control. If the dose doesn't work and the doctor just shrugs her shoulders, say you want a different dosage or drug used. If you encounter resistance, ask that an anesthesiologist be consulted.*

Remember that good pain control and/or amnesia will make a big difference in your child's state of mind during and after treatment.

Emotions may run high after a difficult procedure. Rather than engage in a lengthy discussion about what went wrong, schedule an appointment with the doctor well in advance of the next scheduled procedure to air your concerns and problem-solve.

Because treatment for brain or spinal cord tumors can take many months or years, some children build up a tolerance for sedatives and pain relievers. Over time, doses may need to be increased or drugs changed. If your child remembers the procedure, advocate for a change in the drugs or dosage. It is reasonable to request the services of an anesthesiologist to ensure the best outcome for your child.

> *My 5-year-old has been very hard to sedate for medical procedures such as spinal taps. His oncologist experimented with the commonly used drugs, Versed® and fentanyl, to find a combination that would work. For some recent procedures, he was premedicated with Ativan®. Then he was given Versed® and pentobarb instead of fentanyl. I think we've got it right now, since the last sedation went very well. He still has a full 24 hours of vomiting and headache afterwards (even when he receives antinausea drugs), but at least we don't have to hold him down during spinal taps anymore.*

· · · · ·

> *A new anesthesiologist suggested nitrous oxide before general anesthesia for my young daughter's MRIs. Life around MRIs has never been the same. She is actually excited about scans now as if it is some kind of holiday! The first time with laughing gas she started to go "Wheeeee!!!!" I asked her if she was feeling like she was on a roller coaster, and she said, "No, I feel like I'm on the TILT-A-WHIRL!" The next day she said, "Mommy, I don't want to go to school today, I want to have ANOTHER SCAN!" I can't say I share her anticipation of a scan, but I am thankful for a good attitude and experience. I keep asking them to share the laughing gas, but they won't!*

Your child will not be allowed to eat or drink for several hours prior to procedures that require sedation or anesthesia. After a procedure, your child may eat or drink when she is alert and able to swallow.

Procedures

Knowing what to expect will lay the foundation for months or years of tolerable tests. Because hospitals and practitioners have their own guidelines and preferences, the descriptions of procedures in the rest of this chapter may not exactly mirror your experience, but the fundamentals are the same everywhere. Reading the rest of this chapter may lessen your fears and help you to calm and prepare your child.

Questions to ask before procedures

You need information prior to procedures to prepare yourself and your child. Some suggested questions to ask the doctor include:

- Why is this procedure necessary and how will it affect my child's treatment?
- What information will the procedure provide?
- Who will perform the procedure?
- Will it be an inpatient or outpatient procedure?
- Please explain the procedure in detail.
- Is there any literature available that describes it?
- Is there a child life specialist on staff who will help prepare my child for the procedure?
- If not, are there nurses, social workers, or parents who can talk to me about how to prepare my child?
- Is the procedure painful?
- How long will it take?
- What type of anesthetic or sedation is used?
- What are the risks, if any?
- What are the common and rare side effects?
- When will we get the results?

Accessing catheters

The procedure that occurs most often during treatment—and that can be the most or the least worrisome—is accessing your child's central venous catheter. This procedure is described in detail in Chapter 9, *Venous Catheters*.

> *Mary Margaret had a terrible time having her port accessed. She would scream and cry (probably terrifying the other kids waiting outside the room for their turn!) and I became an expert at holding her down. I'd lie down next to her, holding down her hands, pressing my knee on her legs to keep her from kicking, and with my head on her forehead. It was horrible. I don't think it was particularly painful, just a terrible invasion for her, and she knew she'd feel badly after her treatment. We ended up meeting with the neuropsychologist on staff at the Hem-Onc office. The doctor was wonderful and warm, she talked to MM about why having her port accessed bothered her so much, and we talked about ways that she might cope. The doc made some good suggestions: listening to music, looking at a book, dreaming herself somewhere else, and then accompanied MM and I into the procedure room. MM was calm and completely still through the whole procedure, and never made a fuss again about having her port accessed. I'm very grateful.*

Angiogram

An angiogram is a special x-ray procedure to evaluate the circulation and blood supply in an area of tumor in either the brain or spinal cord. This procedure is performed in the radiology department and requires sedation or general anesthesia, depending on your child's age and temperament. No food or liquids are allowed for a period of time prior to the procedure. A catheter is put in a blood vessel in the groin and then threaded up to the area that needs to be evaluated. Dye is injected and doctors can see the blood supply to the tumor. After the procedure, your child will go to the recovery room until she is awake and then will go back to her room.

Audiogram

Some of the chemotherapy drugs that children receive for treatment of brain or spinal cord tumors can cause hearing loss. Additionally, some children with these tumors experience hearing loss as a result of injury to nerves caused by the tumor itself, or from surgery or radiation. Your child's doctor may order a hearing test, called an audiogram, to monitor for possible hearing problems.

During the audiogram, your child is tested in a soundproof room to prevent outside noises from interfering. You can remain with your child during this procedure. Earphones are placed on your child's ears, through which sounds (such as beeps and tones) are relayed. Your child will be asked to signal when he hears a sound by either raising his hand or pressing a button. Each ear is tested separately. The results of the audiogram are usually displayed in the form of a graph, and the amount of hearing loss is measured in decibels.

Audiograms are repeated throughout therapy to monitor your child's hearing if he is taking drugs that place him at risk.

> Matthew experienced some high-frequency hearing loss from the cisplatin. I think to Matthew, stepping into the soundproof booth and putting on his headset was somewhat like a game. The first few audiograms were done with me sitting in the booth beside him. Eventually, he reached a point where he felt he could do this test on his own.

Blood draws

Frequent blood samples are a part of life during treatment for a brain or spinal cord tumor. Blood specimens are primarily used for three purposes: to obtain a complete blood count (CBC), to evaluate blood chemistries, or to culture the blood to check for infection. A CBC measures the types and numbers of cells in the blood. Blood chemistries measure substances contained in the blood plasma to determine whether the liver and kidneys are functioning properly. Blood cultures help evaluate whether a child is developing a bacterial or fungal infection. (For a list of normal blood counts, see Appendix A, *Blood Tests and What They Mean*.)

A finger poke provides enough blood for a CBC, but blood chemistries or cultures require one or more vials of blood. Children with catheters usually have blood drawn from the catheter rather than the arm or finger. If the child does not have a catheter, blood is usually drawn from the large vein on the inside of the elbow. The procedures for a blood draw are similar to those for placing an IV, which are described later in this chapter. The only difference is that with a draw, the needle is removed as soon as the blood is obtained.

Bone growth test

A bone growth test is a plain x-ray of your child's nondominant hand and wrist. It is performed to determine whether your child's growth is appropriate for her age. Your child's x-ray film will be compared with a series of photographs of wrist films of children of all ages so the radiologist can define your child's "bone age" compared to her chronological age. The results help determine the need for endocrine testing. This test takes only a few moments to perform and is not painful.

Bone marrow aspiration or biopsy

Bone marrow aspirations or biopsies are done as part of the diagnostic workup for several types of brain and spinal cord tumors to see whether the tumor has spread to the bone. They are also done prior to stem cell transplantation.

During a bone marrow aspiration, bone marrow is extracted from bone cavities with a needle. Bone marrow biopsies remove a small piece of bone marrow with a special biopsy needle.

> Melissa (age 5) has had several bone marrow aspirations since her diagnosis. We always use propofol (which I refer to as the "milk of human kindness," because of its milky appearance) before the procedure. After the aspiration is over, Melissa wakes up from a very deep sleep and has felt no pain whatsoever. She's usually hungry and ready to go ASAP. Propofol has worked exceptionally well for her.

Doctors usually take a sample of the marrow from the iliac crest of the hip (the top of the hip bone in back or front). This bone is right under the skin and contains a large amount of marrow. The child lies face down on a table, sometimes on a pillow to elevate the hip. The doctor puts on sterile gloves, finds the site, then wipes it several times with an antiseptic to eliminate any germs. The nurse places sterile paper around the site, then an anesthetic (usually lidocaine) may be injected into the skin and a small area of bone. This causes a burning and stinging sensation that passes quickly. The doctor usually rubs the area to distribute the anesthetic around the site. When she is convinced that the insertion site is numb, the doctor pushes a hollow needle (with a plug inside) through the skin into the bone, withdraws the plug, and attaches a syringe. She then aspirates (sucks out) the liquid marrow through the syringe. Finally, she removes the needle and bandages the area.

Without sedation, bone marrow aspiration is very painful, so almost all centers anesthetize children for this procedure. Do not hesitate to advocate for this at your center. Here are some descriptions from children and adult survivors who have experienced it without sedation:

> It was the worst thing of all. It felt really, really bad.

· · · · ·

> It hurts a lot. It feels like they are pulling something out and then it aches. You know, it hurts so much that now they put the kids to sleep. Boy, am I glad about that. It feels like they are trying to suck thick Jell-O® from inside the bone. Brief but incredible pain.

· · · · ·

> I would become very anxious when they were cleaning my skin and laying the towels down. Putting the needle in was a sharp, pressure kind of pain. Drawing the marrow feels tingly, like they hit a nerve. I always asked a nurse to hold my legs because I felt like my legs were going to jump up off the table.

Brainstem auditory evoked response (BAER)

A brainstem auditory evoked response (BAER) test uses clicking sounds to evaluate the central auditory pathways of the brainstem. This test evaluates a child's hearing when standard audiometric testing is not possible, either because of age or inability to respond. During the test, clicking noises or tone bursts are delivered through earphones. Your child's brain waves are then measured by electrodes placed along the scalp and on each earlobe. The test is not painful and takes about 30 minutes to perform.

> BAER was very easy, quick, and painless. They attached leads to Mary Margaret's head, very gently, and it didn't get tangled up in her hair or anything. Then they put earphones on, and the doctor told her she would hear a series of clicks in one ear, and a whooshing sound in the other, and to just sit still. So she did, and the little lines came out on the computer screen. The doctor duly recorded all the highest humps in the lines, and switched ears. Then they did the TV part, which I think is called VAER. MM stared at a small American flag in the center of a TV screen. She's good at staring at TV, so this was not difficult for her. The rest of the screen is small black and white squares, and they move around as the child stares at the flag in the center. I would say the test took about five minutes of sitting and staring.

Computed tomography (CT)

Computed tomography (CT) is a complex, computer-enhanced procedure for obtaining x-ray images of the body. The machine looks very much like a big donut, and your child will be placed in the hole in the middle. Instead of having a fixed x-ray directed at one part of the body, during a CT scan an x-ray tube rotates around the body, generating hundreds of images as it moves. These images are called "slices," similar to slices in a loaf of bread.

CT imaging allows the doctor to see central nervous system (CNS) structures in great detail. Development of the CT scan was a major step forward in the diagnosis, evaluation, and treatment of brain and spinal cord tumors. CT scans are used to look at the relationship between the tumor and bones. Although magnetic resonance imaging (MRI) is now the gold standard for evaluation of CNS tumors, CT is still a good screening tool.

Before the procedure begins, your child may need to receive a liquid dye, called a contrast agent. The contrast agent is given intravenously for CNS tumors. In the event that your child requires a CT scan of the abdomen or pelvis for another reason, oral contrast will also be given. The technologist will position your child so the area being imaged is inside the opening of the CT machine. The technologist does not stay in the room while the images are taken.

If you plan to remain with your child, you will need to wear a lead apron to protect your body from unnecessary exposure to radiation. Sometimes, if the site being imaged is the chest area, your child may be asked to breathe in and hold her breath for several seconds. It is important that your child remain still during the CT scanning process. Small children who are unable to remain motionless for several minutes at a time are sedated before the procedure. You are usually asked to stay in the department until the images have been reviewed by the technologist to ensure they are adequate and do not need to be repeated.

> The first few scans, they used pentobarb to sedate our son. He was wobbly and sleepy for 24 hours after. Then they switched to propofol to sedate him. He went right to sleep and woke up after the scan without the after-effects. He is now 5 years out off treatment, and he no longer needs sedation for scans. But, one thing that I really appreciate is that the radiologist reviews the scans before we go home. We leave knowing that everything is okay. It breaks my heart that some families need to wait days to find out the results of scans.

Conventional x-ray

X-rays, a type of electromagnetic radiation, provide the doctor with a quick and simple way to view organs and structures inside your child's body. X-rays are performed for many reasons during a child's treatment for a brain or spinal cord tumor. Some of the most common reasons for taking x-rays are because they are:

- Needed before operations

- Needed after your child's central venous catheter is placed to confirm it is in the proper location

- Used to check cerebrospinal fluid shunt placement

- Used as part of a workup for fever to determine whether your child has pneumonia

For an x-ray, your child is positioned by the technologist in a manner that will make it easiest to get the images that are needed. For chest x-rays, your child may be asked to breathe in, hold her breath, and remain perfectly still for a few seconds. The technologist leaves the room during the time the x-rays are taken. As with CT scans, if you are planning to stay with your child, you need to wear a lead apron to protect you from radiation. Your child may also have to wear a lead apron or lead shield to protect specific areas of her body. Pregnant women should not be present in the room when x-rays are taken.

Echocardiograms and electrocardiograms

Spinal radiation and some drugs used to treat brain and spinal cord tumors can damage the heart, decreasing its ability to contract effectively. Many protocols require a baseline echocardiogram to measure the heart's ability to pump before any chemotherapy drugs are given. Echocardiograms are then given periodically during and after treatment to check for heart muscle damage.

An echocardiogram uses ultrasound waves to measure the amount of blood that leaves the heart each time it contracts. This percentage (blood ejected during a contraction compared to blood in the heart when it is relaxed) is called the ejection fraction.

For this test, the child or adolescent lies on a table and a technician, nurse, or doctor applies conductive jelly to the chest. Then the technician puts a transducer (which emits the ultrasound waves) on the jelly and moves the device around on the chest to obtain different views of the heart. He applies pressure on the transducer to obtain clear images; this pressure can be uncomfortable. The test results are videotaped for the technician to see the results as he works and so the radiologist can interpret the findings later.

> Meagan used to watch a video during the echocardiogram. Sometimes she would eat a sucker or a Popsicle®. She found it to be boring, not painful.

An electrocardiogram (EKG) measures the electrical impulses that the heart generates during the cardiac cycle. An EKG can be performed at an office, a lab, or your child's bedside. Before placing the electrodes, the technician cleans the area with alcohol and applies a cool gel under the electrodes. Your child must lie quietly during the test. You can remain with him throughout the procedure, which generally takes less than 10 minutes. Your child will feel nothing during the procedure other than the gel on the electrodes.

Electroencephalogram (EEG)

The most widely used method for diagnosing any type of seizure disorder is the electroencephalogram, or EEG. During an EEG, measures of the electrical activity generated by the brain are taken. There is no health risk from an EEG, with the exception of several very specialized types of EEG (depth and subdural grid EEG), which are discussed below.

To prepare for an EEG, wash your child's hair before the test and avoid conditioner, creams, hairspray, oils, gels, and elaborate hairstyles. Your child should avoid caffeinated drinks for a day before the test. Although the test is not painful, a mild sedative is sometimes used before the test is performed.

For the most common type of EEG test, usually called a scalp EEG, the neurologist or EEG technician will apply 21 electrodes to your child's scalp with gooey, strong-smelling glue. Each disc is strategically placed to capture the brain wave activity from a different region of the brain, and each is attached to a wire called a lead. Because the heart's electrical activity can skew EEG results, it is usually monitored by a separate electrode placed on the chest. The loose end of each lead is attached to the EEG machine itself, which amplifies the tiny amount of sensed activity, making graphing possible. The EEG machine will represent the electrical output of your child's brain on a piece of paper, on a computer screen, or both. The basic type of EEG test lasts between 30 minutes to 2 hours. During the test, the neurologist or EEG technician may try some things that could provoke a seizure. For example, your child may be asked to look at a flashing light (photic stimulation) or breathe rapidly for several minutes (hyperventilation).

> Anna was about 3 and a half when she had one of her first EEGs. The technician we had told her the leads were like a rainbow. He told her the story of the rainbow, what it really means. He had a story for each of the colors, and talked in a very calm and soothing voice. He told her he was going to make her look very important, just like a rainbow. From that time on, she has referred to all her EEGs as "Rainbow Hair." The tech told us he would call it a "clown wig" for the boys. He was great!

Sleep-deprived EEGs are administered after a period of sleep deprivation. Sleep deprivation lowers the seizure threshold dramatically, and deep sleep is a time when some kinds of seizures are more likely to occur. For this test, your child must stay up all or most of the night and then have the scalp EEG performed in the morning. Once the electrodes are hooked up and the neurologist has reviewed the initial brain activity, your child will be allowed to sleep. The dual challenge of sleep deprivation and deep sleep often evokes seizure activity.

Videotaped EEGs are when an EEG is performed while your child is simultaneously videotaped. By comparing your child's visual symptoms with you or your child's reported symptoms with the EEG data, subtle correlations can be made.

The depth EEG requires surgery to temporarily put electrodes into your child's brain. Your child's head will be placed in a frame that is pinned to your child's skull. CT or MRI scanning will then help the doctor decide on positioning of the electrodes. The neurosurgeon will carefully drill through the skull and insert the electrodes into those parts of your child's brain where seizure activity is suspected. Because there are no nerve endings inside the skull, this is not painful; however, some people experience discomfort despite the use of local anesthetic. A post-procedure headache is a common occurrence; your child will have a bandage on her head and her scalp may be sore for up to 4 weeks.

Subdural grid EEG involves placing a grid or strip of electrodes on the surface of the brain. The electrodes do not penetrate the surface of the brain. This type of EEG is most frequently used when seizures occur in areas affecting language or movement. The grid is usually kept in place for 2 or more weeks before being removed during a second operation. As with the depth EEG, your child's head will be sore afterwards and will need time to heal thoroughly.

Electromyogram (EMG)

An electromyogram (EMG) measures the electrical activity of a specific skeletal muscle. The study is generally performed in an EMG laboratory. Your child's position for the examination is determined by the specific muscle being evaluated. Local anesthetic or topical analgesic agents (such as EMLA® cream) are applied prior to the test. A fine, small needle that acts as a recording electrode is inserted into the muscle. In addition, a small skin electrode, such as that used in an electrocardiogram, is placed on the skin's surface. Your child needs to lie still for a baseline reading and then contract the muscle repeatedly for several seconds. The neurologist and technician will then evaluate the monitor readings for evidence of abnormal or diminished function. Sedation is generally not used for this test, because your child's participation is necessary. Your child may experience some discomfort from the needle insertion (similar to an intramuscular injection). You may stay with your child throughout the procedure.

Jessica (age 10) is having treatment for anaplastic astrocytoma, and has a lot of muscle weakness on one side. For the EMG, they put these circuits on her foot and then checked to get a reading while they put a little current there. They shocked her a little each time they did it. They did it on the foot and the knee on the left side, which is her weakest side, and also did a muscle check on her left arm and hand. The doctor was great and had her giggling much of the time. We got to hear what Jessica's muscle sounded like when she moved.

Finger pokes

During the course of treatment, your child will probably have hundreds of finger pokes. Many children cooperate better with this procedure if the finger is first anesthetized with a topical numbing agent to reduce pain. The three topical anesthetics in wide use for pediatric procedures are as follows.

EMLA® cream is a combination of two topical anesthetics, lidocaine and prilocaine. It is available by prescription only. Parents must remember to apply the EMLA® cream at least 1 hour before the scheduled poke. Children with darker skin may need to leave it on longer to achieve the full effect.

To anesthetize the finger, put a blob of EMLA® on the tip of the middle finger, then cover it so the cream doesn't get wiped off. Tegaderm® is a special bandage designed for this purpose, but you can also cover the fingertip with plastic wrap and then tape it on the finger. Another method is to buy long, thin balloons with a diameter a bit wider than the child's finger. Cut off the open end, leaving only enough balloon to cover the finger up to the first knuckle. Fill the tip of the balloon with EMLA® and slide it on the fingertip. Before the finger poke, remove the plastic wrap or balloon, wipe off the EMLA®, and ask the technician for a warm pack. Wrapping this heated pack around the finger for a few minutes opens the capillaries and allows blood to flow out more readily. The finger then should be washed or wiped with disinfectant. Now your child is ready for a pain-free finger poke.

LMX4® is a 4-percent solution of lidocaine in a cream form. It works much like EMLA®, but it is available over the counter. It is important not to wash the child's finger prior to applying LMX4®, because it works best when it mixes with the natural oils on the skin. LMX4® works faster than EMLA®, so in most cases it should not be applied until you arrive at the laboratory or treatment center.

The procedure for applying LMX4® is slightly different than it is for EMLA®. A small amount should be rubbed onto the finger first and left for about 30 seconds, then a thick blob should be applied on top. Cover the finger loosely with tape, a balloon, or Tegaderm®. Remove the wrapping after 30 minutes, clean the site, and proceed with the poke.

Ethyl chloride ("freezy spray") is sprayed on the skin immediately before the procedure by the technician. This medication requires a prescription.

After the skin is numbed by one of the above methods, the technician will hold the finger and quickly stick it with a small, sharp instrument. Blood will be collected in narrow tubes or a small container. It is usually necessary for the technician to squeeze the fingertip to get enough blood. If you have not used a topical anesthetic, the squeezing part is uncomfortable and the finger can ache for quite a while.

> *Even though we use EMLA®, Katy (5 years old) still becomes angry when she has to have a finger poke. I asked her why it was upsetting if there was no pain, and she replied, "It doesn't hurt my body anymore, but it still hurts my feelings."*

Not all treatment centers recommend a topical anesthetic for finger pokes; you may have to advocate for it.

Gallium scan

Gallium scans are performed in the nuclear medicine department. Prior to the scan, your child will be injected with a radiopharmaceutical, called gallium citrate. Your child's venous catheter may be used for the injection, or you may apply EMLA® cream to a peripheral vein site prior to the injection. Usually, the scan is performed 24 to 48 hours after the injection. Gallium localizes at sites of infection and malignancy. The procedure takes about 30 minutes. Your child needs to lie flat on an examination table while the machine scans above her. The machine makes noise but the procedure is not painful. You can stay with your child during this procedure.

Gastrostomy

A gastrostomy is the creation of an external opening in the abdominal wall through which a feeding tube is placed to provide nutrition directly into a child's stomach. This is appropriate for children who cannot eat normally because of chronic swallowing problems or long-term pain in the mouth or throat, or for children who have lost their normal appetite for a prolonged period because of disease or treatment. The stomach end of the feeding tube has a small balloon that prevents it from being accidentally pulled all the way out.

A skilled gastroenterologist or surgeon can perform the procedure in about 10 minutes. Most children have general anesthesia for the procedure and remain in the hospital for 1 to 2 days postoperatively to receive pain medication and make sure they tolerate feedings through the tube. Care of the tube is simple, and after 2 to 3 months the tube may be replaced with an unobtrusive skin-level device called a button. After a short recovery, children may play, bathe, and swim normally.

The tube is used for liquid feedings and medications for as long as the child needs it. If a child no longer requires the tube, it is removed and a bandage is placed over the site. The wound closes spontaneously in a day or two.

Magnetic resonance imaging (MRI)

MRI uses a magnetic field to create two-dimensional images of a cross section of the brain or spinal cord. Your child may need to receive a liquid dye, called a contrast agent, prior to or during the scan. The dye can be administered through your child's central venous catheter or via a peripheral IV. For the MRI, your child lies on a platform that slides into a long tube. Inside the tube is a donut-shaped magnet. A special device, called a surface coil, is then placed around the area of the body that is to be imaged.

> From ages 2 to 5, our son was anesthetized for MRIs. Depending on what they used, he'd either come out acting like a little drunk, or be crabby all day, or sometimes have vomiting. At the children's hospital, they used IV sedation, Versed® and Nembutol®, which often made him sick. Our local hospital used liquid chloral hydrate, which he absolutely hated to take. When he turned 5, the nurse asked me if I thought he could do the MRI without sedation; of course I thought no way. But she asked him, and he said, "I don't have to take the icky medicine? I can do that!" They told him when he could move a little and when he needed to lie perfectly still, and he did it!

• • • • •

> Since the beginning, we've sent each of our MRIs to our pediatric neuro-oncologist for a second opinion. The radiologist will write "no change" on the report. Our neuro-oncologist provides tumor dimensions, mentions how much enhancement compares to last time, mentions structures that are looking the same or are looking different. It can be like night and day in terms of value of the information that you get for long-term follow-up.

The technologist does not stay in the room during the MRI. The MRI machine makes a loud knocking noise as the images are taken. Your child may need to wear special earplugs to help block out this sound. Young children, or any child with a fear of closed-in spaces (claustrophobia), may need to be sedated for the MRI procedure. MRI takes longer to perform than CT scans and requires that your child lie perfectly still to prevent motion artifact in the scan pictures. Although some centers now have open MRI scanners, they are not currently available in the majority of hospitals. Some doctors feel that magnet technology in the open MRI scanners used by some facilities is not yet up to par with older closed machines, which may affect the degree of detail. MRI is considered the best way to image brain and spinal cord tumors.

> We don't run around trying to get copies of scans after the fact (the ones made then aren't as clear anyway and cost money). We ask the technician for a second set of

MRI scans to be made the same day it's taken. That way we always have sets to pull out for consults and other doctor visits. We've also learned that it appears to help with interpreting MRIs to use the same MRI machine, and we also try to get the same technician.

A medical oncologist offers this advice regarding MRI interpretations:

A neuro-radiologist is usually the best person to notice small details or to give interpretations of unusual abnormalities in scans. Any "neuro doctor" who knows your case well—neurologist or neurosurgeon—is likely to be the best person to decide what a change in your scan means in your particular case. This is especially true if the doctor is someone who spends much of his or her time dealing with brain tumors.

Needle aspiration biopsy

Needle aspiration biopsies are sometimes used to obtain a sample of cells from a mass in an accessible area. Prior to the biopsy, children need to fast for several hours. The doctor will first use ultrasound or CT images to determine the exact location of the mass. Once your child has been anesthetized, a needle is guided into the mass and a sample is removed. The sample is then sent to a pathologist, who will view the cells under a microscope. Your child will need to stay in bed for the next several hours with vital signs closely monitored to ensure there is no bleeding.

Neuropsychological testing

Neuropsychological testing encompasses a broad category of oral, written, and performance tests that help define and describe your child's level of functioning. If your child's condition allows, it is best to perform such tests prior to surgery, but sometimes this is impossible. Postoperative and post-therapy testing performed every few years is important for documenting cognitive function and assisting with planning educational and rehabilitative interventions for your child. For more information about neuropsychological testing, see Chapter 18, *School*.

Positron emission tomography (PET) scan

Positron emission tomography (PET) is a type of imaging scan used to identify biochemical changes in the body's tissues. MRI and CT scans provide information about structure and anatomy, but PET scans provide additional information about metabolism, which helps more clearly identify location and extent of tumor and, after treatment, whether masses showing up on CT or MRI are scar tissue, dead tissue, or new growth of disease.

The PET scan involves injection of a radioactive drug (tracer) prior to scanning. The most common drug used is fluorine 18, also known as FDG-18, which is a radioactive version of glucose. The amount of radiation is very small, about the same as a conventional x-ray. After the injection, your child will wait for an hour or so until the tracer has spread throughout the body, and then the scan is done. No anesthesia is used and the entire procedure takes about 2 hours.

Usually, parents are told to not let their child consume any caffeine (e.g., soda, tea, chocolate) for 24 hours before the PET scan. Other than water, your child should not have any food or fluids for 4 hours before the scan. Your child should be told that the scan will not hurt and that he will have to remain very still while in the scanning machine.

Pulmonary function tests

Some of the chemotherapy drugs children receive can damage the lungs. Your child's doctor may order a pulmonary function test to evaluate her respiratory status. The basic pulmonary function test is called a spirogram. Your child will blow into the machine to measure the amount of air she can inhale and exhale. The respiratory technician who administers the test will coach and instruct your child throughout the procedure to ensure she is giving her maximum effort. The test is administered at least three times to ensure the results are reliable. You can stay with your child while this test is done.

Your child cannot take this test if she is agitated, in pain, or too young to cooperate with the procedure. Your child should not take any bronchodilators or use an inhaler for 6 hours prior to the procedure. Also, be sure to have a list of medications your child is currently taking with you, because this is necessary for proper test interpretation.

> Our son didn't like having pulmonary function tests. On the outside, it looks so simple. But blowing into the spirogram was hard for him. He was usually a little tired after the test was complete. We would always make a trip to the hospital gift shop afterwards, because we felt he deserved a special treat for working so hard.

Spinal tap (lumbar puncture or LP)

Due to the blood-brain barrier, systemic chemotherapy sometimes cannot destroy tumor cells in the brain and spinal cord. Chemotherapy drugs may have to be directly injected into the cerebrospinal fluid (CSF) to kill any tumor cells; this is called intrathecal administration. For certain diseases (e.g., medulloblastoma, ependymoma), spinal taps are used to monitor response to treatment. Spinal taps can be diagnostic (done to obtain a specimen of fluid for analysis) and/or therapeutic (done to inject chemotherapy).

Most hospitals sedate children for spinal taps. If a child is not sedated, EMLA® cream is usually prescribed to lessen the pain. Even with sedation, EMLA® may be applied to minimize the sting of the topical anesthetic. To perform a spinal tap, the doctor or nurse practitioner first asks the child to lie on his side with his head tucked close to the chest and knees drawn up. A nurse usually helps hold the child in this position. The doctor, wearing sterile gloves, finds the designated spot in the lower back and swabs it with antiseptic several times. The antiseptic feels very cold on the skin. The nurse then drapes the area with a sterile sheet. The doctor will administer one or two shots of an anesthetic (usually xylocaine) into the skin and deeper tissues. This causes a painful stinging or burning sensation that lasts about a minute. Even if EMLA® was used, the doctor may still inject anesthetic into the deep tissues. It is necessary to wait a few moments to ensure the area is fully anesthetized.

The child must hold very still for the rest of the procedure. The doctor will push a needle between two vertebrae and into the space where CSF is found. The CSF will begin to drip out of the hollow needle into a container. After collecting a small amount of CSF, the doctor attaches a syringe to the needle and slowly injects the medicine. This causes a sensation of coldness or pressure down the legs. The doctor removes the needle, bandages the spot, and sends the CSF to the laboratory to see whether any cancer cells are present and to measure glucose and protein levels.

> *During spinals, Brent listens to rock and roll on his Walkman®, but he keeps the volume low enough so that he can still hear what is going on. He likes me to lift up the earpiece and tell him when each part of the procedure is finished and what's coming next.*

It is important to lie extremely flat for at least 30 minutes after an LP to reduce pressure changes in the CSF. Sitting or standing up too soon can cause severe headaches. If your child develops a persistent severe headache following the procedure that lessens while he lies flat, but throbs when he sits up, notify the doctor or nurse. The nurse will likely have your child lie flat and will offer a high-caffeine beverage (such as Mountain Dew®) to drink. If these measures fail to relieve the headache, an anesthesiologist sometimes does a procedure called a "blood patch," during which your child lies in the same position as for the spinal tap. The anesthesiologist will draw a small amount of blood from your child's arm or central line. She will then inject the blood at the site of the prior spinal tap where CSF may be slowly leaking from the canal into the tissues. If this is the cause of the headache, the relief is immediate. This procedure is generally performed in the recovery room, emergency room, clinic, or inpatient unit. You can stay with your child during the procedure.

Starting an intravenous (IV) drip

Most pediatric hospitals have teams of technicians who specialize in starting IVs and drawing blood. The IV technician will generally use a vein in the lower arm or hand. First, a constricting band is put above the site to make the veins larger and easier to see and feel. The technician feels for the vein, cleans the area, and inserts the needle. Sometimes she leaves the needle in place and sometimes she withdraws it, leaving only a thin plastic tube in the vein. The technician will make sure the needle (or tube) is in the proper place, then will cover the site with a clear dressing and secure it with tape.

The following methods can help when starting an IV:

- **Stay calm.** The body reacts to fear by constricting the blood vessels near the skin's surface. Small children are usually more calm with a parent present, but teenagers may desire privacy. Listening to music, visualizing a tranquil scene (such as mountains covered with snow, floating in a pool), or using the same technician each time can help.

- **Use a topical anesthetic.** Use EMLA® cream, LMX4®, or ethyl chloride, as described earlier in the chapter. However, topical anesthetics are not recommended when giving medications (for example, vincristine) that can burn the skin if leakage occurs.

- **Keep warm.** Cold temperatures cause the surface blood vessels to constrict. Wrapping the child in a blanket and putting a hot water bottle or heating pad on his arm can enlarge the veins.

- **Drink lots of fluids.** Dehydration decreases fluid in the veins, making them harder to find, so encourage lots of drinking.

- **Let gravity help.** If your child is lying in bed, she can hang her arm down over the side to increase the size of the vessels in her arm and hand.

- **Let your child have control, as appropriate.** If your child has a preference, let him pick the arm to be stuck. If he is a veteran of many IVs, let him point out the best vein. Good technicians know that patients are quite aware of their best bet for a good vein.

- **Stop if problems develop.** The art of treating children requires spending lots of time on preparation and not much time on procedures. If a conflict arises, take a time-out and regroup. Children can be remarkably cooperative if they feel you are respecting their needs and if they are given some control over the situation.

> *You'll think I'm crazy, but I'll tell you this story anyway. After getting stuck constantly for a year, my daughter (5 years old) just lost it one day when she needed an IV. She started screaming and crying, just flew into a rage. I told the tech, "Let's just let her calm down. Why don't you stick me for a change?" She was a sport and started a line in my arm. I told my daughter that I had forgotten how much it hurt and I could*

understand why she was upset. I told her to let us know when she was ready. She just walked over and held out her arm.

Traditionally, infants and young children have been restrained on their backs to insert IVs. This technique minimizes the risk of misplacing the IV, but it can cause significant fear and distress. Many treatment centers now allow parents to hold children upright in their laps to minimize stress.

Even though our 6-year-old son seemed okay with IVs and port access during treatment, afterwards he showed lots of aggression, including sticking people really hard with pointy objects, and pinching people's arms. It's gotten better off treatment with some counseling sessions.

Subcutaneous and intramuscular injections

Some medications are given by injection, either under the skin (subcutaneous, or Sub-Q, injection) or into a large muscle (intramuscular, or IM, injection). One drug commonly administered subcutaneously is Neupogen® (G-CSF), a medication that is often used to boost white blood cell counts.

We found that giving 4-year-old Joseph as much power in the process as possible really helped. The shots themselves are non-negotiable, but there are many parts of the process where the child can have some control (where to put the EMLA® cream, where to be sitting for the cream and/or the shot, who holds him, what Beanie Baby® to hold during the procedure, etc.). We also made sure to have a consistent little treat available afterwards, although this became unnecessary after a while. Even at 4, Joseph loved money, so for a long time he kept a pint jar, which would travel to the hospital and back home again, and he'd get to drop in a nickel for each pill successfully swallowed (a huge chore for him) and a quarter for each shot. Of course, adults would look very surprised when we told them we gave Joseph "quarter shots." Something tells me the bar scene will be very confusing to him when he gets to college.

To minimize pain caused by injections, apply EMLA® cream 1 to 2 hours before administration. Parents can also reduce pain by rubbing ice over the site to numb the area prior to injection. Other ideas are available online at *http://webpages.charter.net/drshrink/gcsftips.htm*.

We always used EMLA® cream before our son needed a subcutaneous injection. I think part of the benefit to him was pharmacological, and part of it was psychological. He just seemed to be more at ease with the injections when he knew the EMLA® was applied a few hours before the needle was given.

We eventually gave Matt his Neupogen® shots while he was asleep. At the time, Matt was around 3 years old and we had a night nurse anyway for monitoring his trach and I could not bear the thought of giving him his shots. It is just one of those things that I had to draw the line on. We had the nurse try all different times/ways/ techniques to give the shots. He hated everything about it, which triggered other, more difficult problems (turning blue and passing out). Sometimes Matt would sleep through the shot and other times he would wake up. Once treatment was over, Matt had great difficulty with going to sleep at all. Fought it till the bitter end. The night nurse was here anyway (trach, again) so he stayed up with her. It took a long time to develop a new safe bedtime/wake-up routine and I often wonder if sneaking the Neupogen® in on him was more traumatic than we realized.

Swallowing tests

Swallowing tests are necessary if your child is unable to swallow or does not have an adequate gag reflex. Swallowing tests are performed in the radiology department; your child cannot eat or drink anything prior to the procedure, but will be given a barium-containing "meal" during the test. X-rays are taken and examined to evaluate swallowing. Swallowing tests help determine whether your child can begin to eat and drink more normally following surgery or whether a gastrostomy tube, nasogastric tube, or IV nutrition will be needed for a period of time. You can stay with your child during the swallowing tests.

Taking oral medications (pills and liquids)

As the parent of a child with a brain or spinal cord tumor, one of your most important jobs is to administer each dose of all oral medications to your child on time—every day. Research has proven that children who do not comply completely with the dosing regimen have a lower survival rate than those who do. Your child will need thousands of pills or liquid doses throughout treatment. To accomplish this feat, it is essential to get off to a good start and establish cooperation with your child early in the process.

To teach Brent (6 years old) to swallow pills, when we were eating corn for dinner I encouraged him to swallow one kernel whole. Luckily, it went right down and he got over his fear of pills.

I wanted Katy (3 years old) to feel like we were a team right from the first night. So I made a big deal out of tasting each of her medications and pronouncing it good. Thank goodness I tasted the prednisone first. It was nauseating—bitter, metallic, with a lingering aftertaste. I asked the nurse for some small gel caps, and packed

them with the pills which I had broken in half. I gave Katy her choice of drinks to
take her pills with and taught her to swallow gel caps with a large sip of liquid.
Since I gave her over 3,000 pills and 1,100 teaspoons of liquid medication during
treatment, I'm very glad we got off to such a good start.

Gel caps come in many sizes. Number 4s are small enough for a 3- or 4-year-old child
to swallow. Many pills can be chewed or swallowed whole without leaving a bad taste
in the mouth. Steroid medications (e.g., prednisone, dexamethasone) should not be
chewed, because they have a bitter aftertaste and may cause your child to develop an
aversion to all oral medications. Just remember that different children develop different
taste preferences and aversions to medications, and gel caps are useful for any medication that bothers them.

After much trial and error with medications, Meagan's method became chewing up
pills with chocolate chips. She's kept this up for the long haul.

· · · · ·

I always give choices such as, "Do you want the white pill or the six yellow pills
first?" It gives him a little control in his chaotic world.

For younger children, many parents crush the pills into a small amount of pudding,
applesauce, jam, frozen juice concentrate, or another favorite food. However, your
child may develop a lifelong aversion to these foods after treatment is over. Before mixing with any food, check with the doctor because some foods can negate the effects of
medications.

Jeremy was 4 when he was diagnosed, and we used to crush up the pills and mix
them with ice cream. This worked well for us.

· · · · ·

Our son was 2½ years old when diagnosed. We put the med in an oral syringe and
put very hot water in a tiny glass. Then we would draw a wee bit of the hot water
into the oral syringe and then we would cap it. Then you gently shake the syringe
and turn it back and forth while the med completely dissolves. Then we would take
off the cap and fill it the rest of the way with nice cold Kool-Aid®. Alexander would
get to choose the flavor of Kool-Aid® each day and we would just mix up a couple
different batches of flavors and keep them in the fridge. He felt like he was in control
because he chose the flavor, and it covered up the lousy taste of the medication. We
asked our oncologist about this at the very beginning, and he said it was a great way
to do it because neither the water nor the Kool-Aid® had any unwanted effects on the
medication. Anyway, we never once had any problem with this method.

The method we used for getting Garrett to take his foul-tasting chemo/meds was the mixing agent Syrpalta®. This is a grape-flavored syrup available from the pharmacy. It doesn't react with most meds and the flavor can hide almost anything.

We used quite a bit of the stuff. First, we crushed Garrett's pills with a pill crusher/ cutter, then we mixed them in a cup before putting them in a syringe to squirt in his mouth. (Keep in mind he was only about 15 months old when he got sick.) We had to make sure he got every drop though, since some of the pills were really small and a little bit of syrup could hide a significant portion of the dose.

You should make sure that any med you do this with is safe to crush or mix with Syrpalta® (or chocolate, or anything else for that matter). This particular mixing agent is designed to be "inert," but you can't be too careful. Meds with time-release or slow-release agents should never be crushed. Some meds should never be mixed with milk, for example.

Teens and medication

Teenagers usually have completely different issues around taking pills than young children. Most problems with teens revolve around autonomy, control, and feelings of invulnerability. It is normal for teenagers to be noncompliant, and they cannot be forced to take pills if they choose not to cooperate. Trying to coerce teens fuels conflict and frustrates everyone. If you need help, ask for an assessment by the psychosocial team at the hospital to work out a plan for treatment adherence. Everyone will need to be flexible to reach a favorable outcome.

I think the main problem with teens is making sure that they take the meds. Joel (15 years old) has been very responsible about taking his nightly pills. I've tried to make it easy for him by having an index card for the week, and he marks off the med as he takes it. I also put a list of the meds on a dry erase board on the fridge as a reminder. As he takes the med, he erases it. That way it's easy for him (and me) to see at a glance if he's taken his stuff. The index card alone wasn't working because sometimes he couldn't find a pen or forgot to mark it off.

Taking a temperature

Fever is the enemy during treatment because it signals infection, and children on chemotherapy cannot fight infection effectively, especially when their white counts are depressed. Parents take hundreds of temperatures, especially when their child is not feeling well. Temperatures can be taken under the tongue, under the arm, swiping across the forehead, or in the ear using a special type of thermometer. Rectal temperatures are not recommended due to the risk of tears and infection. Here are a few suggestions that might help.

- Use a glass thermometer under the tongue.

- Use a digital thermometer under the tongue or arm. Some have an alarm that beeps when it is time to remove the thermometer.

    We bought a digital thermometer that we only use under his arm. It has worked well for us.

- Tympanic (ear) thermometers measure infrared waves and are very easy to use.

    When my in-laws asked at diagnosis if there was anything that we needed, I asked them to try to buy a tympanic thermometer. The device cost over 100 dollars then, but it worked beautifully. It takes only 1 second to obtain a temperature. I can even use it when she is asleep without waking her. They are now sold at pharmacies and drug stores, and cost much less.

Before you leave the hospital, you should know when to call the clinic because of fever. Usually, parents are told not to give any medication for fever and to call if the fever goes above 101° F (38.5° C). It is particularly important for parents of children with implanted catheters to know when to call the clinic, as an untreated infection can be life-threatening. It is also really helpful to have a copy of your child's most recent blood counts when you call to notify the doctor about fever issues.

Transfusions (blood)

Cancer treatment can cause severe anemia (a low number of oxygen-carrying red cells). The normal life of a red cell is 3 to 4 months, and as old cells die the diseased or chemo-stressed marrow cannot replace them. Many children require transfusions of red blood cells when first admitted and periodically throughout treatment.

Whenever my son needed a transfusion, I brought along bags of coloring books, food, and toys. The number of VCRs at the clinic was limited, so I tried to make arrangements for one ahead of time. When anemic (hematocrit below 20 percent), he didn't have much energy, but by the end of the transfusion, his cheeks were rosy and he had tremendous vitality. It was hard to keep him still. After one unit (bag) of red cells, his hematocrit usually jumped up to around 30.

One bag (called a "unit") of red cells takes 2 to 4 hours to administer and is given through an IV or catheter. Mild allergic reactions are common. If your child is prone to allergies or experiences an allergic reaction, it may be necessary to premedicate her with an antihistamine such as Benadryl®. Acute allergic reactions are rare, but they do happen. If your child develops chills and/or fever or any difficulty breathing during a transfusion, notify the nurse immediately so the transfusion can be stopped.

There are some risks of infection from red cell transfusions. Because tests have been devised and used to detect the HIV virus in donated blood, the risk of exposure to HIV is minuscule. Although there are excellent tests for the various types of hepatitis, exposure to this disease is still possible (the risk is less than 1 in 4,000). Exposure to cytomegalovirus is also a concern. These risks are the reason transfusions are given only when absolutely necessary.

> My daughter received several transfusions at the clinic in Children's Hospital with no problems. After we traveled back to our home, she needed her first transfusion at the local hospital. Our pediatrician said to expect to be in the hospital at least 8 hours. I asked why it would take so long when it only took 4 hours at Children's. He said he had worked out a formula and determined that she needed two units of packed cells. I mentioned that she only was given one unit each time at Children's. He called the oncologist, who said it was better to give the smaller amount. We went to the hospital, where a unit of red cells was given. Then a nurse came in with another unit. I questioned why he was doing that and he said, "Doctor's orders." I asked him to verify that order, as we had already discussed it with the doctor. He went into another room to call the doctor, and came back and said the pediatrician thought my daughter needed 30 cc more packed cells. I called Children's and they said she didn't need more, so I refused to let them administer any more blood. It just wasn't worth the risk of hepatitis to get 30 cc of blood. Even though I was pleasant, the nurses were angry at me for questioning the doctor.

During transfusions, sometimes the nurse will strap the child's arm to a board for the duration of the procedure. This method of restraint prevents the child from accidentally bending his arm, which can be very painful and can reposition the needle, but the board can be cumbersome.

Transfusions (platelets)

Platelets are an important component of blood. They help form clots and stop bleeding by repairing breaks in the walls of blood vessels. A normal platelet count for a healthy child is 160,000 to 380,000/mm^3. Chemotherapy can severely depress the platelet count. If a child's counts are very low, it may be necessary to transfuse platelets so uncontrollable bleeding does not occur. Many centers require a transfusion when a child's platelet count goes below 10,000 to 20,000/mm^3, and sometimes repeat transfusions are required every 2 or 3 days until the marrow recovers. Platelet transfusions usually take less than an hour.

As with other blood products, an allergic reaction is possible and platelets are capable of transmitting infections such as hepatitis, cytomegalovirus, and HIV. Even though the chance of contracting these viruses is extremely low, platelets are transfused only when necessary.

> *Platelet transfusions are a snap! Platelets are short-lived and boosted Matt's counts for only a few days, just long enough to get over the danger levels during chemo. He often needed them two to three times every cycle. He had a reaction of hives on one occasion, cured with Benadryl®. Ironically, that was one of the last times he needed platelets.*

· · · · ·

> *Three-year-old Matthew had countless platelet transfusions, and only once did he have a reaction. It was an awful thing to watch, but the nurse who was monitoring him was very calm and professional, which helped both of us. Matthew was always premedicated for his platelet transfusions with Benadryl®, which made him very drowsy. Most often he would sleep through the entire transfusion.*

Tumor markers

A tumor marker test examines a sample of blood (obtained from a vein or from a catheter) or CSF (obtained during a spinal tap) for certain substances that help identify specific types of tumors. Tumor markers used to diagnose some germ cell tumors are alpha-fetoprotein (AFP) and beta-human chorionic gonadotropin (β-hCG). To diagnose pituitary tumors, tests may be run to check for the level of alpha subunit pituitary tumor marker.

Urine collections

Certain chemotherapy drugs can cause damage to the kidneys, so sometimes timed urine collections are done to evaluate your child's kidney function. Also, by measuring certain substances in the kidneys, doctors can tell how well the chemo drugs are working. If your child is toilet trained, the collection is done by saving all the urine your child produces in a defined period of hours.

Urine specimens

Chemotherapy requires frequent urine specimens. One way to help obtain a sample is to encourage your child to drink lots of liquids the hour before. If your child has an IV, you can also ask the nurse to increase the drip rate. Explain to the child why the test is necessary. Ask the nurse to show how the dip sticks work. (They change color, so they are quite popular with preschoolers.) Use a "hat" under the toilet seat. This is a shallow plastic bucket that fits under the seat and catches the urine.

> *Turn on the water while the child sits on the toilet. I don't know why it works, but it does.*

As all parents learn, eating and elimination are functions that the child controls. If she just can't or won't urinate in the hat, go out, buy her the largest drink you can find, and wait.

It may be necessary to obtain a sterile specimen, or "clean catch," if infection is suspected. You or your child will need to cleanse the perineal area with soap or an antiseptic towelette, and she will need to urinate into a small sterile container.

If your child is not yet toilet trained, if a clean catch is impossible, or if your child is unable to urinate, it may be necessary to insert a Foley catheter. This procedure can be quite stressful because it involves placing a sterile rubber tube up the urethra and into the bladder. It is definitely appropriate to ask that your child be given a mild sedative or muscle relaxant before the procedure if he is anxious, and to request that the most skilled person available perform the procedure. In skilled nursing hands, the procedure takes less than 5 minutes to perform.

Visual acuity testing

Visual acuity testing is important if your child's tumor involves the optic nerve pathways or an area of the brain, such as the occipital lobes, that controls vision. Children with these types of tumors are routinely followed by a neuro-ophthalmologist or, in some cases, a pediatric ophthalmologist, because vision loss can be a symptom and indicator of tumor growth. When done by an expert, such testing is accurate and fun for your child. Most ophthalmologists who specialize in the care of children employ technology that presents visual stimuli to your child in the form of toys and mechanical games. They usually understand that patience helps produce valid test results. Baseline testing is important prior to surgery and at specified periods throughout treatment.

> *Jamie's eye exams, which happen every 3 to 6 months, involve multiple stops at the children's eye clinic: first, visual field testing with our specialist who checks his fields using handheld toys and a machine with two different size light points. Then we go to our ophthalmologist for acuity testing and eye drops for optic nerve checking. Then one more check with an orthoptist. It used to take most of a day when he was 2, but now that he's a little older, it can be done in one morning.*

Wada test

The Wada test (intracarotid sodium amobarbitol test) is sometimes used to help locate speech and memory centers within the brains of children with low-grade tumors. Sodium amobarbitol is injected into the carotid artery in the neck in such a way that half of the brain is temporarily put to sleep. This allows your child's doctor to perform tests of speech, memory, and other functions while your child can use only one side of her brain. Sometimes an EEG is performed during this procedure. The Wada test is particularly crucial before surgery to ensure that the speech and memory centers are well defined and protected from injury.

Six-year-old Ethan's introduction to procedures started the day he presented with crossed eyes. The MRI that afternoon was no problem for him; our usually perpetual-motion machine was nearly comatose from the increased pressure in his brain. Getting through that scan was difficult only for my peace of mind. His next scan was a day later; now near-manic from steroids, he lay still, occasionally giggling, for the MRI while watching 'Men in Black' through special MRI-safe video goggles. Though he was under anesthesia for his third scan (at that time he was mute, paralyzed on one side, and NOT capable of cooperating with testing), when he regained his power of speech and communication, scans became a not-so-hard routine. Reminded to lie still, he often fell asleep through the jackhammer-like din of the MRI magnet.

Getting to Ethan's blood was, at first, a bit more challenging. After his port was placed, we at first had to hold Ethan down while accessing it. We were told it shouldn't hurt after being anesthetized with EMLA®, but the sight of the needle was scary. The breakthrough came when a child life specialist (what a great addition to pediatrics!!) distracted him and he found that it really did not hurt.

Since that time, with my suggestions, he has devised (often-changing) routines; for accessing the port, he is sitting semi-upright, clutching his left ear with his left hand and holding a parent with his right. For receiving daily GCSF shots, the special Band-Aid® that looks like a tattoo needs to be open on the table; the appropriate site (left or right thigh) agreed upon, pinched, and alcohol-swabbed; a sibling holding one hand and he pinching an ear with the other; on the count of three the QUICK injection, followed as nearly instantaneously as possible by the Band-Aid®. Simple, really, when you know how. No fear and no tears. Audiometry, psychological/ academic testing, and vision checks are just games which he enjoys. Now if we can only get by the hurdle of the eye-drops which sting like the devil.

Chapter 7

Forming a Partnership with the Treatment Team

It is our duty as physicians to estimate probabilities and to discipline expectations; but leading away from probabilities there are paths of possibilities, toward which it is our duty to hold aloft the light, and the name of that light is hope.

— Karl Menninger
The Vital Balance

IT IS VITALLY IMPORTANT that parents and the treatment team establish and maintain a relationship based on excellent medical care, good communication, and caring. In this partnership, trust is paramount. Doctors rely on parents to make and keep appointments, give the proper medicines at the appropriate times, prepare the child for procedures, and monitor the child for signs of illness or side effects. Parents rely on doctors for medical knowledge, expertise in performing procedures, good judgment, compassion, and clear communication. It is a delicate dance that spans years of trauma and emotional upheaval.

Unlike many other diseases, children with brain and spinal cord tumors spend months or years being treated on an inpatient and outpatient basis. In addition, the treatment of brain and spinal cord tumors in children requires a multidisciplinary approach involving many teams of medical, surgical, and rehabilitative specialists. At various points during the diagnosis and treatment journey, the primary responsibility of providing treatment for the child with a brain or spinal cord tumor shifts from one group of doctors to another.

At diagnosis and in the initial stages of treatment, the pediatric neurosurgeon is usually the captain of the multidisciplinary team. This leadership shifts after surgery to the neuro-oncologist, oncologist, neurologist, radiation oncologist, or physical therapy specialist to coordinate the next phase of treatment. Once treatment is finished, the neuro-oncologist or expert in late effects of treatment may assume leadership of the necessary long-term follow-up. It is the parents, however, who bear the responsibility for coordinating the care and communication between members of the multidisciplinary team.

A climate of cooperation and respect between the healthcare team and parents allows children to thrive. This chapter explores ways to create and maintain that environment.

The hospital

Children who are diagnosed with a brain or spinal cord tumor are usually sent to the nearest academic medical center or children's hospital. Most of these centers combine their efforts by participating in clinical studies with other institutions across the country. If you are sent to a local hospital or to an oncologist, rather than to a multidisciplinary team that includes pediatric neuro-oncologists and pediatric neurosurgeons, you should consider going elsewhere. Recent research showed that children treated at major brain tumor centers did significantly better than those treated at local hospitals.

Because most brain and spinal cord tumors require several phases of treatment, you may need to go to different hospitals at different times. For example, your child may get radiation at one hospital and chemotherapy at another, or the neuro-oncologist may see your child in a clinic separate from the hospital.

> We consider our pediatrician and local pediatric oncologist as co-directors of our son's care. At the same time, we make frequent visits to specialists for acuity and visual field testing, endocrine follow-up, and day-to-day seizure management. We've enrolled our child in a post-treatment study at the National Cancer Institute, in Bethesda, Maryland, so we go there twice a year, and we also see a pediatric neuro-oncologist for long-term brain tumor management.

The multidisciplinary team

The first step of treatment for most children with brain or spinal cord tumors involves surgery. It is vital that a pediatric neurosurgeon perform the surgery. A pediatric neurosurgeon is a doctor who has either done a pediatric fellowship (an extra year of training in pediatrics after neurosurgical residency) or devotes at least half of his or her time to operating on children. Most pediatric neurosurgeons are in large teaching hospitals or in children's hospitals in large cities. A list of pediatric neurosurgeons and where they practice is available at *www.aspn.org*. For more information about pediatric neurosurgeons, see Chapter 10, *Surgery*.

After surgery, the responsibility for care of most children with brain or spinal cord tumors shifts to a pediatric neuro-oncologist. Neuro-oncologists are doctors who specialize in the non-surgical treatment of brain tumors. Along with neurosurgeons and neuro-oncologists, children with brain or spinal cord tumors may also see one or more of the following doctors (in alphabetical order):

- **Endocrinologist.** Doctor who monitors hormonal or growth problems.

- **Ophthalmologist.** Doctor who specializes in the eye.

- **Orthopedic surgeon.** Doctor who monitors the spine for any curves (i.e., scoliosis) or changes resulting from surgery or treatment of a brain or spinal cord tumor.

- **Pathologist.** Doctor who determines the type of tumor after surgery by analyzing cells under a microscope.

- **Pediatrician.** Doctor who cares for children in their hometown.

- **Pediatric neurologist.** Doctor who treats seizures.

- **Pediatric neuropsychologist.** A psychologist with a doctoral degree (PhD) who assesses children at various stages of treatment to identify any learning problems that develop from the tumor or treatment.

- **Pediatric surgeon.** Doctor who implants venous catheters used for chemotherapy.

- **Physiatrist.** Doctor who specialize in rehabilitation of nerves, muscles, and bones.

- **Psychiatrist.** Doctor who diagnoses and treats mental or psychological problems.

- **Radiologist.** Doctor who interprets scans at diagnosis and throughout treatment.

- **Radiation oncologist.** Doctor who designs and manages the administration of radiation therapy.

> *We had a pediatric neuro-oncologist meet with us while our son was hospitalized for his neurosurgery. We were on vacation when our son first started having symptoms, so we knew that we would not be receiving treatment under the neuro-oncologist's care, but he educated us about what the treatment options were for us to consider. His level of knowledge about brain tumor treatment far exceeded the expertise of the pediatric oncologists that cared for our son during his treatment, and we might have made the wrong choice about treatment without his input.*

The doctors

At large children's hospitals, there are doctors at all levels of training, from first-year medical students to experienced professors of medicine. It is often hard to sort them all out in the early days after diagnosis. The following section describes each type of doctor you might meet at a training hospital.

A *medical student* is a college graduate who is attending medical school. Medical students often wear white coats, but they do not have MD after the name on their name tags. They are not doctors.

An *intern* (also called a first-year resident) is a graduate of medical school who is in the first year of postgraduate training. Interns are doctors who are just beginning their clinical training.

A *resident* is a graduate of medical school in the second or third year of postgraduate training. Most residents at pediatric hospitals will be pediatricians upon completion of their residencies. Residents are temporary: they rotate into different services every 4 weeks.

A *fellow* is a doctor pursuing post-residency study in a particular specialty. Most fellows you encounter will be specializing in pediatric oncology. Not all teaching hospitals have fellowship programs.

Attending doctors (or simply, *attendings*) are highly trained doctors hired by the hospital to provide and oversee medical care and to train interns, residents, and fellows. Many of them also teach at a medical school.

Consulting doctors are doctors from other services who are brought in to provide advice or treatment to a child in the oncology unit. The attending may ask for consults with other specialists, who may appear in your child's hospital room unexpectedly. If questions arise about who these doctors are and what role they play, you should ask the fellow or attending assigned to your child.

Each child in a teaching hospital is assigned an attending, who is responsible for that child's care. This doctor should be "board certified" or have equivalent medical credentials. This means the doctor has taken rigorous written and oral tests given by a board of examiners in his or her specialty and meets a high standard of competence. You can call the American Board of Medical Specialties at (866) ASK-ABMS (275-2267) or visit *https://www.certificationmatters.org/is-your-doctor-board-certified/search-now.aspx* to find out if your child's attending is board certified.

> Our medical team was wonderful. They always answered our questions and spent the time with us that we needed. We had a group of doctors who were all working together for the patients. I always felt that we were known by each doctor, and that they were on top of Paige's treatment.

If your family is insured by a health maintenance organization (HMO), you probably will be sent to the affiliated hospital, which will have one or more pediatric oncologists on staff. If this hospital is not a regional pediatric hospital or is not affiliated with the Children's Oncology Group, you can go elsewhere to get state-of-the-art care (see the "Choosing a hospital" section later in this chapter). However, make sure your insurance will cover care at the institution you want to use.

The nurses

An essential part of the hospital hierarchy is the nursing staff. The following explanations will help you understand which type of nurse is caring for your child.

An *RN* is a registered nurse who obtained an associate's degree or higher in nursing and then passed a licensing examination. RNs supervise all other nursing and patient care staff (such as nurses aides or nursing assistants), give medicines, take vital signs (e.g., heart rate, breathing rate, blood pressure), monitor IV machines, change bandages, and care for patients in hospitals, clinics, and doctors' offices. Many RNs in the pediatric oncology service have received specialized training in pediatric oncology nursing.

A *nurse practitioner* or *clinical nurse specialist* is a registered nurse who has completed an educational program (generally a master's or doctoral degree) that teaches advanced skills. For example, in some hospitals and clinics, nurse practitioners perform procedures such as spinal taps. Nurse practitioners or clinical nurse specialists are often the liaison between the medical teams and patients and their families. They help parents keep all the different multidisciplinary team members straight and help interpret medical jargon.

An *LPN* is a licensed practical nurse. LPNs complete certificate training and must pass a licensing exam. In some medical facilities, LPNs are allowed to perform most nursing functions except those involving administration of medications. Many pediatric oncology services limit the involvement of LPNs to personal care, such as patient hygiene and monitoring fluid input and output.

The *head* or *charge nurse* is an RN who supervises all the nurses on the floor for one shift. If you have any problems with a nurse, your first step in resolving the issue should be to talk to the nurse involved. If this does not resolve the problem, a discussion with the charge nurse is your next step.

The *clinical nurse manager* is the administrator for an entire unit, such as a surgical or medical floor or outpatient clinic. The clinical nurse manager is in charge of all nurses in the unit.

> *At our hospital, each of our nurses is different, but each is wonderful. They simply love the kids. They throw parties, set up dream trips, act as counselors, best friends, stern parents. They hug moms and dads. They cry. I have come to respect them so much because they have such a hard job to do, and they do it so well.*

The tumor board

Many hospitals have a committee to review surgery, pathology, and radiology findings and discuss potential treatment plans for patients. This committee is called the tumor board. Members consist of representatives from the patient's multidisciplinary team, a pathologist, a radiologist, and other senior specialists who deal with brain and spinal cord tumors. Very often, the consensus opinion from the tumor board is the treatment offered to the family. Many centers present individual cases to the tumor board at various times during treatment, such as after each imaging study or when the effects of treatment need to be assessed as per the protocol.

Finding a neurosurgeon and neuro-oncologist

Sometimes parents do not have the luxury of time in choosing a pediatric neurosurgeon or pediatric neuro-oncologist. Your child may have life-threatening symptoms that require emergency surgery. Or your child might be assigned to the attending or fellow who happens to be on call at the time of diagnosis. However, if it is not an emergency, you probably will have time to check the qualifications of both the doctors and the medical facility where you child was first diagnosed.

> *A medical oncologist sees patients with a wide variety of cancers and blood diseases. It will necessarily have taken him much longer to accumulate respectable clinical experience with brain tumors than would a neuro-oncologist, who sees brain tumor patients exclusively and on a daily basis. What a neuro-oncologist would learn in a single year of practice might take a medical oncologist a decade to grasp. When a situation arises, you want the doctor who calls to mind a hundred similar cases he has seen recently, not the doctor who will rack his brain trying to remember the dozen cases he may have seen or merely read about long ago.*

> *A neuro-oncologist, because of his understanding of the entire brain tumor experience (not just the chemo part), can address questions related to cognitive changes, family tensions, etc., and will have a better handle on interactions among drugs the brain tumor patient is likely to be taking simultaneously. He is also more likely to have the tact and sensitivity needed to deal with the very specific needs of the brain tumor patient and family. The difference between our oncologist and neuro-oncologist was amazing. We considered the original guy fine (and he was), but then someone came in and turned on the light. It was like that moment when Dorothy from* The Wizard of Oz *steps out of the house and the world's in color.*

During treatment, your child will see a myriad of doctors. It is essential that you and your child are comfortable with your child's pediatric neurosurgeon and neuro-oncologist and that your family feels the doctors are competent, caring, and easy to communicate with. When choosing your child's pediatric neurosurgeon and/or neuro-oncologist, here are several traits to look for:

- Board certified in the field

- Establishes good rapport with your child

- Communicates clearly and compassionately

- Skillful in performing procedures

- Uses the latest surgical tools and techniques

- Answers all questions

- Consults with other doctors on complex problems

- Uses language that is easy to understand

- Makes the results of all tests available

- Acknowledges your right as parents to make decisions

- Respects your values

- Able to deliver the truth with hope

If you don't develop a good rapport with your child's doctor(s), ask to be assigned to a different doctor whom you have met on rounds or during clinic visits. Most parents are accommodated, because hospitals realize the importance of good communication and rapport between families and doctors. You will, however, still see different doctors, because many institutions have rotating doctors on call.

> *The neurosurgeon told us that everything looked great on Janet's MRI and to come back and see him in 3 months. He also gave me $10.00 and said if we get down to Biloxi again to play #22 on roulette for him. I asked, "Why 22?" and he said that was the date that he met an individual that helped change his perspective on life, which in turn has allowed him to treat his patients better. He then handed me Janet's chart and pointed to our first appointment date: Sept. 22, 2000.*

• • • • •

> *For 2 months, we were dealing with a doctor who said there was only a "vanishingly small" chance at a cure—NO clinical trials, NO other options, NO, NO, NO. I did my own research, and ended up with a doctor new to our hospital, who gives Danny a "real chance." Not only does his attitude make a difference to my own attitude (it's actually pleasant to be in the same room and talk to him), but I believe he is actively searching out treatment options and in fact has a whole list of things to try. The first doctor came at it from a much more conservative vantage point—if something didn't have a tried and true track record he wouldn't recommend it. The problem in our*

case was that Danny has an incredibly rare brain tumor so there is no track record. One final note: every doctor I spoke with, except, of course, our first one, said that there are always exceptions. They've seen patients 10 years ago who they said would never make it, and they're doing great. I need a doctor who helps me keep my head attuned to the positive.

Choosing a hospital

At diagnosis, you have the option to choose where you would like your child to be treated. Parents can obtain a free referral to an accredited center from either the Pediatric Brain Tumor Consortium (PBTC) or the Children's Oncology Group (COG).

The PBTC is a multidisciplinary cooperative research organization devoted to the study of tumor biology and new therapies for childhood brain and spinal cord tumors. Contact information is available at *www.pbtc.org/public/inst_contact_info.htm*. Member institutions are:

- Children's Hospital Los Angeles (California)

- Children's National Medical Center (Washington, DC)

- Children's Memorial Hospital (Chicago)

- Cincinnati Children's Hospital Medical Center (Ohio)

- Duke University (North Carolina)

- Lucile Packard Children's Hospital Stanford (California)

- Memorial Sloan Kettering Cancer Center (New York)

- National Cancer Institute (Maryland)

- St. Jude Children's Research Hospital (Tennessee)

- Texas Children's Cancer Center

- University of Pittsburgh (Pennsylvania)

The COG is a consortium of more than 200 hospitals in North America, Australia, New Zealand, and Europe that treat children with cancer. Contact information is:

222 E. Huntington Drive, Suite 100
Monrovia, CA 91016
(626) 447-0064
www.childrensoncologygroup.org

Types of relationships

Three types of relationships tend to develop between doctors and parents.

- **Paternal.** In a paternal relationship, the parent is submissive, and the doctor assumes a parental role. This dynamic may seem desirable to parents who are uncomfortable or inexperienced in dealing with medical issues, but it places all the responsibility for decisions and monitoring on the doctor. Doctors are human. If your child's doctor makes a mistake and you are not monitoring drugs and treatments, these mistakes may go unnoticed. You are the expert on your child and you know best how to gauge his reactions to drugs and treatments.

    I once asked a fellow about my daughter's blood work. She literally patted me on the head and said it was her job to worry about that, not mine. I said in a nice voice that I thought it was a reasonable question and that I would appreciate an answer.

Some parents are intimidated by doctors and fear that if they question the doctors their child will suffer. This type of behavior robs the child of an adult advocate who speaks up when something seems wrong.

- **Adversarial.** Some parents adopt an "us against them" attitude, which is counterproductive. They seem to feel the disease and treatment are the fault of the medical staff, and they blame staff for any setbacks that occur. This attitude undermines the child's confidence in her doctor, which is a crucial component for healing.

    I knew one family who just hated the Children's Hospital. They called it the "House of Horrors" or the "torture chamber" in front of their children. Small wonder that their children were terrified.

- **Collegial.** This is a true partnership in which parents and doctors are all on the same footing and they respect each other's domains and expertise. The doctor recognizes that the parents are the experts about their own child and are essential in ensuring that the protocol is followed. The parents respect the doctor's expertise and feel comfortable discussing various treatment options or concerns that arise. Honest communication is necessary for this partnership to work, but the effort is well worth it. The child has confidence in his doctor, the parents have lessened their stress by creating a supportive relationship with the doctor, and the doctor feels comfortable that the family will comply with the treatment plan, thus giving the child the best chance for a cure.

    We had a wonderful relationship with our neuro-oncologist. He perfectly blended the science and the art of medicine. His manner with our daughter was warm, he was extremely well-qualified professionally, and he was very easy to talk to. I could bring in articles to discuss with him, and he welcomed the discussion. Although he

*was busy, he never rushed us. I laughed when I saw that he had written in the chart,
"Mother asks innumerable appropriate questions."*

Another mother relates a different experience:

*We tried very hard to form a partnership with the medical team but failed. The staff
seemed very guarded and distant, almost wary of a parent wanting to participate
in the decisions made for the child. I learned to use the medical library and took
research reports in to them to get some help for side effects and get some drug dosages reduced. Things improved, but I was never considered a partner in the healthcare team; I was viewed as a problem.*

A pediatric oncologist shares her perspective:

*All parents are different and have different coping styles. Some deal best with a lot
of information (lab results, meds, study options) up front, while others are overwhelmed and want the information a little bit at a time. There is no way for the
doctor to know the parents' coping styles at the beginning. (Even the parents may not
yet know!) So if they let the doctor know how much information they want or don't
want, it is very helpful.*

Communication

Clear and frequent communication is the foundation of a positive doctor/parent relationship. Doctors need to be able to explain clearly and listen well, and parents need to
feel comfortable asking questions and expressing concerns before they grow into grievances. Nurses and doctors cannot read parents' minds, nor can parents prepare their
child for a procedure unless it has been explained well. The following are parent suggestions about how to establish and maintain good communication with your child's
healthcare team.

• Tell the staff how much you want to know.

*I told them the first day to treat me like a medical student. I asked them to share
all information, current studies, lab results, everything, with me. I told them, in
advance, that I hoped they wouldn't be offended by lots of questions, because knowledge was comfort to me.*

• • • • •

*If the doctors at Children's told me to do something, I didn't question it because I
trusted them.*

- Inform the staff of your child's temperament, likes, and dislikes. You know your child better than anyone, so don't hesitate to tell the clinic staff about what works best.

  Whenever my daughter was hospitalized, I made a point of kindly reminding doctors and nurses that she was extremely sensitive, and would benefit from quiet voices and soothing explanations of anything that was about to occur, such as taking temperatures, vital signs, or adjustments to her IV.

- Encourage a close relationship between doctor, nurse, and child. Insist that all medical personnel respect your child's dignity. Do not let anyone talk in front of your child as if she is not there. If a problem persists, you have the right to ask the offending person to leave. Marina Rozen observes in *Advice to Doctors and Other Big People:*

  The best part about the doctor is when he gives me bubble gum. The worst part is when he's in the room with me and my mom and he only talks to my mom. I've told him I don't like that, but he doesn't listen.

  $\bullet\ \ \bullet\ \ \bullet\ \ \bullet\ \ \bullet$

  Leeann's doctor here in town has been great. She knows how to talk to kids without talking down to them. She would take the time during her hospital rounds to help Leeann with her homework and laugh at all of our stupid jokes. A good sense of humor was a must for all of us.

- Most children's hospitals assign each patient a primary nurse who will oversee all care. Try to form a close relationship with your child's nurse. Nurses usually possess vast knowledge and experience about both medical and practical aspects of cancer treatment. Often, the nurse can rectify misunderstandings between doctors and parents.

- Children and teenagers should be included as part of the team. They should be consulted about treatments and procedures and be given age-appropriate choices.

- Coordinate communication. If your hometown pediatrician will handle all of your child's outpatient treatments, find ways to facilitate communication between the neuro-oncologist and pediatrician.

  We had a problem with the pediatrician's office not calling me with the results of my daughter's blood work in time for me to call the clinic. This would result in worry for me and a delay in changes to her chemotherapy doses. I told the pediatrician's nurse that I knew how busy they were and I hated having to keep calling to get the results. I asked her if it was possible for them to give the lab authorization to call me with the results. They thought it was a great idea, and it worked for years. The lab would fax the doctor the results, but call me. Then I would call the clinic and get the dose changes. The clinic would then fax that information to the pediatrician's office. It was a win/win situation: the pediatrician's office received no interruptions, they got copies of everything in writing, and I got quick responses from the clinic on how to adjust her meds to her wildly swinging blood counts.

• Go to all appointments with a written list of questions. This prevents you from forgetting something important and saves the staff from numerous follow-up phone calls.

• Ask for definitions of unfamiliar terms. Repeat back the information to ensure you understood it correctly. Writing down answers or recording conferences are both common practices.

• Some parents want to read their child's medical chart to obtain more details about their child's condition and to help in formulating questions for the medical team. Sometimes the doctor or nurse will let the parents read the chart in the child's hospital room or in the waiting room at the clinic, but some hospitals have policies that prohibit this. Most states and provinces have laws that allow patient access to all records. You may have to write to the doctor asking to review the chart and pay any duplication costs.

• If you have questions or concerns, discuss them with the nurses or residents. If they are unable to provide a satisfactory answer, ask the fellow or attending doctor assigned to your child.

> *We found that sitting down and talking things over with the nurses helped immensely. They were very familiar with each drug and its side effects. They told us many stories about children who had been through the same thing and were doing well years later. They always seemed to have time to give encouragement, a smile, or a hug.*

• The medical team includes many specialists: doctors, nurses, physical therapists, nutritionists, x-ray technicians, radiation therapists, and more. At training hospitals, many of these people will be in the early stages of their training. If a procedure is not going well, the parent has the right to tell the person to stop and to request that a more skilled person do the job.

> *While I truly supported the teaching hospital concept, it was difficult to deal with a first-year resident who couldn't do a spinal tap or insert an IV. We had a tendency to lose patience rather quickly when our child was screaming and the doctor was getting impatient. More than once we requested a replacement and had someone else do the test.*

- Know your rights—and the hospital's. Legally, your child cannot be treated without your permission. If the doctor suggests a procedure you do not feel comfortable with, keep asking questions until you feel fully informed. You have the legal right to refuse the procedure if you do not think it is necessary.

> One day in the hospital, a group of fellows came in and announced that they were going to do a lung biopsy on Jesse. I told them that I hadn't heard anything about it from her attending, and I just didn't think it was the right thing to do. They said, "We have to do it," and I repeated that I just didn't think it needed to be done until we talked to the attending. They seemed angry, but we stood our ground. When the attending came later, he said that they were not supposed to do a biopsy because the surgeon said it was too risky of an area in the lung to get to.

However, if the hospital feels you are endangering the health of your child by withholding permission for treatment, they can take you to court. All parties must remember that the most important person in this circumstance is the child. Don't let problems turn into grievances.

- Use "I" statements. For example, "I feel upset when you won't answer my questions," rather than, "You never listen to me."

- If it helps you feel more comfortable, keep track of your child's treatments to check for mistakes.

> Few children were on the same protocol at the time my daughter was being treated. The attendings always knew exactly what was supposed to be done, but the fellows sometimes made mistakes. I was embarrassed to correct them, but I just kept reminding myself that they had dozens of protocols to keep track of, and I had only one.

> • • • • •

> It was important for us to make sure that we were educated about all aspects of this disease without fear. The more we read and researched the better equipped we were to make decisions. It's important to know the bad news also. An added benefit to constant research was that I stumbled upon more and more survivors of PNET and medulloblastoma. This gave us hope and it only came from continuous research. In our family, I left my job and became the main researcher and home/care coordinator, while my husband continued to work.

- Be specific and diplomatic when describing problems. For example, "My son gets very nervous if we must wait a long time for our appointment, which makes him less compliant with the doctor. Could we call ahead next time to see if the doctor is on schedule?" rather than, "Do you think your time is more valuable than mine?"

- If you have something to discuss with the doctor that will take some time, request a conference or a family meeting. These are routinely scheduled between parents and doctors and should be scheduled to allow enough time for a thorough discussion. Grabbing a busy doctor in the hallway is not fair to her and may not result in a satisfactory answer for you.

> One technique I use to keep from forgetting what I want to say at the doctor's appointment is to type out an agenda for the appointment. I also make a copy for the doctor. This helps me stay calm and focused on the agenda, and it gives me and my doctor a written record of what our concerns were, and what was discussed during the appointment.

- Do not be afraid to make waves if you are right or to apologize if you are wrong.

> When my daughter was in the hospital one time, the nurse came in with two syringes. I asked what they were, and she said immunizations. I said that it must be a mistake, and the nurse said that the orders were in the chart. So I checked my daughter's chart, and the orders were there, but they had another child's name on them.

- Show appreciation.

> I sent thank-you notes to three residents after my daughter's first hospitalization. The notes were short but sweet. I wanted them to know how much we appreciated their many kindnesses.

· · · · ·

> I always try to thank the nurse or doctor when they apologize for being late and give the reason. I don't mind waiting if it is for a good cause, and I feel they show respect when they apologize.

· · · · ·

> Erica's doctor would sometimes call up just to say, "How's my little chickadee?" He really cared. It touched me that he took the time to call, and I told him that I appreciated it.

· · · · ·

> Early in my daughter's treatment, we changed pediatricians. The first was aloof and patronizing, and the second was smart, warm, funny, and caring. He was a constant bright spot in our lives through some dark times. So every year during my daughter's treatment, she and her younger sister put on their Santa hats and brought homemade cookies to her pediatrician and nurse. This year was the first time she was able to walk in, and she looked them in the eye and sang, "We Wish You a Merry Christmas." Her nurse went in the back room and cried, and her doctor got misty-eyed. I'll always be thankful for their care.

Getting a second opinion

There are times during your child's treatment when a second opinion may be advisable. Parents are sometimes reluctant to request a second opinion because they are afraid of offending their child's doctor or creating antagonism. Conscientious doctors will not resent a parent seeking a second opinion. If your child's doctor does resist, ask why. Second opinions are a common and accepted practice, and they are sometimes required by insurance companies.

There are two ways to get a second opinion: see another specialist or ask the child's doctor to arrange a multidisciplinary second opinion. Many parents seek a second or third opinion at the time of diagnosis. Do not do this in secret. Explain to your child's pediatric neurosurgeon or neuro-oncologist that, before proceeding, you would like additional viewpoints. To allow for a thorough analysis, arrange to have copies of all records, scans, and pathology slides sent ahead to the doctor(s) who will give the additional opinions. It is often helpful to get an opinion from a neuro-oncologist and one from a neurosurgeon.

> *Personally, I feel there is nothing wrong with getting a second opinion from another major center. If you like and feel comfortable with your current team, that's great, but I definitely do not like when a doctor tells the patient there's "no reason" to go elsewhere, "they can't do anything we don't do," and so forth. Many people choose to go elsewhere and have great results when a first doctor may have told them "no surgery," "it's hopeless," whatever the case may be. Many people travel great distances to get treatment at another facility whose treatment philosophy they prefer. And, granted, that is their choice. We chose to take our son to a top neurosurgeon about 3 hours away and, let me tell you, it has been the best thing that we have done for him. Now, your second opinion doctor may look at your child's MRIs and say, "Your team is doing exactly the right things; stick with them," or they may tell you something totally different and then you can make your own decision on what to do. It is always wise to get more than one opinion when dealing with something as serious as a brain tumor.*

Multidisciplinary second opinions incorporate the views of several different specialists. Parents who would like to get various viewpoints can ask to have the child's situation discussed at a tumor board, which usually meets weekly at major medical centers. These boards include medical, surgical, and radiation oncologists, as well as pathologists, radiologists, fellows, and residents. Your child's pediatric neurosurgeon or neuro-oncologist will present the facts of your child's case for discussion. Ask him to tell you what was said at the meeting.

Conflict resolution

Conflict is a part of life. In a situation where a child's life is threatened, such as when a child has a brain or spinal cord tumor, the heightened emotions and constant involvement with the medical bureaucracy guarantee conflict. Because clashes are inevitable, resolving them is of paramount importance. A speedy resolution may result if you adopt Henry Ford's motto, "Don't find fault; find a remedy."

Following are some suggestions from parents about how to resolve problems:

- Treat the doctors with respect, and expect respect from them.

  I always wanted to be treated as an intelligent adult, not someone of lesser status. So I would ask each medical person what they wished to be called. We would either both go by first names or both go by titles. I did not want to be called 'Mom.'

- Expect a reasonable amount of sensitivity from the staff.

  During our little boy's first MRI, I was very emotional, and wondered out loud if he could feel or hear what was going on even though he was sedated. The MRI nurse caught me completely off-guard by banging loudly on the side of the transport bed without getting any reaction from him. "See, he's out," she said. I was too startled then, but I wished I had told her how much that bothered me.

- Treat the staff with sensitivity. Recognize that you are under enormous stress, and so are the doctors and nurses. Do not blame them for the disease or explode in anger. Be an advocate, not an adversary.

  Doctors must deal with this disease over and over again. They can never really escape unless they change their careers. And, many, many times, they lose yet another patient. Our treatment for PNET/medulloblastoma lasted less than a year. While our subconscious is still filled with fear, at least the actual act of going to the hospital and receiving treatment is finite. If we lose our child, that also is a finite act. The doctors must deal with pain over and over again. In some ways it is so dreadful for them because they are the ones we look to for a cure. So, doctors now hold a very special place in my heart!

- If a problem develops, state the issue clearly, without accusations, and then suggest a solution.

  I found out late in my daughter's treatment that short-acting, safe sedatives were being used for many children at the clinic to prevent pain and anxiety during treatments. Only parents who knew about it and requested it received this service. I felt that my daughter's life would have been incredibly improved if we had been able to remove the trauma of procedures. I was angry. But I also realized that although I thought that they were wrong not to offer the service, I was partially at fault for not expressing more clearly how much difficulty she had the week before and after a procedure. I called the director of the clinic and carefully explained that I thought that poor staff/parent communication was creating hardships for the children. I suggested that the entire staff meet with a panel of parents to try to improve communication and to educate the doctors on the impact of pain on the children's daily lives. They were very supportive and scheduled the conference. From then on, children were sedated for painful procedures. This is a classic example of how something good can come out of a disagreement, if both parties are receptive to solving the problem.

- Recognize that although it is hard to speak up, especially if you are not naturally assertive; but it is very important to solve the problem before it grows and poisons the relationship.

- Most large medical centers have social workers and psychologists on staff to help families. One of their major duties is to serve as mediators between staff and parents. Ask for their advice about problem solving.

- Monitor your own feelings of anger and fear. Be careful not to dump on staff inappropriately. On the other hand, do not let a doctor or nurse behave unprofessionally toward you or your child. Parents and staff members all have bad days, but they should not take it out on each other.

- Do not fear reprisal for speaking up. It is possible to be assertive without being aggressive or argumentative. If you are worried, practice what you have to say with a trusted listener before approaching the treatment team.

- There are times when no resolution is possible; but expressing one's feelings can be a great release.

My son and I waited in an exam room for over an hour for a painful procedure. When I went out to ask the receptionist what had caused the delay, she said that a parent had brought in a child without an appointment. This parent frequently failed to bring in her child for treatment, and consequently, whenever she appeared, the doctors dropped everything to take care of the child. When the doctor finally came in, an hour and a half later, my son was in tears. The doctor did not explain the delay or apologize, he just silently started the procedure. After it was finished, I went out of the room, found the doctor, and said, "This makes me so angry. You just left us in here for hours and traumatized my son." He told me that I should have more compassion for the other mother because her life was very difficult. I replied that he encouraged her to not make appointments by dropping everything whenever she appeared. I added that it wasn't fair to those parents who played by the rules; she was being rewarded for her irresponsibility. After we had each stated our position, we left without resolution.

Changing doctors

Facing childhood cancer is one of life's greatest struggles. A skilled doctor you trust, who communicates easily and honestly with you, can greatly ease this struggle. If the doctor adds to your family's discomfort rather than reducing it, you may have to change doctors. Changing doctors is not a step to be taken lightly, but it can be a great relief if the relationship has deteriorated beyond repair. It is a good policy to exhaust all possible remedies prior to separating and to examine your own role in the relationship to prevent the same problems from arising with the new doctor. Mediation by social service staff and improved communication can often resolve the issues and prevent the disruption of changing doctors.

Although there are many valid reasons for changing doctors, some of the most common are:

- Lack of qualifications

- Grave medical errors being made

- Poor communication skills or refusal to answer questions

- Serious clash of philosophy or personality; for example, a paternalistic doctor and a parent who wishes to be informed and share in decision making

> It was late on a Friday night when our 2-year-old son was diagnosed with medulloblastoma at a local hospital in NYC. We were told that we had to move quickly on surgery, although we were not comfortable with the neurosurgeon on their staff who had a pompous demeanor and wasn't a very good communicator. One of our friends, a pediatrician, took us aside and recommended the best pediatric neurosurgeon in the city. We called the doctor's office and he arranged for a neurosurgery fellow to meet us first thing on Sunday morning to review the scans. It was that Sunday afternoon that the neurosurgeon called us from his home to discuss our son's case. He was warm and caring and, we later found out, one of the top people in the country. We arranged for the transfer to his hospital on Monday and were greeted by an experienced neurology and neurosurgery team. We were lucky to find this out so soon after diagnosis since those first days were such a blur.

Many parents, fearing reprisal, choose to continue with a doctor in whom they have no confidence. Such reprisals rarely happen at large, regional children's hospitals. Although there may be lingering bitterness or anger between parents and doctors, the child will continue to benefit from the best-known treatment. Children may actually suffer more from the additional family stress caused by a poor doctor/parent relationship than from changing doctors.

In a small treatment center like Group Health, there are only two pediatric oncologists. When parents change doctors, the situation becomes very tense because the terminated doctor still cares for their child nights, weekends, and when he is on call. I would not recommend changing doctors if there are only two doctors in the clinic. It's probably better to change treatment centers if possible.

Once the decision to change doctors is made, parents must be candid. Either verbally or in writing, they should give an explanation for the change and make a formal request to transfer records to the new doctor. Doctors are legally required to transfer all records upon written request.

We've had wonderful docs, mediocre docs, and one who made a terrible mistake. We've had warm, compassionate docs, ho-hum docs (on a good day they're nice, on a bad day they're neutral), and we've met a couple of world-class jerks. Sounds pretty much like a slice of humanity, right?

Parents hold doctors to a different standard because the stakes are so high—our kids' lives. But the reality is they are usually overworked, exhausted, and deal with newly diagnosed families on an almost daily basis, day after day, week after week, year after year. I can't even begin to imagine the emotional toll that must take.

I tell my kids all human relationships are like a goodwill bank. If you make lots of deposits, an occasional withdrawal won't be so noticeable. I tell my docs and my kids' docs whenever things go right. I like to write, so I send many thank-you notes. When our pediatrician went on sabbatical, he took me into his office and showed me every mushy Christmas card I'd sent him lined up on the back of his messy desk.

I also have been known to bring in brownies for the office staff. We did this on my daughter's last day of radiation and several people brushed away tears when they saw the thank-you note she drew—a picture of herself holding a Snow White and the Seven Dwarves audiotape. She listened to that during every radiation session because I'd promised that day's radiation treatment would be over before the dwarves appeared.

I recently asked one of my favorite doctors (a pediatric oncologist who has incredible compassion) how many thank-you notes she had received from parents over the years. She said she could count them on two hands. I asked how many complaints, and she said, "You wouldn't want to know."

So, while I think docs should be called out for bad behavior and bad medicine, I also think we should continually acknowledge good medicine and good behavior. I'd like to encourage the good ones to stick around—new little innocents keep getting cancer every day.

CHAPTER 8

Hospitalization

Every day is a journey,
and the journey itself is home.

— Matsuo Basho

THERE ARE FEW THINGS in life more uncomfortable than rising from a lumpy pull-out couch to face another day of your child's hospitalization for cancer. Hospitals are noisy bureaucracies that run on a time schedule all their own. Staff members wake children in the middle of the night to check temperature, pulse, and blood pressure or to draw blood. For a child, being hospitalized means being separated from parents, brothers, sisters, friends, pets, and the comfort and familiarity of home. A child's hospitalization can rob both parent and child of a sense of control, leaving them feeling helpless. With a little ingenuity, however, you can make the most of the facilities, liven up the atmosphere, and even have some fun.

The room

Because kids on chemotherapy are at increased risk of infection, many hospitals give them private rooms. This means more space for the child, the parents, and visitors; it also means much more freedom to personalize and decorate the room. Covering the walls with big, bright posters of interest to your child can brighten up the room immensely.

> *The first thing we put up in Meagan's room was a huge poster of The Little Engine That Could saying, "I think I can, I think I can."*

· · · · ·

> *We were away from home for surgery, and I wanted to be sure to have lots of family pictures around for Anthony to see when he woke up. We covered the walls with them.*

Cards can be displayed on the walls, hanging from strings like a mobile, or taped around the windowsills. You can display pictures of your child engaged in her favorite activity, and add photos of her friends. Most hospitals don't allow flowers on oncology floors because they can grow a fungus that can make children sick; but it's fun to have bouquets of balloons bobbing in the corners. Younger children derive great comfort from having a favorite stuffed animal, blanket, or quilt on their bed. If your child likes certain scents, make the room smell good with potpourri or aromatherapy oils.

> *I went and bought a travel bag on wheels. It is so much easier than trying to carry several handle bags when Zach is admitted. It has several pockets to carry stuff. I love it and wished I had done it 2 years ago when we started this!*

> *I take these things to the hospital: flavored creamer for my coffee (a little treat for me); a book for us to read together so I don't go crazy from Cartoon Network (we are reading the Narnia series, and Zach begs me to read to him. I snuggle up with him in his bed while we read); his favorite pillow from home; little airplanes and parachuters to drop from the third floor at night when the lobby is empty (if he's feeling well enough); my thermometer so I can check his temp anytime I want to; lots of Legos®; phone numbers of friends; canned ravioli; toaster strudels; story tapes (Adventures in Odyssey®); and music CDs with earphones.*

To personalize visits, some parents bring a guestbook for people to sign. Others put up a medical staff sign-in poster, which must be signed before examinations begin or vital signs are taken. Another variation of the sign-in poster is to have each staff member or visitor outline his or her hand and write his or her name within the handprint. If your budget allows, a digital camera can help identify the many staff members involved in your child's care and can provide a fun activity for your child.

> *In my position as a parent consultant, I suggest that a journal (possible titles are Book of Hope, Book of Sharing, My Cancer Experience, and Friends Indeed) be kept in the child's room for any visitor, family member, or medical caregiver to write in at any time. Leaving a message if the child is sleeping or out of the room for procedures can be a nice surprise. Later, a surviving child and her family, or the family of a child who has died, have a memory book of those who have touched their lives.*

Some children who have undergone surgery for a brain or spinal cord tumor have difficulty communicating for a period of time after surgery. If your child loses the ability to speak, you can request and use a communication board (a felt or plastic board with pictures and movable figures) until his speech is more understandable. During that time it is important to let your child know that you understand that he sees and understands all communication around him although his ability to acknowledge that is not present. As your child recovers, the ability to communicate will return.

> *My son Alex was diagnosed with medulloblastoma when he was 6 years old. He came out of surgery speaking and then 2 days later couldn't say a word. He was mute for about 2 months and then very slowly he could pronounce things again. His voice and his muscle movements (swallowing and coughing) were okay, but he just*

couldn't say anything. All he would do is shake his head for yes and no or he would cry. It was so frustrating for him. He couldn't laugh. He would just stare into space. You know what brought him around, the show "America's Funniest Home Videos"! He had such a belly laugh and after that he started saying words again. My husband and I would practice words with Alex after he made an effort to talk, and before that we just had a system where he would squeeze our hands for yes or no. We also used flashcards for "hungry," "bathroom," "lights on/off," and for different kinds of food.

Bringing music will help block out some of the hospital noise, as well as help everyone relax. An iPod® or other portable device with headphones makes the time pass more quickly.

My daughter's preschool teacher sent a care package. She made a felt board with dozens of cutout characters and designs that provided hours of quiet entertainment. She also included games, drawings from each classmate, coloring books, markers, get well cards, and a child's tape player with earphones. Because we had run out of our house with just the clothes on our backs, all of these toys were very, very welcome.

The floor

As soon as possible after admission, ask for a floor tour. Find out if a microwave and refrigerator are available, learn what the approved parent sleeping arrangements are, and ask about showers and bathtubs for both patients and parents. Ask about available laundry facilities. Obtain a hospital handbook if one is available. These booklets often include information about billing, parking, discounts, and other helpful items.

Either my husband or I stayed with Delaney the entire time she was in the hospital. To improve the comfort of the fold-out chair that the hospital provides for the sleep-in parent, we used a self-inflating camping mat. When it is rolled out, it self-inflates with a one-way valve. The straps can be used to secure it to the vinyl chair. It makes the chair much more comfortable and allows your muscles to relax. When it is not in use, it can be rolled up with straps and set in the corner.

Many children's hospitals have in-room or portable DVD players available. You can sign out DVDs from the hospital media library or bring from home a favorite funny movie or DVD of a TV show. Humor helps, so joke books and things that make kids laugh (such as Silly String®) are great items to pack. Most hospitals have wireless Internet for connection to social media for older children and adolescents. This keeps them connected to their friends at home and also provides a way to stream movies and other videos for children of all ages.

> *A friend brought in a bag from the local dime store. He included a water pistol (good for unwelcome visitors or unfriendly interns), Play-Doh®, a Slinky®, checkers, dominos, bubbles, a book of corny jokes, and puzzles.*

Although many hospitals provide brightly colored smocks for young patients, most children and teens prefer to wear their own clothing if at all possible. This can pose a laundry problem, so find out whether the hospital has laundry facilities for families to use.

Food

Buying meals day after day in the hospital cafeteria is expensive. Check with the hospital social worker to find out whether the hospital has food discount cards or free meals for parents. Some hospitals deliver meals to families via a meal cart or provide sandwiches in a family lounge at meal times. Check to see if the floor has a refrigerator for parents' food and stock it with your favorite items from home. Remember to put your name in a prominent place on your containers.

> *Our hospital provides vouchers for the cafeteria that can be used instead of ordering food for the room. For us, they have been a godsend. The food on the tray is much worse than what is in the cafeteria. Also, oncology patients have no spending cap on the vouchers, so we can get a few extras. When our son is not able to go to the cafeteria, we go down and bring the food back to his room.*

Many hospitals have cooking facilities for families where they can cook or microwave favorite meals brought from home. Family and friends can bring food when they visit, and some parents order extra items to come up on their child's tray. Ordering out for dinner can also be a nice change of pace for you and your child. As long as there are no medical restrictions, there's no reason why food from local restaurants can't be delivered to the hospital. You can check with the nurses to see if they have menus from local restaurants.

> *Just the smell of food nauseated my daughter. I'll never forget taking the tray out in the hall and gobbling the food down myself. I always felt so guilty, and thought that the staff viewed me as that parent who ate her kid's food. But it saved money and prevented her meals from going to waste. I also did not want to leave her side for the few minutes it took to go to the cafeteria although, in hindsight, the walk would have done me some good.*

Parking

Many parents of children with cancer have unpleasant memories of driving around in endless loops looking for a parking space while their child was throwing up in a bucket in the back seat (or even worse when the bucket was left at home). The hospital might have both long-term and short-term parking arrangements. The nurses and other parents will know whether parking passes are available or where the cheapest parking is located. Some hospitals have valet parking, which may be as inexpensive as self-parking for a short appointment.

> *I had no idea that the hospital gave out free parking passes to their frequent customers. Now I tell every new parent to check as soon as possible to see if they can get a parking pass. It will save them lots of money that they would have spent on meters and parking tickets, and time that they would have spent running out to move the car out of the emergency parking spot.*

The endless waiting

Everything seems to take forever in the hospital, so parents must learn the art of waiting patiently or they will go nuts. For example, the nurse might tell you not to go to the playroom because someone will be "right up" to take your child for an echocardiogram. "Right up" can easily mean 2 hours or more. Many parents find themselves getting nervous or angry while waiting for the doctors to appear during rounds each morning (when the attending physicians, residents, and interns move from room to room in a large group), then feeling let down when the visit lasts only a few moments. If you have questions to ask the doctors, write them down and tell the doctors when they come in that you would like a moment to discuss concerns or ask questions.

> *You don't have to go too crazy. Make sure you watch the videos or eat the popcorn or flirt with the nurses or taunt the residents or leave notes for the cleaning lady or chat with the security guard or make coffee for all the parents or pretend you like puking or show the nurses how to hack into the hospital mainframe or paint your face with Butt Paste. Or, all of the above, if you like. Just do something.*

It helps for both caregiver and child to come prepared for long waits each time they go to the hospital. Some well-supported institutions have iPads®, DVDs, videogames, toys, and games available, but you might need to bring your own entertainment such as favorite card games, board games, computer games, drawing materials, and books. Some children will take comfort from having a favorite blanket or pillow along with them for a day in the clinic or during a lengthy hospitalization. If your child is scheduled for surgery, you can bring a good book, a model airplane project, your holiday card list, or a jigsaw puzzle that several people can work on together.

> *Our emergency bag had two sides. The most important was mine, because our hospital provided nothing for parents. I would pack deodorant (plus an extra set of clothes), a book I had not read (I survived on romance novels that I bought at the*

used bookstore, four for a dollar), decent lighting, a soft sweatshirt top and bottom to wear at night, paper and pen for taking notes, and clean socks. You might laugh, but I can deal with a scared, irritable kid for a L-O-N-G time as long as I have clean, soft socks!

On the kids' side was an art kit with Play-Doh®, crayons, pencils, markers, scissors, glue, finger paints, clay, and reams of paper. It also had plastic cutlery, and some cookie cutters for the Play-Doh®. I always brought the game Trouble®, since it's self-contained and the dice are enclosed in the little bubble. The pieces fit nicely in a plastic sandwich bag (or medication bag). The lifesaver was video games. They provided hours of enjoyment. We also brought a Lego® table with blocks. Since Matthew is usually neutropenic, or in isolation for some mysterious complication, we bring our own games. Monopoly® and Battleship® are both long games that can take an entire morning to play.

We also made it a habit to always bring Matthew's special blanket on any clinic or ER visits. I cannot imagine trying to have him in the hospital without it. He does not carry it around, but it is always there at bedtime.

I also kept a box of stuff for me to do in case of incarceration at Club Children's. In particular, the box had pictures and photo albums. One nurse remarked how organized I was, but I pointed out that the album I was putting together was of Matthew's first birthday. (He was almost 6 at the time.)

Working with the staff

There are wonderful and not-so-wonderful people employed by hospitals, but it helps to remember that working in the pediatric oncology service is extremely stressful and that most of the staff are working hard on behalf of the children. Even the tiniest effort on your part to ease their burden or empathize with their circumstances will go a very long way toward establishing a cooperative and friendly relationship. For example, if parents change soiled bedding, take out food trays, and give their child baths, it can free up overworked nurses to take care of medicines and IVs. If you are making a run to the coffee shop, ask whether you can bring them something, too. Simply remembering to thank them every day will make a big difference. Chapter 7, *Forming a Partnership with the Treatment Team*, contains many suggestions to enhance your relationship with the staff.

Having cancer strips children of control over their bodies. To help reverse this process, parents can take over some of the nursing care. Children may prefer to have their parents help them to the bathroom or clean up their diarrhea or vomit. Making the bed, keeping the room tidy, changing dressings, and giving back rubs helps your child feel more comfortable and lightens the burden on the nurses. However, some children and teens may feel better if the nurses provide these services, and for younger children whose parents work it may be necessary for the nursing staff to provide these services.

It helps to learn about the shift changes on the oncology floor. If you need to leave during the day or night, don't leave a request with one nurse if another will be coming on duty soon. If you have a request or reminder, you can post it on your child's door, on the wall above the bed, or on the chart.

> Parents should not have to worry about helping the staff or whether the staff is stressed. They have enough on their plate to worry about. But families often feel like they're so helpless, and they think, "What can I do, how can I get in control of this situation?" Many parents find comfort in changing the bed; they very often feel so completely overwhelmed, because they can't give the medicines, and they can't make the cancer go away. So they do what they can do for their child. Look at the staff as a team. You are part of that team. But no one can be your child's parent but you.

In addition, parents and staff can help children regain some control by encouraging choices whenever possible. Older children should be involved in discussions about their treatments, while younger children can decide when to take a bath, which arm to use for an IV, what to order for meals, what position their body will be in for procedures, what clothes to wear, and how to decorate the room. Some children request a hug or a handshake after all treatments or procedures.

> Our son is almost 6. He prefers to talk first with the nurse or technician about fun stuff, like his trains, before he allows any kind of IV or blood draw. Most good techs don't mind; they try to do that anyway. He definitely prefers it when I step back, stay quiet, and let him lead.

It is often helpful to post a schedule for each day that identifies when your child will receive therapies such as chemo, recreation therapy, physical therapy, occupational therapy, or speech therapy. The medical team, social workers, and child life therapists can help you set up the schedule.

It also helps to find out whether there are support groups for parents, patients, and siblings. These groups help family members of newly diagnosed children understand the diagnosis and treatment, as well as provide much-needed support.

Being an advocate for your child

Hospitals can be frightening places for children. Fear can be prevented or lessened if parents are there to provide comfort, protection, and advocacy for their child. Most pediatric hospitals are quite aware of how much better children do when a parent is allowed to sleep in the room. Sometimes small couches convert into beds, or parents can use a cot provided by the hospital.

> *Whenever my husband couldn't be at the hospital at bedtime, he would bring in homemade tapes of him reading bedtime stories. Our son would drift off to sleep hearing his daddy's voice.*

· · · · ·

> *Sometimes you can create your own fun with just a little imagination. On one particular occasion, Matthew was feeling especially bored. With a little ingenuity, we soon discovered that four unused IV poles and as many blankets as we could "steal" from the linen cart made for one pretty cool tent. We then used the mattress from a roll-away cot, and spent the night "camping" in his hospital room. He had a wonderful time.*

Of course, sometimes it isn't possible to stay with your child if you are a single parent or if both parents work full time. Many families have grandparents, older siblings (over age 18), or close friends who stay with the hospitalized child when the parents cannot be present. Older children and teenagers may not want a parent in the room at night, but they may need an advocate there during the day just as much as the preschoolers.

> *Our hospital did not allow parents into the MRI suite. We worked with the head of that department, and now it is permitted for all families. This avoided the use of general anesthesia, so it was good for everyone involved. You don't need to take "no" for an answer.*

Some families find staying at the hospital day and night to be too stressful. An oncologist made the following suggestion:

> *When people are subject to stress, some people cope by focusing on all the details. For these people, being there all the time reduces their stress level. In other words, they would be more stressed if they were at home or work because they would be worrying all the time. Other people cope with stress by blocking out the details and trying to make life normal. I think that you need to think about how your family can best cope with this process and make your decisions based on that. Have a family meeting to sort out these issues, and don't feel bad if you decide what is best for your family is different from what other people say you should do.*

Whenever a family member is not present, children who are old enough should have a smartphone or be taught to use the telephone in the room. Tape a phone number nearby where a parent can be reached and have the child call if anyone tries to do procedures that are unexpected. The hospital staff should be informed that any changes in treatment (except emergencies) need to be authorized by a parent.

Everyone makes mistakes and hospital workers are no exception. Parents can help out by checking before any medications or blood transfusions are given. For instance, check that the name of the drug and the dose match what the protocol says should be given; if you weren't given a copy of the protocol (sometimes called the "roadmap"), you can ask the hospital staff for a copy. You should feel free to ask questions or point out any deviations from prescribed treatment. Parents are the last line of defense against mistakes.

> *Know every drug your child takes. Write down the name of the drug and the dosage. Watch that the name on the drug matches what YOU are expecting your child to get, and ask if it isn't something you recognize. Watch that the name on the unit of blood is your child's name. Watch everything.*

Playing

Children need to play, especially when hospitalized. The hospital might have a recreation therapy or child life department that has toys, books, dolls, and crafts, and is staffed by specialists who really know how to play with children. These staff members also provide many therapeutic activities, such as medical play with dolls, which helps children express fears or concerns about what is happening to them. By encouraging contact with other children in similar circumstances, recreation therapy helps children feel less alone and less different from other children.

The fun-filled activities and smiling staff people in the recreation therapy rooms are a cheerful change from lying in a hospital bed. If your child is too ill or if her counts are too low to go to the play area, arrangements can be made for a recreational therapist to bring a bundle of toys, games, and books to the room. Music therapists may also come to the bedside. This can give the parent time to go out to eat or take a walk.

> *When I wanted to have a conference with the oncologist about Katy's protocol, I called recreation therapy and they sent two wonderful ladies to the clinic. The doctor and I were able to talk privately for an hour, and Katy had a great time making herself a gold crown and decorating her wheelchair with streamers and jewels.*

Exercise is important, too. For kids strong enough to walk, exploring the hospital can be fun. Even if they can't walk, you can wheel them around or pull them in a wagon if they feel up to it. (This is also a great workout for you.) Plan a daily excursion to the gift shop or the cafeteria. Go outside and walk the entire perimeter of the hospital if weather and the neighborhood permit. Don't feel limited by an IV pole; it can be pushed or pulled and will feel normal after a while. Many children stand on the base of the IV pole with a parent pushing them down the hall at a good clip. Physical and occupational therapists can help your child incorporate exercise into the daily routine.

Tori was in the hospital recently for fever and positive blood cultures. She has a great time in the hospital. I had been trying to get her out on a pass as she was to have Grandparent's Day at school. We only would have been gone for a couple hours but no go. We came up with a plan to videotape the school part and have her do it with the tape for her grandparents at the hospital. In addition, child life got another videotape and we made a video for the school about the hospital at the same time. She was able to go all over the hospital (the play room, PT and OT gym, McDonalds®). It was great and I think I am going to treasure the copy.

Tori and I also went reverse trick or treating. She had wanted to do it Halloween week but we were not in clinic. We were inpatient, but I had promised, so we did it anyway. I brought in her witch costume and she ran around the hospital giving out candy to her therapists, nurses, and doctors. It was fabulous. She looked so cute. People in the halls did think it was a little weird but everyone from oncology under-stood that you do what makes you happy. Just call November 16th Halloween and everyone just pretends it is.

Any action that parents, family members, and friends take to support and advocate for the child with cancer buoys the spirit. Courage is contagious.

It becomes second nature. Step, shuffle, shuffle. Step, shuffle, shuffle. Sometime between two and five o'clock in the morning—somewhere between the nurse's station and the bathrooms—your gait, pulse, and breath synchronize into a rhythm of surprising calm. Step, shuffle, shuffle.

The Walk. That's what we call it. It's a milestone of sorts. A sign of acceptance and perseverance. A notice to the rest of the Club that you have put in sufficient hours of hospital vigil to find solace in simple movement. Hurried paces, strident races to the pay phones are far behind you. Tearful staggers and despairing stumbles are also long gone. Long stretches of hospital hallway lay before you, endless miles to be traversed while waiting and watching. Step, shuffle, shuffle: the comforting drag of the bottom of your feet against industrial linoleum.

I round the corner and modify my slide to catch up with the woman in front of me. "Hey, Susan."

"Hey, Gigi." Her Walk is smooth and practiced. I suspect it follows her home. We move down the corridor together, clutching empty water pitchers, cutting a path through beeps, moans, and rustles that issue from the doors on each side. Each of us is only partly in the space our body inhabits—our essential selves are back in our assigned rooms watching over little boys in huddled sleep.

I am in the Club. I am allowed direct questions. "How's Matthew doing?"

"Shunt infection, I.V. antibiotics, you know."

I nod. My son has a shunt, too. It drains excess fluid from the brain.

"Heparin for the clot in his leg," she continues. "Feeding tube still in. And they want to increase the steroids." Too many complications for such a little guy. My heart gets tight and I am fervently glad not to be Susan. An instant later, I am ashamed of my thoughts and blurt out some hopeful babble. "But he's sleeping okay?"

Susan raises her eyes to mine. The Look is there, much more developed than mine—she's had 4 months longer to perfect it. It is calm (with a dead-hold over hysteria), it is knowledgeable (endless hours of research masterfully synthesized and assimilated), it is forgiving (of COURSE you don't want to be me). Look to Look, my shame fades away. She smiles and squeezes my arm. "Yeah. He's sleeping okay."

We stop briefly in front of the water dispenser and then head back the way we came. The tan plastic pitchers sweat coldness over our hands, but we don't hurry. That's one thing about the Walk. It buys you time—alone time, out-of-the-room time. A chance to look at something other than the disease that is breaking your heart.

"And Ben?" she asks as we reach my corridor.

"Pretty good. This chemo cycle doesn't seem as rough on him."

"Great!" She means it. Good news for anyone in the Club is good news for all of us. Small victories add up.

I veer off to the left. "See ya."

"See ya," she calls back. Step, shuffle, shuffle. Step, shuffle, shuffle. Our feet take us quietly back to battle.

Chapter 9

Venous Catheters

Do what you can, with what you have,
where you are.

— Theodore Roosevelt

MANY CHILDREN WITH BRAIN OR SPINAL CORD TUMORS require intensive treatment, including surgery, chemotherapy, intravenous (IV) fluids, IV antibiotics, blood and platelet transfusions, frequent blood sampling, and sometimes IV nutrition. Venous catheters provide a very effective method for allowing entry into the large veins for intensive therapy. Venous catheters eliminate the difficulty of finding veins for IVs and allow drugs to be put directly into the heart, where they are rapidly diluted and spread throughout the body. They also reduce stress and discomfort for the child by eliminating the need for hundreds of needle sticks.

The three types of venous catheters are: external catheters, subcutaneous ports, and peripherally inserted central catheters (PICC). Other names for a venous catheter include: venous access device, right atrial catheter, implanted catheter, indwelling catheter, central line, Hickman®, Broviac®, PORT-A-CATH®, Medi-port®, and PICC line.

External catheter

The external catheter is a long, flexible tube with one end in the right atrium of the heart and the other end outside the skin of the chest. The tube tunnels under the skin of the chest, enters a large vein near the collarbone, and threads inside the vein to the heart (see Figure 9-1). Because chemotherapy drugs, transfusions, and IV fluids are put in the end of the tube hanging outside the body, the child feels no pain. Blood for complete blood counts (CBC) or chemistry tests can also be drawn from the end of the catheter. With daily care, the external catheter can be left in place for years.

The tube that channels the fluid is called a lumen. Some external catheters have double lumens in case two drugs need to be given at the same time. External catheters are usually put in under general anesthesia. Once the child is anesthetized, the surgeon makes two small incisions. One incision is near the collarbone over the spot where the catheter will enter the vein, the other is the area on the chest where the catheter exits the body.

To prevent the catheter from slipping out, it is stitched to the skin where it comes out of the chest (see Figure 9-1). There is a plastic cuff around the catheter right above the exit site (under the skin) into which body tissue grows. This further anchors the catheter and helps prevent infection. After healing is complete, normal activities can resume.

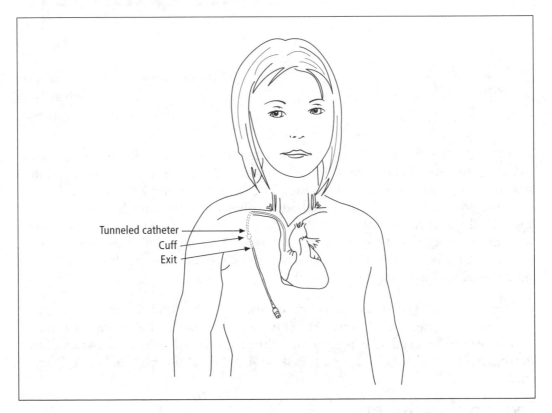

Figure 9-1: External catheter

Daily care

The external catheter requires careful maintenance to prevent infection or the formation of blood or drug clots. It is necessary to frequently clean and bandage the site where the catheter exits the body (schedules range from daily to weekly). Procedures and schedules for daily cleaning and bandaging vary from one institution to another. Some pediatric oncology centers also place a small antibiotic-impregnated disk around the catheter at the exit site. The site should be checked daily for redness, swelling, or drainage.

To prevent clots, parents or older children are taught to flush the line with a medication called heparin that prevents blood from clotting. Each institution uses its own flushing schedule, and nurses at the hospital teach parents and children how to care for the catheter. Both parent and child should be given lots of time to practice with supervision and should not be discharged until they are comfortable with the entire procedure. At discharge, parents can arrange for home nursing visits to provide further help.

> We were very grateful for Matthew's Hickman® line. Like a lot of children, he was terribly afraid of needles. The maintenance that was necessary to keep his line working properly became second nature to me. After his diagnosis, and again after his relapse, he had a Hickman® implanted. In total, he had his external catheter for more than 4 years.

Risks

The major complications of using external catheter are infections—either in the blood or at the insertion site—and the formation of clots in the line or the vein where the catheter is placed. Rare complications include kinking of the catheter, the catheter moving out of place, or breakage of the external part of the catheter.

Infections

Even with the best care, infections are common in children with external lines. Children who have low blood counts for long periods of time are at risk for developing infections anyway, and each time the line is flushed or cleaned, there is a chance of contamination. Usually, it is a bacterium called staphylococcus epidermidis—which lives on the skin—that is the culprit, although a host of other organisms can cause infections in children receiving chemotherapy.

If your child develops a fever over 101° F (38.5° C), redness or swelling at the insertion site, or pain in the catheter area, you should suspect an infection. This is a life-threatening situation, so call the doctor immediately. To determine whether bacteria are present, blood will be drawn from the catheter to culture (i.e., grow in a laboratory for 24–48 hours). Treatment will start whenever an infection is suspected and will end if the culture comes back negative. If the culture is positive, treatment usually continues for 10–14 days. Some physicians require that the child be hospitalized for antibiotic treatment, while others allow the child to receive treatment at home. Treatment with antibiotics is usually effective. However, if the infection does not respond to treatment, the catheter will need to be removed.

> When my daughter had a line infection, I wanted to use the antibiotic pump at home. It was hard, though. It took 2 hours per dose, three doses per day, for 14 days. I would get up at 5 a.m. to hook her up, so that she would sleep through the first dose.

The second dose I would give while she watched a TV show in the early afternoon. Then I would hook her up at bedtime so she would sleep through it. I had to wait up to flush and disconnect, so I was very tired by the end of the 2 weeks.

• • • • •

We used the IV infusion ball when Joseph needed a 3-hour vancomycin infusion because he didn't have to sit chained to a pump. The IV infusion ball is cool because if you have a sweatshirt with front pockets, you can make a tiny hole in the back of the sweatshirt to put the tubing through and stash the ball in the pocket so you can go about your business while your IV is infusing and no one has to know a thing! It's handy for pain meds, too. He even used it at school, as long as I was there with him. An awesome invention—brilliantly simple. Here's the website that describes it: www. iflo.com/prod_homepump.php.

Clots

Even with excellent daily care, some external catheters develop blockages or clots. If the catheter becomes blocked with a blood clot, it will be flushed with a drug to dissolve the clot, such as activase, urokinase, and streptokinase. These agents are given in the clinic or hospital, and the child usually needs to remain nearby for 1–2 hours. On rare occasions, the catheter becomes blocked by solidified medications, which can occur if two incompatible drugs are administered simultaneously. In those cases, a diluted hydrochloric acid solution may be used to dissolve the blockage.

Two months before the end of Kristin's treatment, her line plugged up. We tried several maneuvers at home unsuccessfully. We had to bring her in for the IV team to work on it. I think the bumpy ride to the hospital loosened it because at the hospital they were able to dislodge the clot just by flushing it with saline.

Kinks

Rarely, a kink develops in the catheter due to a sharp angle where the catheter enters the neck vein. In such cases, the fluids may go in the catheter but it is hard to get blood out. Parents and nurses are often able to work around this problem by experimenting with different positions for the child when the blood is drawn. The nurse may ask your child to bear down as if having a bowel movement, take a deep breath, cough, stretch, or laugh.

My son is 16, and was diagnosed January 2001 with PNET. His Hickman® was giving the nurses problems, so they planned to do a dye study. They didn't even have to inject the dye, the x-ray showed the line had come out and was clear across the opposite side of his chest and kinked! I don't think it had been out long. But it was a little scary to think of that chemo maybe going everywhere. They did a procedure where they go in with a special catheter line and grab the IV and pull it back into place. It was still attached to the vein, so the chemo hadn't been going amok. We are all so happy they got it fixed without surgery.

Catheter breakage

Breaks in the line do happen, but they are extremely rare. If a break or rupture of the line inside the body occurs when the line is not in use, only heparin will leak into surrounding tissues (not a major problem). If the break occurs when corrosive chemotherapy drugs are flowing through the catheter, they may leak and cause damage to surrounding tissue. The risk of an internal line leaking is far lower than the chance of leakage from an IV in a vein of the hand or arm.

The external portion of the catheter can also break. If this occurs, clamp the line between the point of breakage and the chest wall, cover the break in the line with a sterile gauze pad, and notify the doctor immediately. In most cases, the line can be repaired. Many institutions send a catheter repair kit home with parents.

I think it is important for parents to obtain clamps from the treating institution to carry with them. The preschool or school the child attends should also have one, in case something happens to the external line above the clamps that exist on the catheter. Younger children should wear a snug tank top that helps hold the catheter in place. Pinning it to the shirt is not the best solution for an active or younger child.

Other factors to consider

The proper care and maintenance of an external catheter requires motivation and organization. The site needs to be cleaned and dressed frequently, and heparin must be injected using sterile techniques. If your child's skin is quite sensitive, or if she cries when tape or Band-Aids® are removed from her skin, the external line may not be the best choice because the dressing must be taped to the skin.

One of my most difficult times was learning to change the dressing for Ben's catheter. I am totally freaked out by syringes, and anything like that, and here we were given a 10-minute demonstration in the hospital and an instruction book and that was it. I was petrified of doing something wrong to hurt my son. My husband tried, but he does not have very good balance, and he could not get the sterile gloves on without contaminating them. I went into panic mode the first week home from the hospital. I felt like the most inadequate mother in the whole world. Since neither of us could do what had to be done, my husband called a home health agency and they sent a nurse.

Kathy was the most wonderful person on earth. She told me that even though she had been a nurse for 20 years, she didn't think she could change the dressing on her own child, and she perfectly understood my fears. She had me watch her over and over again until I was comfortable enough to do it with her watching, and then finally on my own. She also talked to our insurance company numerous times to explain why she had to change the dressing instead of the family, and they ended up paying for her services! It was totally amazing. In addition, she helped my mental mood immensely, always telling me how good Ben was doing and sharing stories with me. I could tell her anything and she always understood. After I no longer needed her, she still stopped by about once a month to see how Ben was doing. She was my guardian angel.

The external line is a constant reminder of cancer treatment and can cause changes in body image. Both parent and child need to be comfortable with the idea of seeing and handling a tube that emerges from the chest. It is noticeable under lightweight clothing and bathing suits, but not under heavier clothing such as sweaters or coats. If a younger sibling might pull or yank on the catheter, the Hickman® or Broviac® might not be the appropriate choice.

On the other hand, the reason external lines are chosen so frequently is that there are no needles and no pain. This is a very important consideration for any children or teens who are scared of needles and/or pain. Some treatment protocols require double lumen access and the external catheter is the only option. For instance, children who need a stem cell transplant use double-lumen external venous catheters. But in most cases, families have a choice of which type of catheter to use.

Ben was diagnosed at age 5 with medulloblastoma, had a full resection, radiation to whole brain and spine, and one year of chemo. He had a double-lumen Broviac-Hickman®, a long tube with two ends that came out of his chest just above his right nipple. When not in use, it was curled and taped against his skin. I hated this thing. It made him Borg-like. I had to clean it every day for more than a year, and flush both ends of the tube. This hated thing, however, was what kept Ben from having to be stuck with needles several times a week. It was direct access to his blood supply, for tests, medication administration, and chemotherapy. One day Ben told me he had "made friends with his tubies." They had names, "The red one was Ralph, and the white one was Henry." He liked his tubies, he said, because they kept him from getting "ouchies." I was speechless. His matter-of-fact example showed me that the sooner I made friends with Ralph and Henry, the better off I'd be.

Children with external catheters have restrictions about contact sports, swimming, use of hot tubs, and sometimes bathing and showering, although care protocols vary by institution.

Subcutaneous port

Several types of subcutaneous (under the skin) ports are available. The subcutaneous port differs from the external catheter in that it is completely under the skin. A small metal chamber (1.5 inches in diameter) with a rubber top is implanted under the skin of the chest. A catheter threads from the metal chamber (portal) under the skin to a large vein near the collarbone, then inside the vein to the right atrium of the heart (see Figure 9-2). Whenever the catheter is needed for a blood draw or infusion of drugs or fluid, a needle is inserted by a nurse through the skin and into the rubber top of the portal. Usually a topical numbing agent such as EMLA® is used to make the needle insertion less painful.

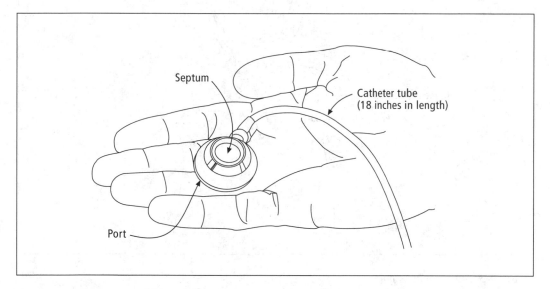

Figure 9-2: Parts of the subcutaneous port

How it's put in

The subcutaneous port is implanted under general anesthesia in the operating room during a procedure that generally takes less than an hour. The surgeon makes two small incisions: one in the chest where the portal will be placed, and the other near the collarbone where the catheter will enter a vein in the lower part of the neck. First, one end of the catheter is placed in the large blood vessel of the neck and threaded into the right atrium of the heart. The other end of the catheter is tunneled under the skin where it is attached to the portal. Fluid is injected into the portal to ensure that the device works properly. The portal is then placed under the skin in the right side of the chest and stitched to the underlying muscle. Both incisions are then stitched closed. The only evidence that a catheter has been implanted are two small scars and a bump under the skin where the portal rests.

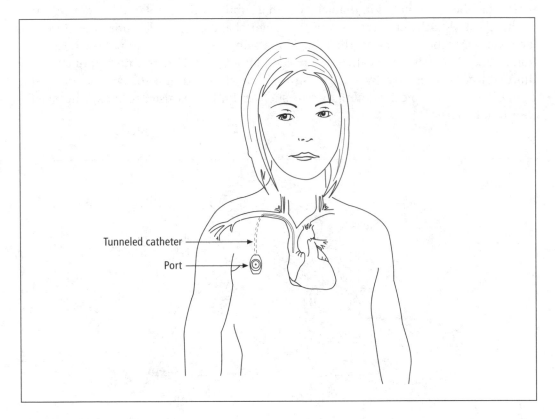

Figure 9-3: Subcutaneous port

Before my child's surgery to have a port implanted, I saw other children being wheeled into the operating room screaming and trying to climb off the gurney to return to the parents. It broke my heart. When it was Jennifer's turn, I asked them to give her enough premedication so that she was relaxed and happy to go. I also insisted that I be in the recovery room when she awoke.

• • • • •

Christine had her port surgery late at night. The resident gave her some premedication, then the chief resident ordered him to give her more. She felt so silly that she looked at me, giggled, and said "Mommy has a nose as long as an elephant's." I asked the surgeon if I could be in the recovery room before she awoke, and he said,

"Sure." When I told the nurse that I had permission to go in recovery, she refused. When I persisted, she became angry. I told her that my child was expecting to wake up seeing my face, and I wanted to be there. I suggested that she go in and ask the surgeon to resolve the impasse. When she came out, she let me in the recovery room.

How it works

Because the entire subcutaneous port is under the skin, a needle is used to access it. The skin is thoroughly cleansed with antiseptic, then a special needle is inserted through the skin and the rubber top of the portal. The needle is attached to a short length of tubing that hangs down the front of the chest. A topical anesthetic cream (see Chapter 6, *Coping with Procedures*) can be applied 1 hour before the needle poke to anesthetize the skin, or ethyl chloride ("freezy spray") can be sprayed on right before the poke. Subcutaneous ports have a rubber top (septum) that reseals after the needle is removed. It is designed to withstand years of needle insertions, as long as a special "non-coring" needle is used each time. Fluid will leak into the tissues if the wrong needle is used.

If the child is in a part of treatment that requires using the line every day, the nurse will attach the tubing to IV fluids or will close the end off with a sterile cap after flushing the line with saline solution. A transparent dressing will be put over the site where the needle enters the port. The port can remain accessed in this way for up to 7 days. After that time, to avoid the risk of infection, the needle should be removed and the port reaccessed when necessary. If the needle and tubing are to be left in place, it is important to tape them securely to the chest to avoid accidents.

Molly (3 years old) hated tape removal, so we did not secure the IV tubing to her stomach or chest. On one of her many trips to the potty, we accidentally tugged on the tubing and caused a very small tear in the skin around the needle. It became infected. We did home antibiotics on the pump and felt very fortunate that we were able to clear the line with antibiotics. We were glad our doctor was not too quick to remove the line, but it did require 2 weeks off chemotherapy.

If the port is only needed infrequently, the sequence of events is: clean the site, put in the needle, rinse the line with saline, give the drug or draw blood, rinse the line with saline, add heparin to the line, withdraw the needle, and place an adhesive bandage over the site.

Care of the port

The entire port and catheter are under the skin and therefore require no daily care. The skin over the port can be washed just like the rest of the body. Frequent visual inspections are needed to check for swelling, redness, or drainage. Signs of infection include redness, swelling, pain, drainage, or warmth around the port. Fever, chills, tiredness, and dizziness may also indicate that the line has become infected. You should notify the doctor immediately if any of these signs are present or if your child has a fever above 101° F (38.5° C).

The subcutaneous port must be accessed and flushed with saline and heparin at least once every 30 days, which might coincide with clinic visits or blood checks. This procedure is done by a nurse or technician. The port system requires no maintenance by a parent.

> My 3-year-old was being treated for a low-grade astrocytoma, and had a port inserted for a period of about a year and a half. His port survived all kinds of normal kid wear and tear. I remember that kids with external lines were discouraged from swimming, but with a subcutaneous port, there weren't any restrictions in activity or special precautions, which meant one less thing for us to worry about.

Risks

The risks for a subcutaneous port are similar to those for the external catheter: infection, clots, and, rarely, kinks or rupture. If the needle is not properly inserted through the rubber septum, or if the wrong kind of needle is used, fluids can leak into the tissue around the portal.

> My son (8 years old) has had a PORT-A-CATH® for 33 months with absolutely no problems. He uses EMLA® to anesthetize it prior to accessing. He hates finger pokes so much that he has his port accessed every time he needs blood drawn.

· · · · ·

> We had a few unusual problems in the beginning with the catheter. It was a bit kinked where the catheter went under the clavicle (collarbone) and would not easily draw. This caused more stress than anything in the hospital, because their middle-of-the-night blood draws were always an ordeal for our daughter. They needed to wake her up and try multiple manipulations. Once we were familiar with its idiosyncrasies and were outpatient, we worked it out much better. Then about halfway through treatment, her catheter broke at the kink and travelled into her heart. To make a long story short, it was retrieved by a cardiologist without major surgery, and she got a new one placed, this time with the catheter going down from her neck. It works like a dream.

Infections

Most studies show that the infection rate for subcutaneous ports is lower than that of external catheters. If the subcutaneous port does become infected, it is treated the same as an infected external catheter is treated.

> Katy had two infections in her PORT-A-CATH® during treatment. One occurred when the tape loosened during a blood transfusion. She developed a fever the next day and required 14 days of vancomycin. Eighteen months later, we went in for her monthly chemo, and she became ill in the car on the way home. Her skin became white and clammy, and she felt faint and nauseated. She spiked a 102° temperature, which only lasted for 2 hours. The blood culture both times grew staphylococcus epi.

Kinks, clots, ruptures

These events rarely occur with the subcutaneous port. If they do occur, they are treated as described in the external catheter section.

> My son had a very bad blood clot in his PORT-A-CATH.® In fact, he had two. He was put on Lovenox® (low molecular weight heparin) for 3 months (twice a day). We went for an ultrasound last week and it showed that the clots are mostly gone now.

· · · · ·

> When we got to clinic for weekly chemo, no matter what gravity-defying positions we tried (raising arms, lying down, standing up), our nurse couldn't get the line to flush. Adrienne's port was clogged. Luckily, they were able to clear the line with an injection of streptokinase, although it meant entertaining her in clinic for more than an hour while we waited for it to work. They did tell us that if this didn't work we'd have to go in overnight for slow infusion of chemo, but the line cleared, and we did chemo outpatient.

Peripherally inserted central catheter

A peripherally inserted central catheter is also referred to as a PICC line. This type of catheter is placed in the antecubital vein (a large vein in the inner elbow area) and is threaded into a large vein above the right atrium of the heart (see Figure 9-4). Unlike other catheters, a PICC line can be inserted by an IV nurse, rather than by a surgeon.

The PICC line can remain in place for many weeks or months, avoiding the need for a new IV every few days. PICC lines can be used to deliver chemotherapy, antibiotics, blood products, other medications, and IV nutrition. When the PICC line needs to be accessed, an IV line is connected to the end of the catheter. When it is not in use, the IV is disconnected and the catheter is flushed and capped.

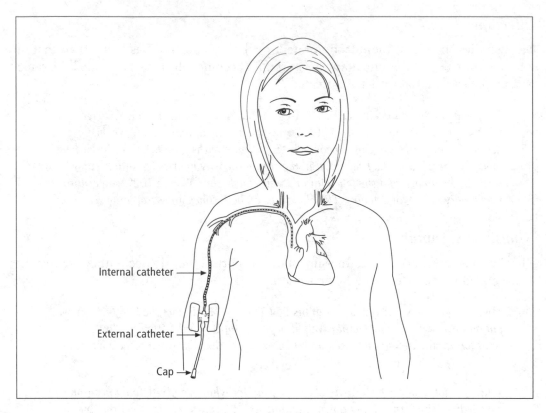

Figure 9-4: Peripherally inserted central catheter (PICC) line

How it's put in

The PICC line can be inserted in your child's hospital room by a nurse or doctor. Your child will be positioned on a flat surface, and he will need to keep his arm straight and motionless during the procedure. An injection to numb the area is given to decrease discomfort during insertion. A special needle is used to place the PICC line into the arm vein. The catheter is then threaded through the needle. Once the line is in place, a chest x-ray is taken to ensure that it is positioned properly. Some children may require light sedation during the procedure.

Care of the peripherally inserted central catheter

The PICC line, like the external catheter, requires care to prevent problems. The nurses will teach you how to change the dressing, flush the line, change the injection cap, and inspect the site for possible signs of infection. The dressing covering the exit site is changed once a week, or if it becomes wet or is exposed to air. The line must be flushed after every use, or every day. You should get plenty of practice under the supervision of a nurse until both you and your child are comfortable with caring for the line. The care required for your child's PICC line may be slightly different from what has been described in this section, because institutional preferences vary.

> Kelsey had a PICC line in her right arm, and she would not straighten it out, but kept it a little bent. I definitely think she was protecting it, and also I think when she tried to straighten it, it pulled on the suture and on the dressing in an uncomfortable way that could have been painful, so she just wouldn't try. I had to do a heparin flush every day and change the dressing twice a week. She could not tolerate Tegaderm®, so we used another kind of porous adhesive bandage, and doused it with Detachol®, which dissolved the adhesive within a few minutes, allowing us to get the bandage off quite easily. The Detachol® was a godsend for her, as removing the adhesive was like pulling teeth and a source of unnecessary pain. [For more information about Detachol®, see the section "Adhesives" later in this chapter.]

Risks

The problems associated with a PICC line are similar to those of any external catheter. Veins may become irritated, infection can occur, or the line can be accidentally torn or moved.

Irritated veins

Within the first few days of insertion, the vein where the catheter is located may become irritated. Signs of irritation include swelling or pain in the area. Often, the discomfort can be alleviated by placing a warm, moist cloth or a carefully monitored heating pad on the vein. Elevating the arm on a pillow is also sometimes helpful.

Infections

Meticulous care using sterile techniques is extremely important to reduce the risk of infection. The dressing over the exit site should be changed every week, or if it becomes wet or exposed to air. Injection caps must also be regularly changed using sterile techniques when the line is not in use, and the line must be flushed on a regular basis. Signs of infection include redness, swelling, pain, drainage, or warmth around the exit site. Fever, chills, tiredness, and dizziness may also indicate that the line has become infected. You should notify the doctor immediately if any of these signs are present or if your child has a fever above 101° F (38.5° C).

Torn catheter

Accidents sometimes happen, and a hole or tear in the line can occur. Careful handling of the catheter can help prevent these accidents. You should suspect a torn catheter if fluid leaks out of the line, especially during an injection. If a tear is found, you should find the hole, fold the line above the tear, tape it together, cover it with sterile gauze, and immediately notify your child's doctor.

Displaced catheter

As with other external catheters, a PICC line must be securely taped to the exit site to prevent movement. Signs of a displaced catheter include chest pain, burning or swelling in the arm above the exit site or in the chest, fluid leaking around the catheter, or pain when fluid is injected into the line. If you suspect that the line has moved, you should tape the catheter in place and immediately notify your child's doctor.

Cost

The external catheters and PICC line require supplies for cleaning, dressing, and irrigating the line, but the subcutaneous port does not. The port itself, however, is usually more costly than the external catheter and PICC line. The external catheter and the subcutaneous port require operating room time and the services of a surgeon and an anesthesiologist to insert, but PICC lines are usually inserted in the hospital room by a doctor or nurse. External catheters can be removed in the clinic with only IV sedation, but subcutaneous ports can only be removed in the operating room. A good rule of thumb to consider is that if the lines stay in place at least 6 months, the overall costs are almost equal.

Most insurance plans will cover the placement of any central venous catheter and the services of the surgeon, anesthesiologist, and operating room facility. Many plans, however, will not cover the cost of the supplies to maintain the line, and this can be an additional financial hardship for families.

Choosing not to use a catheter

Many doctors automatically schedule surgery for catheter implantation as soon as a child is diagnosed with a brain or spinal cord tumor. A few, however, do not recommend using implanted catheters in their pediatric patients. If your child's doctor recommends not using one, ask the reason why and and discuss it thoroughly if you are uncomfortable with the options presented.

Stephan (6 years old) has no catheter. Sometimes I wish he had one. It seems like it would be easier. We were told he didn't need it. He is running out of usable veins and it is getting harder and harder.

Some children and teens prefer IVs to an implanted catheter.

My son had a port for a very short time, and due to frequent fevers (with no evidence of infection) and because he had a blood clot form in his heart, they pulled the port. He had IVs for the remainder of treatment and was much happier with the IVs than with what he called "that foreign object in my chest."

To help you make the best decision for your particular situation, the table below outlines the pros and cons for each type of catheter. There is no right or wrong choice; different options are available because each child, each parent, and each family is unique.

Things to Consider	External Catheter	Subcutaneous Port	Peripherally Inserted Central Catheter
Infection rate	Higher	Lower	Higher
Maintenance	Daily	Monthly	Daily
Body image	Changes: tube outside body	Changes: small lump under skin	Changes: tube outside body
Pain	Dressing changes	Needle poke to access (use EMLA®); dressing changes when accessed	Needle poke to insert the line; dressing changes
Anxiety	Low to high	Low to high	Low to high
Cost	• Insertion cost: moderate • Maintenance cost: high	• Insertion cost: highest • Maintenance cost: low	• Insertion cost: lowest • Maintenance cost: high
Risk of drugs leaking into tissues	Lowest	Low	Low

Making a decision

After obtaining information about your options, talk with the doctor about the merits of each type of catheter and ask for her opinion. Talk about the pros and cons with your child if she is old enough. Then make the rounds of the oncology unit, asking both parents and children which type of catheter they chose and why. You will probably hear many opinions about the benefits and drawbacks of each catheter.

The nurses in the clinic and on the unit are another source of valuable information. They will have seen dozens (or hundreds) of children with catheters, and they can give excellent advice, given your family situation. There is no right or wrong choice, just different options for each unique child.

> When we asked one of the young children on the ward which catheter she had, she pulled up her shirt with a big grin to show us her Hickman®. She had a coil of white tubing neatly taped to her chest. My husband's face turned as white as her tubing.

· · · · ·

> My 4-year-old daughter loved ballet and was extremely interested in her appearance. Her younger sister was very physical, and we were worried that if we chose the Hickman® she would grab and pull on the tubing. We chose the PORT-A-CATH® so that she could wear her tutus without reminders of cancer, and so the children could play together without mishap.

· · · · ·

> We chose the Hickman® for Shawn because we didn't want any needles coming at him. He spent almost the whole first year in the hospital, so it saved him from so many pokes. The line was a blessing. He went 3 years and 3 months with no infections. We thought it was just a beautiful thing.

Adhesives

Whether your child has a subcutaneous port, external catheter, or PICC line, dressing changes will be necessary. Some children don't mind having the Tegaderm® or tape pulled off. For others, it is traumatic every time. Parents have many suggestions for ways to make it easier for kids. These suggestions also work for removing tape used to hold plastic wrap over EMLA®:

• Don't use Tegaderm® if it bothers your child or reddens the skin. Try plastic wrap cut into a square and use paper tape or tape with perforations.

- Try Hypafix®, a dressing retention material that looks like gauze with a sticky side. Usually, several sterile 2x2 gauze pads are put over the needle entry site, then Hypafix® is applied to hold them in place.

  I like Hypafix® because when it's time to take it off, you can use the adhesive dissolver where it's stuck to the skin, and even without the dissolver, it comes off more easily and gently than the Tegaderm®. The nurses at our oncology clinic use this all the time. Our local clinic and hospital do not use Hypafix®, so I bought a roll and take it with me whenever we have to go locally for a port access so we don't have to use the Tegaderm®.

- When it's tape removal time, use an effective adhesive remover such as Detachol® (an orange-colored product made by Eloquest Healthcare®—*www.eloquesthealthcare.com/products-3/removal-of-tapes*). If you douse the paper tape with adhesive dissolver and wait a couple of minutes, it will usually pull right off with no pain.

- Ask for expert advice.

  Apryl has had skin tears and reactions from the adhesives as a result of using Tegaderm®. We were using Primapore® dressings for a while, but after a year she started having the same reaction. When she had her line replaced, I asked for a consultation with the skincare nurse. She recommended All-Dress®. It is a waterproof dressing with non-stick gauze in the center surrounded by Hypafix® tape. Apryl changes hers once every 3 days, whether it gets wet or not. She also has this pink tape that has zinc oxide in the adhesive to protect the skin. These two have worked out great.

- Once you have found a routine that works well, negotiate with nursing staff to remove the tape yourself or to have them follow your system.

  Using adhesive dissolver (or peeling off tape or Tegaderm® millimeter by millimeter) takes a bit of time—it's not just a swipe—and it works. It has to sort of soak in and takes some time to dissolve the sticky stuff. I know the nurses are really busy and under pressure to keep on time schedules, so it's probably a conflict for them. I deal with this by always being the one to get the Tegaderm® off. This took some "muscling in" with nurses who were used to doing it, but it works much, much better. I try to make a joke of it: "I have a deal with my kid that I'm taking off the Tegaderm®. It might take a while and I wouldn't want you to fall asleep waiting on us—how about if I holler out the door when it's off and we're ready?" That way they don't have to stand around and wait, and you don't feel like you need to hurry your child.

Catheters are usually removed as soon as treatment ends; this process is explained in Chapter 22, *End of Treatment and Beyond*.

When Scott (age 3) was diagnosed, his doctor gave us a choice of which central line we could use. He showed us a mannequin with a Broviac® and a PORT-A-CATH®. He also told us the pros and cons of each type, then asked us to decide. We chose the Broviac®, and feel it was the best decision for Scott. The day it was installed was the end of a lot of unnecessary pain (from needle sticks) for Scott.

Scott finished all his treatments 3 months ago, and yesterday he had his Broviac® removed. It went extremely smoothly. He had only one cuff and it was halfway out already. And to think I fretted and worried about the removal all week!

He has lots and lots of energy. His hair is coming back in and he actually has color in his face. He looks so healthy! I love it!

Chapter 10

Surgery

Ring the bells that still can ring
Forget your perfect offering
There is a crack in everything
That's how the light gets in
— Leonard Cohen

SURGERY HAS A CENTRAL ROLE in the treatment of brain and spinal cord tumors. At each new treatment stage, surgery is considered as an option. Surgery is used to take a sample of a tumor (called a biopsy), remove all or part of a tumor, place a shunt or endoscopic bypass to treat hydrocephalus, or insert a central venous catheter. Surgery is usually the first treatment considered after your child has been diagnosed with a brain or spinal cord tumor.

This chapter describes the importance of consulting a pediatric neurosurgeon to obtain an opinion about surgical options for your child's tumor. Next, it explains the advances in technology that have improved the surgical treatment of children with brain or spinal cord tumors. Information is provided on the evaluation before surgery and what happens in the operating room. Finally, caring for your child after surgery is discussed.

The neurosurgeon

Pediatric neurosurgery developed as a subspecialty in the 1980s. Generally, neurosurgeons who operate 50 percent of the time or more on children are considered pediatric neurosurgeons. Today most pediatric neurosurgeons complete 1 year of fellowship with an established pediatric neurosurgeon in a program approved by the American Board of Pediatric Neurological Surgery. There are approximately 225 board-certified pediatric neurosurgeons in the United States (see *www.abpns.org* for their names and locations). Surgeons who devote the majority of their practice to children usually provide the most aggressive surgical approach to try to cure the child.

> *A few hours earlier, we had come to the children's hospital to determine what was bothering Mia. I thought it would be a sprained muscle, a pinched nerve, maybe a herniated disk; never in a million years did I imagine she had a tumor and we'd be*

discussing brain surgery. A team of doctors came by and one doctor said it was a tumor and it was pretty big. He said that she needed surgery right away because the tumor was causing fluid in her brain to accumulate. My head was spinning. I needed to understand. Ask questions. What was the neurosurgeon's background? How long did it take? How many times had he done this? Did the children always live? Could he promise me she would live?

She was in surgery for hours, and my mom, my aunt, and I sat in the waiting room. Then I saw the green jumpsuit, a little green hat, white beard, and small eyes. We jumped up and the neurosurgeon said, "She's fine. We're done and she is sleeping. Come with me." We walked into a small room and before he could close the door, I asked him, "Is it malignant? He said he had good news and bad news. He told us the tumor was malignant and was called medulloblastoma. The good news was that he believed he had removed all of it.

If your child does not require emergency surgery, you have time to locate a board-certified pediatric neurosurgeon with significant experience operating on children with brain or spinal cord tumors. Results of the most recent research studies indicate that the amount of tumor removed by the surgeon directly affects a child's chances of survival and cure. Research has also confirmed that children operated on by pediatric neuro-surgeons have more tumor removed than those operated on by adult neurosurgeons. Therefore, it is best to have your child's surgery performed by a pediatric neurosurgeon with extensive experience operating on children with cancer. A senior pediatric neuro-surgeon suggests:

The most important advice I would offer to a family is logical but not necessarily widely accepted. Quite simply, be certain that your child is cared for by a surgeon who is experienced in caring for children. Children are not simply "little adults." There is no rationale in assuming that the surgeon who cares largely for adults is equally qualified to look after a newborn baby or young child. This has nothing to do with intelligence, but is simply a logical extension of the meaning of experience in any facet of life. A carpenter who builds bookshelves will probably do it better than a carpenter that has spent his life building houses. A pilot of a space shuttle is not trained to be an airline pilot.

Surgical treatment is only one aspect of overall care. Therefore, when a major surgical procedure is planned, it is essential that it be carried out in a children's hospital that uses a team approach. With a team approach, pediatricians, pediatric anesthesiologists, pediatric radiologists, pediatric nurses, child life specialists, and social workers are all part of an integrated group that is devoted to a single goal: the recovery of your child.

Types of surgery

Surgery is performed at different times during treatment. Varying amounts of tumor are removed—from a small biopsy to the whole tumor. This section describes several of the most common surgeries used to treat children with brain or spinal cord tumors.

Biopsy

An area that looks abnormal on an MRI scan is not always a tumor, so a biopsy is usually necessary before major surgery or other treatment begins. In some situations, a biopsy is not possible because of tumor location or it is not recommended because of the damage the procedure could cause. For example, biopsies are not often done for pontine gliomas.

A biopsy involves taking a tiny sample of tissue through a small incision. When the pathologist evaluates the tissue removed in a biopsy, she determines whether the lesion is a tumor and, if so, what type of tumor it is.

> Jordan was 3 years old when she was diagnosed with an inoperable pilocytic astro-cytoma. Since she was not using her right hand, our pediatrician told me to take her to a pediatric neurologist. But, because of insurance, our first visit was to a local neurologist. Now this doctor was used to seeing adults, so when he saw her MRI, he told us to give her a happy 6 months. He referred us on to the pediatric doctors at a children's hospital 3 hours away. They took a biopsy and told us there were treatments available.

You should have your child's biopsy done at a pediatric center that uses MRI and/or CT scans to guide the surgeon to the site of the tumor. The scans are used as a roadmap so the neurosurgeon can obtain the biopsy from the center of the tumor (called a stereotactic biopsy). If the biopsy doesn't obtain adequate tissue, a diagnosis is sometimes not possible. In other cases, the piece of tumor obtained by biopsy is not representative of the whole tumor. Some tumors have areas that are very aggressive ("high grade"); other areas appear "low grade."

If a stereotactic biopsy does not provide a diagnosis, an open biopsy may be considered. In this case, an operation is done to directly view the tumor and to obtain an adequate sample. MRI and CT guidance can also be used with this approach.

Special tools called endoscopes are used by neurosurgeons to biopsy tumors that are located in the fluid spaces called ventricles. These telescope-like tools contain a camera that allows the surgeon to see the tumor with one channel and to use a separate channel to biopsy the tumor.

Debulking

Surgical debulking is the partial removal (usually 40 to 90 percent) of the tumor. This type of procedure is done for tumors that are deep within the brain, next to large blood vessels, or growing from the brainstem. In these areas, the risk is too great to allow total removal. Instead, the goal of surgery is to relieve any symptoms caused by the tumor, especially increased intracranial pressure. A debulking procedure is often done prior to giving either radiation or chemotherapy, because these treatments are sometimes more effective on smaller tumors.

A debulking procedure may also slow or stop the growth of a slow-growing tumor for a period of time, thus delaying the need for other treatments.

> Anthony was just over 2 years old when he was diagnosed with an optic nerve glioma. Radiation was not recommended, because of the risks of serious long-term side effects. We agreed that the pediatric neurosurgeon should debulk as much of the tumor as possible. She removed most of the low-grade tumor that extended into the temporal lobe. Chemotherapy was not needed for several years.

Delaying treatment, if possible, has several advantages. For instance, studies have shown that children who have radiation to the brain at an older age have fewer long-term effects than children who have radiation before age 5. Slowing tumor growth for several years can also allow time for the discovery of newer and more effective methods of treatment.

> My brain tumor is located in the midbrain, and my neurosurgeon told us at diagnosis that it was inoperable. Since it was diagnosed though, I have had numerous surgeries to shrink it. So, even though they say it is inoperable, they can still go in and reduce its size. My neurosurgeon has always said that the medical field is an ongoing research area. What they couldn't do yesterday, they can do today.

Surgical resection

The goal of surgery for most brain and spinal cord tumors is to remove the entire tumor (called maximal safe surgical resection). It is important to understand what this term means. Unlike a tumor in the intestine, where the surgeon can cut a wide margin on either side of the tumor to ensure that no tumor cells are left behind, brain and spinal cord tumors can't be removed with large margins because there are vital structures throughout the brain and spinal cord. Surgeons usually remove a brain or spinal cord tumor by working from the inside of the tumor out, coring out the cavity. Some tumors are removed and require no more treatment.

> In 2008, I suffered a mild seizure. A CT scan revealed a lesion, and a nervous, bow-tied neurologist added the word "suspicious" to the findings. Oops, time for a

second opinion. This led me to a renowned pediatric neurosurgeon who diagnosed a low-grade, benign juvenile pilocytic astrocytoma (JPA) tumor on the frontal left lobe of my brain. The thought of a tumor made my insides shake. While the slow-growing tumor was in a quiet part of the brain and did not pose an immediate threat, if not removed, it would eventually affect my speech and other neurological functions. My surgery was scheduled for the following week. Suddenly reality hit—I was 14, and instead of spring break and boys, I was thinking about mortality.

No matter how hard I tried to be cool, the day of my surgery was probably the most terrifying day of my life. As the anesthesiologist prepared the IV, I held on tightly to my mother's hand and drifted away with the prayers of my friends and family in my heart. A night in intensive care and one in the pediatric oncology unit followed the surgery. By the third day, I was ready to go home. Less than a week later, the surgical staples were removed and I returned to school and all activities.

It has been almost 3 years since my surgery. From a medical point of view, I am a healthy statistic that will be cited when another person is diagnosed with the same grade JPA. There is an empty cavity where the tumor was removed because brain matter does not regenerate. Reality has taught me to never take anyone or anything for granted. Today I am preparing for college, dealing with my parents' divorce, working, volunteering and dancing competitively. Although I accept my flaws more graciously now, embracing my strengths and weaknesses is still a work in progress. Mostly, I am grateful just to be me.

Recent studies have indicated that the best chance for long-term survival and cure occurs with total, or near total, removal of the tumor. This may not be possible if the tumor is deep within the brain or near a part of the brain responsible for a vital function (for example, near the area that controls breathing). A maximal surgical resection, however, is now possible in many areas within the brain and spinal cord due to new technology in operating equipment and monitoring. The majority of tumors in the frontal, parietal, temporal, and occipital lobes and the cerebellum can be totally, or almost totally, removed. Similarly, most spinal cord tumors can also have maximal surgical resections.

John Michael was 11 years old at the time of surgery. He has a brain tumor located in the thalamus. We were told that it was inoperable by our local neurosurgeon. Then we found a more experienced pediatric neurosurgeon. He did indeed have surgery to remove about 85 percent of his golf ball-size tumor, and he has no lasting deficits.

· · · · ·

Exactly 3 weeks after being diagnosed with a pilocytic astrocytoma almost the size of an orange in the cerebellum, Christopher went back to school! The tumor was benign and located in the most accessible place possible, so he arrived at school with a full head of hair, no residual effects from surgery, and a bigger smile than he left with 3 weeks before.

It is common for children to undergo more than one surgical procedure during the treatment process. Total, or near total, removal of the tumor is often achieved by operating in more than one stage and/or from different approaches. For example, if an MRI scan after surgery reveals a lump of tumor remaining and the surgeon feels he can remove it safely, a second surgery is performed. Similarly, a deep tumor may be approached surgically from above and then during a separate operation from the side. Tumors that are very slow growing are debulked and the remaining tumor monitored with MRI scans every 3 to 6 months. A second surgery is performed months or years later if the tumor grows.

> *About 2 weeks following surgery, I had to return to the hospital for a post-op check-up and MRI to check the residual tumor. The MRI showed that the pediatric neurosurgeon removed about 50 percent of the tumor, but he informed us that he could see himself going in from another direction to obtain more of the tumor. We left the office feeling a little peace of mind, because we now knew that the tumor was smaller.*

The results from a number of clinical trials support a second-look operation after a phase of treatment (chemotherapy or radiation) if tumor is still visible on the MRI scan. During a second-look surgery, a piece of the remaining tumor is obtained and sent to a pathologist to see if the treatments have injured or killed the tumor cells. Occasionally, on second look, an abnormality thought to be tumor on the MRI scan turns out to be scar tissue. The results of the second-look surgery provide information to the treating physician that helps him plan the next step of treatment. In some cases, children have special imaging studies done (e.g., positron emission tomography [PET] scan or MRI spectroscopy) rather than a second-look surgery to evaluate treatment effect.

> *Our 10-month-old daughter was diagnosed with medulloblastoma. Her first surgery took about 9 hours to remove the baseball-sized tumor. The pathology showed that it was malignant. She had chemotherapy that she tolerated very well. The first MRI after chemo showed a shadow where the tumor had been. So, they did a second-look surgery, which thankfully, only showed scarring. That surgery didn't take as long as the first since they had nothing to remove. After a week in the hospital, we went home. Kristin is now 13 years old, with no late effects from treatment. She is mentally and physically on par with her friends—whom she spends a lot of time talking with on the phone and computer!*

Intraoperative monitoring

Intraoperative monitoring involves watching the electrical nerve impulses as they travel from an area of the brain to another part of the body, such as the arms, legs, or face and eyes. Electrodes are placed on the scalp and on the extremities (similar to an electroencephalogram [EEG]) to monitor the brain's electrical impulses. By using this technology during an operation, the surgeon can determine the location of a tumor in relation to important body functions. This technology helps the surgeon remove the tumor while preserving as much function as possible. Intraoperative monitoring is most often used for tumors in the frontal and parietal lobes adjacent to the motor strip or the brainstem. Intraoperative monitoring is also vital for surgery in the spinal cord, because the monitoring allows the surgeon to remove the tumor while observing the nerve activity from the brain down the spinal cord and out to the arms and legs.

Another type of monitoring uses electrodes to locate seizure activity in the brain. This type of EEG involves placing a grid or strip of electrodes on the surface of the brain after a tumor has been removed. It monitors the tumor cavity and surrounding brain to determine whether seizure-generating tissue is still present. If the place where the seizure starts is not in a vital area, then that seizure-generating tissue is also removed to try to reduce or eliminate the seizures. If the tumor is near the speech center, this procedure is done while the child is awake. By having the child awake, the surgeon can converse with him during the tumor removal, ensuring that the speech center remains uninjured. The child has to be mature enough to cooperate, and this is usually not possible until at least early teen years.

> An attempt to awaken my son Michael during his first awake craniotomy for a mixed tumor of JPA [juvenile pilocytic astrocytoma] and PNET [primitive neuroecto-dermal tumor] failed. He was only 12, but more importantly, I think the person who was talking with him was cold and aloof, as was his surgeon. As he came out of the anesthetic, he tried to move his head while in the cage, was very confused, and they ended up just putting him back to sleep.

> The second surgery was a whole different story. Now he was 15, and we used a major neurosurgery center. Both the pediatric neurosurgeon and his assistant took the time to really talk to Michael, get to know him well, and goof around with him (making him feel comfortable with them). When they woke him up, they chatted to him about gymnastics (his first love), his best friend Alex, his desire to be third in his class (to escape having to make a speech at graduation), and so on. The awake surgery was a super success—the surgeon was able to go deeper, get all of the tumor, and yet know that Michael's speech would remain intact.

Computer-guided surgery

Until recently, neurosurgeons had only an MRI picture to refer to during surgery. Now it is possible to use the MRI along with a computer in the operating room to help the surgeon localize and remove the tumor. An MRI is performed prior to the surgery. The information from the MRI is transmitted to a computer in the operating room, which serves as a navigational system. The surgeon then uses a pointer aimed at various reference points on the child's head and the computer generates a three-dimensional picture of the brain and tumor location. This technology allows removal of the tumor through a much smaller incision.

> My son had a late effect from radiation called a cavernous angioma. It is an abnormal collection of blood vessels that is not a problem unless it gets big and/or it starts to bleed. Six years after my son's initial treatment, this was diagnosed on a follow-up MRI and 3 months later it had grown quite large and had some signs of having bled, so our local vascular neurosurgeon felt that surgery was necessary. Unfortunately, the location of the angioma was quite poor, deep in the frontal lobe on his dominant side, so very near the speech center. My son was 12 at the time, and I really wanted to find a pediatric vascular neurosurgeon, someone who would think that my son's brain looked quite large, rather than an adult neurosurgeon who might think it a bit on the small side from his experience.
>
> This is a rare thing in children, so I did some investigation. I asked my local neurosurgeon for a name for a second opinion. I also asked other parents in my brain tumor support group, and I did a literature search to see who had published an article on this complication. There was one name that came up more often than others, and I contacted him by email. He was very responsive and kind to me immediately. When we met with him, he told us what we wanted to hear, that he could perform this surgery without any danger of our son losing his ability to talk. He told us to be prepared for a week in the hospital, but my son was up talking immediately, and he was walking within 6 hours of surgery. He ate a breakfast burrito 8 hours after surgery and we were discharged less than 24 hours after surgery. He had just a small bandage, otherwise you would not know that he had undergone a major operation.

Preoperative MRI scans that use a technology called diffusion tractography generate a picture that shows the child's vital motor or visual pathways, which helps the surgeon plan her route to the tumor. MRI scans are also used with the guidance system to minimize the risk of injury during the surgery.

Surgeons are also working with MRI companies to develop MRI scanners for the operating room. An intraoperative MRI scanner allows the surgeon to obtain an MRI scan during the surgery to show him how much tumor is left. This technology has faced some challenges in development and is only available in a small number of pediatric centers.

Another new method to help neurosurgeons safely remove tumors is intraoperative ultrasonography, which uses ultrasound probes to guide the surgical approach. Ultrasonography is also used to examine the ventricles during surgery to look for collections of cerebrospinal fluid (CSF) or cysts.

Surgical treatment of hydrocephalus

Hydrocephalus is the buildup of fluid in the brain caused when a tumor blocks the normal flow of CSF. The surgeon can insert a tube (called a drain or ventriculostomy) prior to or during the tumor removal surgery to remove excess CSF. The tube shunts fluid from the brain to a collection bag outside the body. The drain is usually removed a few days after surgery.

> We were fortunate to be located near one of the most experienced pediatric neurosurgeons in California. They put Megan, who was just 20 months old, in the hospital for 2 days on Decadron® to reduce brain swelling before doing surgery. The tumor, an anaplastic ependymoma, was huge, and they did a gross total resection. They told us ahead of time that she might have language retrieval/word finding issues and loss of mobility on the right side, but that didn't happen. She did have an external drain after surgery, and they said she might need a permanent shunt because of the tumor's size, but the temporary drain worked well and came out without any fluid buildup, so they didn't need to do that.

Occasionally, part of the tumor remains or blood from the surgery scars the normal sites of CSF reabsorption and the hydrocephalus persists after surgery. In this case, a shunt surgery is performed. The shunt functions as a drain inside the body. The tube diverts the excess fluid from the brain into another space in the body—abdomen, chest, or a large vein in the heart. The fluid is then absorbed by the body. If your child has persistent hydrocephalus, an excellent resource is the Hydrocephalus Association (*www.hydroassoc.org*).

> Tori had a regular ventriculostomy that had a tube that drained out to a bag at the bedside. The reason that they do this is that she had impressive hydrocephalus and they wanted to decrease the pressure during the surgery to resect the medulloblastoma. There was great hope that she might not even need a shunt. They tried for 10 days (intermittently clamping the tube) but once they clamped the bag to see if her body could handle the fluid, it started to drain out her incision site. Even if it is only a teaspoon a day that the body cannot handle, the child must have a shunt as it will build up. This was one of the hardest things for me; I really did not want a shunt. It meant to me that she would be a medical device kid her entire life. We could never leave this experience behind. Funny thing—our shunt has been blissfully easy so far. Not a problem at all.

Like the plumbing in your house, shunts can block and back up. This blockage is called a shunt obstruction or shunt malfunction. Buildup of proteins or debris from surgery that circulates in the CSF can prevent the fluid from draining properly through the shunt. Symptoms of a shunt problem are the same as the symptoms of hydrocephalus (headaches, vomiting, double vision). When this happens, the surgeon replaces the entire shunt or repairs the part of the shunt that is obstructed. Rarely, shunts fracture or become disconnected. Surgical repair is also the treatment for this problem.

An infection in the shunt can also cause a blockage. In this situation, intravenous antibiotics are given to treat the infection. The bottom end of the shunt is brought outside the body and connected to a drainage bag while the infection is treated. Daily cultures of the fluid are sent to the laboratory to confirm that the antibiotics are working. Once three negative cultures have been obtained, the entire shunt system is removed and a new clean one is surgically inserted.

> I was 16 when I had my first surgery, when a VP shunt was placed for a large amount of fluid buildup. Then I had a second surgery to remove part of the tumor. About a month later, I started having severe headaches again. This time I could not raise my head up without becoming ill. I was rushed back to the emergency room, and another MRI was done. My neurosurgeon explained that the MRI was showing fluids back in the head again. He said that this was unusual, since I did have the shunt, and the shunt appeared to be working when he completed the last surgery. He performed some tests to see if he could figure out why the fluids were building up in the head. The next day, he told us that he wanted to go back in to check the shunt. He went in and discovered that my shunt had shut down due to a buildup of scar tissue around a valve on the shunt. He replaced the valve so that the shunt began working again. My stay in the hospital this time was about 7 days.

Hydrocephalus caused by a tumor that blocks the flow of CSF is sometimes treated with a procedure called an anterior third ventriculostomy (also called an endoscopic bypass or an endoscopic third ventriculostomy [ETV]). The surgeon uses an endoscope (a long tube with a camera at the end) to make an opening in the floor of the third ventricle. This new opening is a detour for the fluid around the obstruction caused by the tumor. The opening creates a pathway from inside the brain's fluid spaces to the outside circulation. Here the fluid can be absorbed normally by the subarachnoid space without the need of a shunt tube.

> Although Molly (14 months old) had no outward symptoms of hydrocephalus, the main concern at diagnosis was surgery to relieve the pressure on her brain from the pineoblastoma. We were given the option of either a shunt, or something called a third ventriculostomy. This would create a hardware-free channel for the extra cerebrospinal fluid to leave her brain. This sounded like the best option for Molly, so surgery was scheduled for the next afternoon. Surgery went very well, and she was released the following afternoon. Molly is now 3 years old, she is followed regularly, but she hasn't had any more problems with pressure in the brain.

Palliation

Palliation is a type of health care that focuses on relieving or preventing suffering. Surgery is sometimes used to improve the quality of life of terminally ill children. Some tumors that do not respond to radiation or chemotherapy grow and cause painful pressure. Surgeons can remove parts of the tumor that are causing the pain. The insertion of a shunt or an ETV also may be considered to temporarily improve the quality of life in a child who develops hydrocephalus because of tumor growth.

> Surgery was the only thing that made Laura feel better. She wanted to have the tumor operated on each time it came back. Before the last operation, she spoke to the surgeon and asked him to take it out one more time so that she could enjoy her summer.

Vascular access

Children with brain or spinal cord tumors have to endure many months or years of treatment. To avoid the pain of repeated needle sticks, many children receive a surgically implanted catheter. Direct access to a blood vessel allows the administration of chemotherapy, antibiotics, blood products, and hyperalimentation (IV nutrition) and avoids the pain of repeated needle sticks for the child. For more information, see Chapter 9, *Venous Catheters*.

Enteral access

Adequate nutrition plays an important role in children's overall well-being and prognosis. Children who are unable to eat or drink a liquid diet sometimes need enteral access, a method that delivers nutrients directly to the gastrointestinal tract. Enteral access can be accomplished in several ways, including the insertion of a nasogastric tube (a tube passed down the nose to the stomach) or the surgical installation of a gastrostomy tube (a tube placed through the abdominal wall into the stomach). For more information, see Chapter 20, *Nutrition*.

Presurgical evaluation

Soon after the diagnosis of a brain or spinal cord tumor, parents meet with the pediatric neurosurgeon to discuss the surgery. The consultation is important because it provides the surgeon with background information about your child, including your family's medical history. It is also important for the family because the surgeon will explain the procedure to you, answer questions, and address any concerns you have. Only an experienced, board-certified pediatric neurosurgeon is equipped to handle the intricacies of treating a pediatric brain or spinal cord tumor.

My son had several surgeries at different points in his treatment. Each time we had a long discussion with his surgeon to review the procedure and to talk about the possible complications. It made me feel scared when I thought about my little boy lying on an operating table being cut with a knife. Still, I'm glad that the surgeon was so thorough in explaining everything to us. I think that if I didn't know what was going to happen, my imagination would have really given me a hard time.

The following is a list of questions you can ask before signing a consent form for surgery:

- What percentage of your practice is pediatrics?
- How many other children with this type of tumor have you operated on?
- What is the purpose of the surgery? What are the expected findings?
- What are the common and not-so-common deficits that my child might develop after surgery?
- Is this a new procedure? If so, how many other children have had it?
- How much of the tumor do you expect to remove?
- Where will the incision (cut) be?
- How large will the incision be?
- How much hair will be shaved?
- How long will the operation take?

Our son was admitted for surgery to have his tumor resected early on a Monday morning. The surgery took 5 hours. We stuck close by in a waiting room, although the hospital had beepers to call us if we wanted to leave the area. It was an unbearable wait, but we were given updates every hour or so.

- What are the possible complications of the surgery?
- What types of tubes will my child have after surgery (i.e., number of IV lines, nasogastric tube, catheter in bladder, drain, or shunt)?
- Will blood transfusions or blood products be required?
- Will my child remain on a ventilator (breathing tube) afterwards? For how long?

When my child had surgery, the doctor said that there was a possibility that he would need to stay on the ventilator for a few days. Thankfully, that never happened, and he came from the recovery room breathing completely on his own.

- How long will my child need to stay in the intensive care unit (ICU) after the surgery?
- How long will my child need to stay in the hospital after leaving the ICU?
- How much pain will my child have after the surgery? How will it be controlled?

- When will my child be able to eat?

- How long will it take my child to recover?

- Will I need to learn how to care for her operation site after she is discharged?

- How long do the stitches or staples stay in?

- What are the possible long-term effects of this procedure?

- Will the scar be very noticeable?

> *Our son's surgery was at a major center. I hadn't expected that the incision line that curved along the side of my son's head would at first be raised like a fold, but eventually, the line thinned and flattened, then faded to white. It's not indented or jagged-looking, and his hairline hides it pretty well.*

Your child may undergo many tests before the operation, depending on the type of surgery and your child's medical condition. This is usually called presurgical testing. Some of the tests that are frequently ordered are blood work, urinalysis, x-rays, electrocardiogram, echocardiogram, and pulmonary function tests. If computer-assisted surgery is planned, an MRI is done a few hours before the surgery. Your child's surgeon should explain what tests are necessary.

It is important that the pre-operative preparation includes explaining the upcoming surgery to the child. Most large centers have a child psychologist, child life therapist, or nurse practitioner who can help you prepare your child for surgery. A simple, age-appropriate explanation can be given to the child during the pre-operative testing or, in some cases, just prior to surgery.

> *The psychologist on our team suggested that we think up age-appropriate, honest descriptions about what was going to happen. The idea was to give our 5-year-old son some vocabulary so he could think about his situation and maybe process things without being afraid of the unknown. The day before his surgery, we told him that he needed an operation. We explained, "An operation is where they open the skin to fix something. This time, they will be taking the tumor out. A special doctor will give you medicine that puts you to sleep, but it's really more than sleep; while the medicine is working, you can't feel anything. After the surgery, you'll feel very sleepy. If you have a headache, a nurse will give you medicine to make it go away." We reassured him that we would stay in the hospital with him, and we were clear about the whereabouts of each family member. "Mommy will be here when you wake up, but Daddy will sleep on the couch in the room with you."*

The older the child, the more detailed the explanation should be. However, follow your child's lead and give brief but clear answers for each question. Then ask if there is anything else he would like to know. If you don't know the answers, write down the questions and ask the surgeon or nurse practitioner at the next appointment. Make sure you and your child have all of your questions answered prior to surgery.

Anesthesia

The anesthesiologist is a key member of the surgical team. It is her responsibility to ensure that the child is properly anesthetized and monitored during the operation. Prior to the surgery, you will have a consultation with the anesthesiologist, during which she will ask you about your child's medical history and any allergies to medications. Take this opportunity to ask any questions you have or to express concerns. For instance, if your child is very frightened, ask the anesthesiologist if she could prescribe a pre-surgical sedative.

The following is a list of questions you can ask the anesthesiologist before the surgery:

- How will my child be put to sleep (mask or intravenous medication)?

- Will my child be sedated prior to the operation?

- What are the common side effects of the anesthesia drugs?

> *Surgery was a scary time for me. My mother and sister don't do very well under anesthesia, and we were afraid that Sean might react badly to it also. Sean did very well and came through the procedure without any complications.*

- Will I be able to stay with my child until he is anesthetized?

> *For our son's brain surgery, we weren't able to attend the hospital's children's tour for surgery, and he wasn't that well-prepared. But, we had a great experience for his port insertion at our local tertiary care center. We were invited to attend an evening tour of an operating room by Maureen, from Child Life. Our son sat in a circle with other kids while the whole anesthesia process was explained. They all tried on masks and practiced breathing deeply. On the day of surgery, the anesthesiologist spent time talking to our son. My husband, Jim, suited up in scrubs, our son was presedated, and they went off together down the hall to the O.R. chatting with the anesthesiologist.*

- Will my child need to remain on a ventilator afterwards? For how long?

You will be asked to sign a consent form prior to the administration of any anesthesia. The anesthesiologist will answer any questions or concerns you might have and may explain some of the ways children can react when coming out of anesthesia.

> *Anesthesia recovery is horrible for my son. He stands, hits, screams, cries, tries to leave, refuses to leave, you name it. Or rather, I should say his body does these*

*things. The thinking part of him is still anesthetized or dealing with a whopper of a
headache. Eventually I get my son back.*

. . . . .

*Brendon has been in and out of treatment for the last 10 years. He's had numerous
surgeries, radiation, and chemo. When he was little he was sedated for all of his
scans. I can't count the number of times he's been anesthetized. And he never had a
problem. He bounces right back so easily each time. I think that it helps that he is
always joking with the staff and thinking up funny pranks.*

The surgery

The surgical technique used to remove your child's tumor depends on several factors,
including the type and location of the tumor, your child's general medical condition,
and the type of procedure needed. However, some principles apply to all operations
requiring a general anesthetic. Children are usually given anesthesia through a breathing mask, an intravenous injection, or both. A breathing tube is placed in the trachea
(windpipe) and connected to a ventilator that will breathe for the child every few seconds. Your child will be anesthetized before the breathing tube is inserted.

During the operation, your child will be connected to many different monitors to ensure
there is an adequate supply of oxygen in the blood and that fluids are maintained at
proper levels. Blood pressure, heart rate, and other functions are carefully monitored.
Your child may also be connected to special monitoring to watch electrical impulses
controlling movement of the face, arms, and legs. Brain wave monitoring is sometimes
used to detect the presence of seizure activity.

> *The surgery was handled very well. Paige was treated with kindness and prepared,
> so she wasn't too scared. We were informed of her progress while surgery was taking
> place, and the surgeon explained the outcome as soon as he could.*

Once the child awakens from the anesthesia, clear liquids are given first and solid foods
are offered after the neurosurgeon feels it is safe. Some children are not able to drink
and/or eat for several days, depending on the surgery. These children are given nutrition
through an intravenous line or through an NG tube through the nose to the stomach.

> *Michelle had a number of major surgeries and more minor ones than I remember.
> She hated waking up to a liquid diet of Popsicles®, Jell-O®, and juice. One day she
> pleaded with the doctor to have something else. The doctor replied, "If you can think
> of anything else that's clear, you can have it." Michelle thought and thought, and she
> finally came up with jelly, no seeds. So on her next liquid diet tray were little packets
> of clear grape jelly.*

Most children who have brain surgeries do not experience serious complications. Many children are awake and hungry by the evening of surgery and are out of bed and walking the next day. The risk of complications in children is usually lower than in adults, because children recover from postoperative symptoms and weakness at a much faster rate than adults.

> My son was anxious to start moving about a few hours after he had his surgery to remove his tumor. He really amazed me. His mobility was limited for a few days, but he didn't let the operation stop him from trying to do most activities.

A small number of children with brain or spinal cord tumors experience significant complications from the surgery. These are discussed in the next section.

Postoperative complications

Postoperative problems are very stressful for the child and family. Symptoms that the child had prior to surgery are usually worse following the operation because of swelling or surgical trauma. This is normal. Less common complications after surgery are:

- Paralysis in arm(s) and/or leg(s)
- Seizures
- Loss of blood supply to an area of the brain (stroke)
- Hydrocephalus that requires another surgery to place a shunt or make a detour via an anterior third ventriculostomy
- Loss of bowel and bladder control
- Leakage of fluid from the incision
- Infection at site of incision
- Memory problems

> My son Darren is 12, although very mature for 12, and also a whiz at math. Several weeks after surgery when he had recovered enough to talk, we found that his short-term memory had been disrupted. He could not remember all of the letters of the alphabet or what certain numbers were. He also had trouble with word retrieval—he knew what he wanted to say but just couldn't think of the word he wanted to use. For example, he wanted to ask for pain medication, but could only ask us, "Make hurt less." This lasted just over 6 weeks or so, and I'm happy to say that he is now just as smart as he once was.

The majority of postoperative complications are not permanent; they can be reversed with additional surgical, medical, or rehabilitative treatment.

*My son had complications that were worse than the norm. It would have been help-
ful to me to know that all kids are referred to physical and occupational therapy
after brain surgery. Knowing that they expect physical impairment after surgery
would have given me some before-surgery perspective.*

Three less common but more serious complications are discussed next.

Aseptic meningitis

Aseptic meningitis can occur in the first few weeks following surgery, usually when
steroids (medications used to decrease swelling and inflammation) are reduced. It is
thought that aseptic meningitis is caused when blood and cells from the tumor removal
get into the CSF, causing chemical irritation. Symptoms of aseptic meningitis include
fever, headache, and stiff neck. If your child has any of these symptoms, the doctor usually asks for a sample of CSF to test for a bacterial infection. This sample is obtained
from a spinal tap (see Chapter 6, *Coping with Procedures*) or from fluid near the incision.
All cultures that test for the presence of bacteria are negative if your child has aseptic
meningitis. The symptoms usually improve when the child is given a short course of
additional steroids.

Cranial nerve deficits

Cranial nerves control movement of the eyes, face, and throat. The control center for
the cranial nerves is located in the brainstem. Problems with the cranial nerves can
be caused by tumors in the brainstem, tumors pressing on the brainstem, or hydrocephalus. Surgery in the posterior fossa (cerebellum or brainstem) can also result in
temporary or permanent cranial nerve problems. Some of the deficits that may develop
include:

• Double vision

• Bouncing of eyes

• Inability to look up or to one side

• Inability to close one eyelid

• Pain in the jaw

• Weakness, droop, or asymmetry of face

• Hoarse or raspy voice

• Difficulty swallowing and coughing

• Respiratory problems, such as difficulty breathing, pneumonia, and frequent respiratory illnesses

If these symptoms are present prior to surgery, they may get worse after surgery. However, recovery of cranial nerve function is possible over a long period of time. If eye and facial cranial nerve problems persist, surgery can correct some of them. Children who can't swallow are given nutrition through an NG or gastrostomy tube. Children with severe respiratory problems have a tube inserted into their throat (tracheostomy) that is connected to a respirator to help them breathe.

Posterior fossa syndrome

Posterior fossa syndrome (also called cerebellar mutism) is a complication of posterior fossa (cerebellum or brainstem) surgery. The most common tumors in this area are medulloblastomas, astrocytomas, and ependymomas. Most children wake up from the surgery moving their arms and legs and responding to questions. In some cases, 24 or more hours later the child stops talking, may develop weakness of arms and legs, and cranial nerve deficits appear. Emotionally, the children seem disconnected from their environment and may respond by simply crying.

These symptoms improve over a period of days in the minimally affected child, but improvement may take months in the severely affected child. Physical, occupational, and speech therapy should be started immediately. Children who have severe posterior fossa syndrome require transfer to an inpatient rehabilitation facility to facilitate quicker recovery.

> Tori developed posterior fossa syndrome and cerebellar mutism after surgery. These were slow to improve, but after months in rehab, she was eventually able to see and to form short sentences. We have come a long way, and now she is an active 5 year old in regular private kindergarten. She has, however, been basically on a feeding tube for the last 10 months since surgery. We occasionally try to have her eat, but usually after a week it needs to go back in because she is getting on the dry side (dehydrated). The tube often is one of the most obvious things that makes her look "sick," so this has had its ups and downs.

· · · · ·

> Ayla (32 months) was diagnosed with medulloblastoma, a 5x5 cm tumor in the posterior fossa, cerebellopontine angle, fourth ventricle, and arising from the brainstem. When all of this happens, you are not necessarily in the position or frame of mine to get all opinions. In retrospect, we know we had an excellent pediatric neurosurgeon who removed as much as he felt he could without causing additional deficits. He was very compassionate. When Ayla came out of it after surgery, she said, "I want pasta and salmon with paprika on it." Then she noticed the balloons that we there for her, and she wanted to make sure her sister Jasmine got one. We didn't notice it right away, but she couldn't walk at first and she couldn't drink liquids without choking. All that lasted about a week. They didn't tell us ahead of time about posterior fossa syndrome, though we feel she came out of surgery relatively unscathed.

Our son had radiation late this summer (2.3 Gy craniospinal and a boost to the tumor bed) and is about to start round two (of eight) of chemotherapy (cisplatin, cytoxan, and vincristine). He was mute for 2½ months post-op, and had a right hemiparesis as well as a gaze palsy. He is back to his hyperactive self in terms of speech, but the physical return has been slower. His vision has improved, but he may still need a surgical correction. However, while he remembers even the worst of his impairments, he has a "today is today" attitude—no complaints, no frustration. He is the youngest of four, and I think the attention he has garnered has made him feel special and loved (he claimed he was "Moses, Prince of Egypt" just 2 weeks ago). Chemo every 3 weeks, all the testing, at-home hydration, meds and mouth care, port accessing, G-CSF [granulocyte-colony stimulating factor], etc., has just become routine for him. I am trying to catch up to his good spirits.

Rehabilitation

Rehabilitation services are necessary for the majority of children with brain or spinal cord tumors. The tumor itself or the effects of treatments may impair use of or coordination in the arms or legs. Speech, language, and comprehension problems may occur. Problems with swallowing and breathing also sometimes happen. If these problems occur while your child is hospitalized, he should see a pediatric physiatrist—a medical doctor who evaluates children's physical function and then writes the orders for physical, occupational, and/or speech therapy.

The initial evaluation occurs soon after surgery, and periodic re-evaluations focus on revising the long- and short-term goals of therapy. After discharge from the hospital, most children can receive rehabilitation services on an outpatient basis. Occasionally, an intensive inpatient rehabilitation program is needed for children with many deficits. Physical, occupational, recreational, and speech therapy are all components of rehabilitation.

I have made it quite clear what I think is best for my daughter. My approach is that I am the CEO of the company "My Tori has a Brain Tumor, Inc." and that essentially everyone else is consultant and that I do have options. I definitely don't know everything, but no one else knows my daughter, my family, or our ethos better than me, and that has to count for a lot. You may be bothersome, but guess what, it is your child, and you have that right.

When my Tori came out of surgery for a multicentimeter, standard risk medulloblastoma, she was blind, mute, her right eye turned all the way in, she had right facial droop, was unable to swallow, she was paralyzed in the right leg and both arms, incontinent, irritable and very hypotonic (floppy): essentially the severe end of cerebellar mutism with several regular neuro complications thrown in. They initially did not want to send her to a rehab facility and I got the feeling that they did not think that she was a promising rehab candidate.

The rehab doc and our neuro-oncologist (independently) told us it would be about 3 years until she could walk again, and the rehab doc added that that might even be a little optimistic. Well, essentially we did a lot of stuff ourselves using the therapist as guides. We got tapes to play for her so she could listen to music and stories. We read books. We described everything going on in the halls. I brought in a little shopping cart from a local store (one of the heavy metal ones) that she could use as a walker when her left arm came back (she couldn't use a walker because her right side was too weak and she wouldn't tolerate the arm being strapped in). She was able to guide the shopping cart by putting her left arm in the middle of the bar and pushing.

I actually had a box of sand in the room for her to dig through and find treasures (one with about 25 pounds of sand). She also had shaving cream to play with and we had syringe battles (like squirt guns). I got bath sponges and we made a shield from cardboard (that I velcroed on her arm). We had battles throwing the bath sponges. It is not quite 18 months later, and she has regained her sight and speech (albeit a little nasal and often slow). She is able to walk on just about any surface, play on a play-ground independently, swing, slide, and climb ladders. She goes on the trapeze bar and she can do chin-ups and flip over. She finally is not tube fed and she can write. Hospital staff need to believe that these kids can come back and go on to do normal kid things.

Physical therapy

Physical therapy involves using exercise and motion to improve the body's strength and movement. If an arm or leg is not moving at all, the physical therapist moves the limb through the entire range of motion to prevent the muscles from tightening during recovery. When the arm or leg begins to recover, the physical therapist devises strengthening exercises for the affected limb. Physical therapy uses equipment such as tilt tables, stationary bicycles, and treadmills. Therapy in a pool (also called aquatic therapy) is another form of physical therapy used to strengthen affected limbs.

Our son was diagnosed with medulloblastoma when he was 2 years old. He was inpatient for most of the first 6 months, then on outpatient chemo for 18 months. He had intensive rehab while in the hospital. When we were at home, I accessed the city early intervention program. He had physical therapy, occupational therapy, speech therapy, and an itinerant teacher each twice a week until he was 5 years old, when he became ineligible. Now we get the services he needs through the school system.

Occupational and recreational therapy

Occupational therapy focuses on recovering or maintaining the ability to participate in activities of daily life. For example, occupational therapists help children regain the fine motor skills needed to tie shoes, hold a pencil, eat, and dress themselves. They also evaluate the child's need for any special equipment to maximize independence such as an adaptive holder to help the child write with a pencil or a computer if handwriting is not a realistic goal.

Recreational therapy also works on activities of daily living, as well as working on social and cognitive functioning, developing coping skills, and integrating children back into community settings. Examples of methods used by recreational therapists are creative arts (e.g., painting, dance, drama), sports, and leisure activities.

> *Alissa's had multiple operations for an astrocytoma. One of her best friends at the hospital is Julie, a recreation therapist. One time, Julie came in with some paints. She just started painting, quietly, and then Alissa started painting. They've bonded and Julie always comes by now to work with Alissa. All the recreation therapists come to see Alissa when she's in for an operation. They come see her right before surgery and stay with her until she goes in. Alissa's taking oil painting, taught by adults, once a week. She is using her hands, using the parts of her body that work, and she is doing very well.*

Speech therapy

Speech therapy improves children's speech and language skills. Some young children may need therapy because of delays in speech development. Other children require this therapy if the tumor or its treatment affects the speech and language areas of the brain. Some survivors of brain or spinal cord tumors have trouble interpreting speech or difficulty actually getting the words to come out. Children with slurred, halted (referred to as ataxic) speech benefit greatly from speech therapy. Speech therapists also work with children who have difficulties with swallowing.

Accessing therapies in school

Rehabilitation helps many children make a full, or near full, recovery. These children will have the rehabilitation services slowly phased out. Other children have disabilities that require long-term rehabilitation to maximize and maintain function. Once a child re-enters the school environment, it is best to get rehabilitative services within the school. However, schools provide educationally relevant therapies (i.e., speech therapy and occupational therapy) and not all rehabilitation therapies. For information about therapies provided by schools, see Chapter 18, *School.*

Therapeutic activities in the community

Formal rehabilitation in the outpatient or school setting is frequently enhanced by recreational activities. Community and school athletic teams are excellent therapy for children who can participate in them. Additionally, the arts, such as music, art, drama, and dance, are excellent therapy alternatives.

Last Friday, Tori had her dance recital (tap and ballet). For me, it was a completely overwhelming experience. In the fall, I looked around for a place that was willing to take her since she was fairly disabled from her treatment for medulloblastoma. Finally, I found that the YMCA would enroll her in their Saturday morning program. Although she was 6, I put her with the 4- and 5-year-olds. She is tiny and no one really knew the difference.

When we started, she did most everything from a chair and often would just sit and watch. Later, I would kneel behind her and hold her waist as she tried to do the front and back points. Over winter, I had to decide whether she would be in the spring recital. It was hard: getting up to get there by 9 a.m. every Saturday, watching how hard it was for her, hoping that she would be able to go on stage and not be frustrated or embarrassed. During dress rehearsal the doubts multiplied. Would she be too cold in the skimpy outfit (beautiful but sleeveless and very, very short)? Would she slip and fall as she only wore the tap shoes once before? Would she go on in front of 200 people or so? Would the sound system bother her? Would the bright lights make her shield her eyes? When the curtain opened, there she was standing so poised and absolutely stunning. She did the entire routine. She didn't look different than any of the other kids. Most people in the audience had no idea how incredibly fantastic it was, how she could weight shift, point her toes, jump, move side to side and all in tap shoes! It was truly a moving moment.

· · · · ·

Our 6-year-old son has slower speed than his peers. He also has a visual field cut and partial seizures. Our local Jewish Community Center has an excellent swimming and camp program. Our son was assigned an experienced counselor for a swimming buddy at camp. They also provided lessons in soccer, archery, and tennis. Our son sat out any activities when he was too tired. There was no pressure, and it was very supportive. The nurse handled the few partial seizures quite well.

· · · · ·

My Anjulie, who had a diffuse brainstem glioma, had aquatherapy and it benefited her greatly. Not only did the water calm and soothe her, but it provided her with much needed freedom to move. The water pressure also helped her digestive system and lungs, too. Anjulie loved swimming and she worked hard at all of her games while in the pool.

Many communities have formal or informal therapeutic activities. Some have sports teams for disabled children and teens. Other children participate in Special Olympics or Easter Seals programs. Many communities have therapeutic riding programs for children with medical challenges.

A new girl approaches. The same lilting gait as my daughter who had a brain tumor removed 3 years ago. The new girl lifts her face to the horse. She turns her head to see him better. The child steps forward and wraps her arms around the middle of the horse, not the head of the horse. She buries her face there and lingers. As a part of WE CAN, a parent support group for families of pediatric brain tumors, we invite other survivors to meet our horse and learn to ride.

"You brush the way the hair grows," my daughter says, showing her how to move her hand. "Before you can ride, you have to pick the horse's feet." She leaned over beginning below the knee, squeezing her fingers down the length of the horse's hock until he lifted his foot. The other child stood by the leg trying to mimic the movement. Together they run their hands down the length of the horse's leg, which yields easily this time.

The new girl's mother said, "With all of the tests we've been through and the surgeries, sometimes it's difficult to be normal. Being here in the dirt, having something to talk about, feels like we are mending something between us."

I knew what her mother meant. I had also found that my daughter's riding, her self-induced therapy so to speak, gave her something that made her feel good about herself. In a way I felt the riding was re-circuiting her brain's functions, repairing the damage to the left side of her body, damage from the encroaching tumor and surgery. For her it was simply the smell of horse, the feel of it, the fact that he would be there to listen if she needed him.

Discharge

When your child is discharged from the hospital after surgery, you are given written instructions about home care that should include instructions for care of the incision or directions about dressing changes. The most important thing to remember when caring for the operation site is to wash your hands thoroughly with soap and water before changing dressings. Most neurosurgeons recommend cleaning incisions with regular showers, including shampooing, beginning as soon as 3 days after surgery.

You may also need to ensure that your child does daily physical therapy exercises. Before discharge, the physical therapist will discuss this with you and give you written directions for helping your child do the exercises properly. Sometimes a physical therapist comes to your home, or you will take your child to physical therapy appointments several times a week.

We had some physical therapy as soon as he could tolerate it in the hospital, but the doctor didn't feel he needed it at home. Our child was under 3 and eligible for early intervention services (which is available to all children younger than school age who have the potential for delayed development) because of his diagnosis, so we asked for and received some physical therapy from them for a period of time.

· · · · ·

Our neurosurgeon told me not to worry about Michael playing soccer (he scored a goal in his first game back—a diving head ball!), that his metal plate was screwed in with titanium screws and wasn't about to move.

At discharge, you will receive a follow-up appointment with your child's surgeon to have any staples or stitches removed. Your surgeon should let you know the next step in the treatment process and which member of the multidisciplinary team is in charge of that phase of treatment.

Chris was born with a condition called gelastic epilepsy, caused by a hypothalamic hamartoma, a rare congenital tumor which can cause intractable seizures, behavior rages, early puberty, and cognitive decline. Surgery to remove this tumor has had to be the most emotional and most difficult experience of my life. Everything was running through my head, both negative and positive thoughts. Of course, there was the overwhelming fear that something might go wrong. I had experienced this in the weeks leading up to surgery, and had tried to prepare myself more for this time, but the intense feelings were so strong, it is hard to explain. I kept telling myself that we had to go through with it because this was his real chance.

I left Chris asleep in the anesthetic room. I came out in tears and continued to battle with my emotions. Our neurosurgeon came to see us and assured us that things would be all right. He was going to take good care of him. I felt a deep inner sense of comfort about this man, that he truly did love and care for all the children he operated on. This helped a lot and we began to settle down a little. The neurosurgeon's associate came up to the ward a few hours later to tell us that he had got the tumor out. We then went down to the parent recovery waiting room and our neurosurgeon came out to talk with us and tell us more about the surgery in detail—the beaming smile on his face said it all.

It was like a dream, there we were, sitting and being told that this terrible thing was no longer inside our son's head. All of a sudden there was this tremendous weight taken off my shoulders and I felt a strange sense of peace within.

Chris slept more or less the whole night and most of the following day. We watched over him as he was constantly checked for responsiveness, blood pressure, signs of seizure, and fluid input and output. That evening he developed a high temperature, we were told to expect this might happen, and it settled down.

Next morning at around 4 a.m., Chris woke up and asked, "Dad, can I have some cola?" You cannot imagine how I felt: I had my son back, he was going to be okay.

Chapter 11

Chemotherapy

The first wealth is health.
— Ralph Waldo Emerson

THE WORD CHEMOTHERAPY IS DERIVED from a combination of the words "chemical" and "therapy" (meaning treatment). During chemotherapy, drugs are used individually or in combination to destroy or disrupt the growth of tumor cells without permanently damaging normal cells.

This chapter explains how chemotherapy drugs work, how they are given, and how dosages for children and teens are determined. It then describes the most common drugs used to destroy brain and spinal cord tumor cells, as well as medications used to prevent nausea and treat pain. Numerous stories are included that show the range of responses to different chemotherapy drugs. A brief discussion of complementary and alternative treatments is also included.

Reading about chemotherapy's potential side effects can be disturbing. However, by learning what to expect from the various drugs, you may be able to recognize symptoms early and report them to the doctor so swift action can be taken to make your child more comfortable. On rare occasions, side effects may be life-threatening and some can persist throughout life. However, most are merely unpleasant and subside soon after treatment ends.

Not all children respond to these drugs in the same way. Some children develop serious side effects from certain drugs, but others are unaffected. In most cases, it is impossible to predict how an individual child will tolerate chemotherapy.

How chemotherapy drugs work

Normal, healthy cells divide and grow in a well-established pattern. When these cells divide, an identical copy is produced. The body only makes the number of normal cells it needs at any given time. As each normal cell matures, it loses its ability to reproduce. Normal cells are also preprogrammed to die at specific times.

In contrast, tumor cells reproduce uncontrollably and grow in unpredictable ways. They invade surrounding tissue and cause disruptions in the functions of the normal brain and spine.

All chemotherapy drugs work in some way to interfere with the cancer cells' ability to live, divide, and multiply. Some of the types of drugs used to treat brain and spinal cord tumors are:

- **Alkaloids.** These drugs, derived from plants, interrupt cell division through a variety of mechanisms, including interfering with DNA and specific enzyme activities. They also disrupt the membrane (outer wall) of the cancer cell, causing cell damage or cell death.

- **Alkylating agents.** All cells contain DNA and RNA, which provide the instructions needed by cells to make exact copies of themselves. Alkylating agents poison cancer cells by interacting with DNA or RNA to prevent cell reproduction.

- **Antibiotics.** This type of drug prevents cell growth by blocking reproduction, weakening the outer wall of the cell, or interfering with certain cell enzymes.

- **Antimetabolites.** These drugs starve cancer cells by replacing essential cell nutrients that are necessary during the synthesis phase of the cell cycle (growth in preparation for cell division).

- **Hormones.** These drugs create a hostile environment that slows cell growth. They can also signal to cancer cells that it is time to die.

- **Immunotherapeutic agents.** These substances, usually used in targeted therapies, either encourage the cancerous cells to die or help the body destroy them. (For more information, see Chapter 3, *Types of Tumors*.)

- **Protein inhibitors.** These drugs interfere with tumor cells' ability to reproduce by depriving the cells of specific proteins necessary for cell growth and division.

- **Anti-angiogenesis agents.** Drugs in this category have the ability to disrupt the blood supply to the tumor, depriving it of nutrients necessary for growth.

How chemotherapy drugs are given

The five most common ways to give chemotherapy drugs during treatment for childhood cancer are:

- **Intravenous (IV).** Medicine is delivered directly into the bloodstream through a venous catheter in the chest or an IV in the arm or hand. IV medicines can be administered in a few minutes (through IV injection or push) or as an infusion over a number of hours.

- **Oral (PO).** Drugs, taken by mouth in liquid, capsule, or tablet form, are absorbed into the blood through the lining of the stomach and intestines.

- **Intracavitary/Interstitial/Implanted.** Drugs are delivered directly into a body cavity through a catheter, or they are placed in a tumor bed in a form that will slowly dissolve (e.g., wafers).

- **Intramuscular (IM).** Drugs that need to seep slowly into the bloodstream are injected into a large muscle such as the thigh or buttocks.

- **Intrathecal (IT).** Doctors perform a spinal tap and inject the drug directly into the cerebrospinal fluid (the fluid surrounding the brain and spinal cord).

- **Subcutaneous (Sub-Q).** Drugs that need to enter the bloodstream at a moderately rapid rate are injected into the soft tissues under the skin of the upper arm, thigh, or abdomen.

- **Sublingual (SL).** Several drugs are now available as lozenges that dissolve quickly when placed under the tongue.

Dosages

Dosages vary among protocols, but most are based on your child's weight or body surface area (BSA). BSA is calculated from your child's weight and height and is measured in meters squared (m^2). Doses of medications your child is scheduled to receive should be recalculated by the doctor at the beginning of each new phase of treatment. Recalculating doses more frequently is necessary if your child experiences significant weight gain or loss (more than 10 percent of his initial weight).

You do not need to do the calculations, but it is important to know the appropriate dosage for each drug and how you should give it to your child. Most families write the dosages for each drug on a calendar and cross them out after each dose has been given to make sure they don't forget a drug or accidentally repeat a dose.

Variability in response to medications

Children's bodies have a wide range of responses to medications, some of which are due to their genes. Some children inherit genes that do not allow them to break down (metabolize) certain drugs, or that allow them to break the drugs down very slowly. If a child cannot metabolize a drug or metabolizes it slowly, it can build up in the blood stream and cause excessive toxicity.

Tumor cells also show dramatic variability in how they respond to different chemotherapy drugs. The tumor cells in one child's body might be extraordinarily sensitive to a specific chemotherapy drug, while the tumor cells in another child's body might be very resistant to that same drug.

Therefore, the combination of variability in children's ability to metabolize drugs and variability in how sensitive their tumor cells are to certain drugs causes a big range in the effectiveness of standard doses of medications. How much of this variability is due to genetics is not well understood. However, researchers are identifying ways to test children's ability to metabolize certain drugs and are tailoring treatments based on that genetic information; this area of science is called pharmacogenetics. Following are two examples of genetic characteristics that are used by doctors to tailor treatments to a child's unique genetic makeup.

CYP2D6. A genetic variation currently being investigated concerns CYP2D6, which affects the metabolism of codeine. Approximately 10 percent of people do not get pain relief from codeine, because they are genetically not able to metabolize the codeine into morphine. Because codeine products are often used for painful side effects of treatment (e.g., vincristine neuropathy), some institutions test all children with cancer for this genetic variation so appropriate pain medications can be prescribed.

Methlyenetetrahydrofolate reductase (MTHFR). The chemotherapy drug methotrexate is used to treat some children with brain and spinal cord tumors. A common genetic variation—MTHFR C677T—increases some children's sensitivity to methotrexate, resulting in liver toxicity, excessively low blood counts, and other side effects. Children who have these reactions while receiving methotrexate are sometimes tested for this genetic variation.

Questions to ask the doctor

Before giving your child any drug, you should be given answers to the following questions:

- What is the dosage? How many times a day should it be given?
- Should the drug be given at a particular time of day or under specific conditions (e.g., on an empty stomach or before bed)?
- What are the common and rare side effects?
- What should I do if my child experiences any of the side effects?
- Will the drug interact with any over-the-counter drugs (e.g., Tylenol®), foods, or vitamins?
- What should I do if I forget to give my child a dose?

- What are both the trade and generic names of the drug?

- Should I buy the generic version?

- Will you give my teen detailed counseling about the risks associated with drinking alcohol, smoking cigarettes or marijuana, or getting pregnant while using this drug?

Guidelines for calling the doctor

Sometimes parents are reluctant to call their child's neuro-oncologist with questions or concerns, so here are some general guidelines about when you should call:

- A temperature above 101° F (38.5° C)

- Shaking or chills

- Shortness of breath

- Severe nausea or vomiting

- Unusual bleeding, bruising, or cuts that won't heal

- Pain or swelling at a chemotherapy injection site

- Any severe pain that cannot be explained

- Exposure to chicken pox or measles

- Severe headache or blurred vision

- Constipation lasting more than 2 days

- Severe diarrhea

- Severe headaches

- Painful urination or bowel movements

- Blood in urine

Parents should not hesitate to bring their children to the hospital if they are ill and their blood counts are low, as this can be a life-threatening emergency. Any time your child is sick and you are concerned, call the doctor.

Chemotherapy drug list

Drugs used to treat children with brain and spinal cord tumors are known by various names, which can get very confusing. You may hear the same drug referred to by its generic name, an abbreviation, or one of several brand names, depending on which doctor, nurse, or pharmacist you talk to. The list below provides the generic name of the most commonly used chemotherapy drugs for newly diagnosed chidren and some of the most common brand names.

Drug Names	Brand Name(s)
Bevacizumab	Avastin®
Bleomycin	Blenoxane®
Busulfan	Busulfex®
Carboplatin	Paraplatin®
Carmustine BCNU	BiCNU®
Cyclophosphamide	Cytoxan®, Cytoxan Lyophilized®, Neosar®
Dacarbazine	DTIC-DOME®
Dexamethasone DEX	Decadron®, Hexadrol®, and multiple other brand names
Etoposide VP-16	VePesid®, Toposar®
Gemtuzumab	Mylotarg®
Ifosfamide	Ifex®
Interferon-alpha	Intron®
Irinotecan	Camptosar®
Lomustine CCNU	CeeNU®
Methotrexate MTX	Trexall®
Prednisone	Sterapred®
Procarbazine	Matulane®
Temozolamide	Temodar®
Thalidomide	Thalidomid®
Thiotepa	Tepadina®, Thioplex®
Topotecan	Vesanoid®, Hycamptin®
Vinblastine	Velban®
Vincristine	Oncovin®, Vincasar PFS®

Chemotherapy drugs and their possible side effects

This section contains both common and infrequent side effects of anticancer drugs, along with parent and survivor experiences and suggestions. You may be overwhelmed by reading about all the potential side effects of each drug. Please remember, each child is unique and will handle most drugs without major problems. Most side effects are unpleasant, but not serious, and subside when the medication stops. The parent experiences included here may provide insight, comfort, and suggestions should your child have an unusual side effect. If you have any concerns after reading these descriptions, consult with your child's neuro-oncologist.

Remember to keep all chemotherapy drugs in a locked cabinet away from children and pets.

Side effects terminology

Many of the side effects caused by the drugs described in this chapter have medical names that may be unfamiliar to you. This table defines those terms so you can understand what the members of your child's treatment team mean when they discuss side effects.

Medical Name	Description (most of these conditions are temporary)
Alopecia	Hair loss
Amenorrhea	Absence of a menstrual period
Anemia	Low red blood cell count, which causes weakness, fatigue, and paleness
Arrhythmia	Abnormal electrical rhythm in the heart; the term is usually used to describe an abnormal heartbeat
Aseptic necrosis	Death of bone tissue, caused by reduced blood supply
Bowel perforation	A hole that develops in the stomach or intestine
Conjunctivitis	Inflammation or infection of the membrane that lines the eyelids (eyes can be red, irritated, crusty, and watery; vision may be blurry)
Dyspnea	Shortness of breath; breathing difficulties
Dystonia	Muscle contractions that result in repetitive twisting or movement of a limb or other body part, which may be painful
Dysuria	Painful urination
Hematuria	Blood in the urine
Hemorrhagic cystitis	Inflammation of the bladder; characterized by pus or blood in urine, pain with urination, and decreased urine flow
Hyperglycemia	Increased blood sugar
Hypoglycemia	Decreased blood sugar

Medical Name	Description (most of these conditions are temporary)
Hyperpigmentation	Darkening of the skin
Hyperproteinuria	Too much protein in the urine
Hypertension	High blood pressure
Hypotension	Low blood pressure
Jaundice	Yellowish discoloration of the skin or eyes, caused by too much bilirubin in the blood; jaundice may indicate liver toxicity
Mucositis	Inflammation and ulceration of the mucous membranes lining the digestive tract
Myelosuppression	Decreased bone marrow activity, resulting in lowered counts of all blood components (red blood cells, white blood cells, and platelets)
Neutropenia	Not enough neutrophils (white blood cells that fight infection); this condition increases the risk of infection
Pancreatitis	Inflammation of the pancreas, normally associated with abdominal pain, nausea, or vomiting
Pancytopenia	Reduction in the number of all kinds of blood cells (red blood cells, white blood cells, and platelets)
Peripheral neuropathy	Pain, numbness, tingling, swelling, or weakness, usually in the hands, feet, or lower legs; caused by damage to the nerves that transmit to the extremities; usually temporary, but occasionally permanent
Petechiae	Small red spots under the skin caused by bleeding in tiny blood vessels
Photosensitivity	Sensitivity to the sun; can cause sunburn, rash, skin discoloration, hives, and itching
Somnolence	Sleepiness, drowsiness, and lethargy
Stomatitis	Inflammation or irritation of the membranes of the mouth; mouth sores
Thrombocytopenia	Not enough platelets, resulting in poor blood clotting, bleeding, bruising, and petechiae
Veno-occlusive disease (VOD)	A blockage in the veins of the liver; symptoms include weight gain, liver pain or swelling, and increased bilirubin levels in the blood

Chemotherapy drugs

This section lists drugs commonly used to treat brain and spinal cord tumors.

Bevacizumab (bev-a-SIZ-u-mab)

How given: Intravenous (IV) injection; intrathecal (IT) injection

How it works: Bevacizumab is an angiogenesis inhibitor that inhibits the growth of new blood vessels.

Precaution: Children must be monitored closely for signs of bleeding or kidney toxicity.

Common side effects:

- Nosebleeds
- High blood pressure
- Dry skin
- Back pain
- Headaches
- Irritation of the nose

Infrequent side effects:

- Bowel perforation
- Serious bleeding
- Wound healing problems
- Kidney problems

Bleomycin (blee-oh-MY-sin)

How given: Intramuscular (IM), subcutaneous (SQ), intravenous (IV), intracavitary

How it works: Bleomycin binds with DNA to stop cell growth.

Precautions: A small percentage of children are allergic to this drug. Lung function tests are used to detect possible lung toxicity.

Common side effects:

- Hair loss
- Mouth sores

- Nausea, vomiting
- Weight loss and loss of appetite
- Darkening of the skin
- Thickening of skin on palms, fingers, soles of feet
- Fever, with or without chills

Infrequent side effects:
- Lung toxicity (potentially permanent)
- Allergic reactions
- Joint swelling

Hints for parents: Plan on staying with your child during the short time that the drug is given in case an allergic reaction occurs. Promptly report any shortness of breath, cough, or other breathing difficulties to the nurse or doctor.

Busulfan (byoo-SUL-fan)

How given: Pills by mouth (PO)

How it works: Busulfan is an alkylating agent that interferes with DNA to prevent cell division.

Precaution: The child should have lung function tests for early detection of possible toxicities.

Common side effects:
- Low blood counts, which may increase risk of infection or bleeding, and cause weakness, fatigue, and paleness
- Patchy darkening of the skin
- Nausea, vomiting, and diarrhea (usually mild)
- Fever
- Loss of appetite
- Mouth sores
- Dry mouth
- Liver damage (temporary)

Infrequent side effects:

- Lung toxicity (potentially permanent)
- Cataracts (with long-term use)
- Blurred vision
- Mental confusion
- Seizures

Hints for parents: Giving your child the medicine at bedtime often decreases nausea and vomiting. Promptly report any respiratory, visual, or neurological symptoms to your child's doctor or nurse. Schedule your child's pulmonary function tests the week prior to starting a new cycle of therapy so that test results will be available for your physician to review.

Carboplatin (car-bo-PLAT-un)

How given: Intravenous (IV)

How it works: Carboplatin inhibits DNA replication, RNA transcription, and protein synthesis.

Precautions: The child may be given extra fluids to prevent possible kidney toxicity. Mannitol, a diuretic medication, is sometimes given with this drug to increase urine output. Children are also usually given a baseline hearing test and then another hearing test before each dose.

Common side effects:

- Low blood counts, which may increase risk of infection or bleeding and cause weakness, fatigue, and paleness
- Nausea and vomiting
- Altered taste

Infrequent side effects:

- Ringing in the ears
- Hearing loss
- Numbness or tingling in fingers and toes
- Kidney damage

Hints for parents: Make sure that you have adequate antinausea medication at home after your child receives this drug. Taste distortion may alter your child's food preferences. Promptly report to the doctor any hearing problems, such as ringing in the ears, problems hearing in the classroom, or background noise interference. Also report any fine motor coordination problems, such as difficulty buttoning clothes, writing, or picking up small objects.

> *Our son did experience ringing in his ears and had some questionable hearing tests during treatment with carboplatin, but a recent thorough hearing test after we finished showed his hearing is near perfect.*

Carmustine (CAR-mus-teen)

How given: Intraveneous (IV)

How it works: Carmustine is an alkylating agent that disrupts DNA and RNA replication, resulting in cell death.

Precautions: Give through central venous catheter or newly placed peripheral IV. Baseline pulmonary function tests are necessary.

Common side effects:

- Low blood counts, which may increase risk of infection or bleeding and cause weakness, fatigue, and paleness
- Nausea and vomiting
- Hair loss that is not permanent
- Patchy brown discoloration of the skin
- Low blood pressure if rapidly infused
- Irritation along the vein if given through a peripheral IV

Infrequent side effects:

- Diarrhea
- Inflammation of the esophagus
- Clots in blood vessels in the liver
- Permanent lung damage
- Permanent kidney damage
- Second cancer (cancer that occurs as a result of treatment)
- Facial flushing and dizziness

Hints for parents: The serious side effects of this drug are generally only seen at the high doses used as part of a stem cell transplant. Report any shortness of breath or dry, nonproductive cough to your child's physician promptly. Your child should have pulmonary function tests performed prior to starting therapy with this drug and at specified intervals thereafter. The drug is reconstituted in alcohol, and some children act intoxicated after a high dose is given.

Cisplatin (sis-PLAT-un)

How given: Intravenous (IV)

How it works: Cisplatin is a platinating agent that inhibits DNA replication, RNA transcription, and protein synthesis.

Precautions: The child should be given large amounts of IV fluids while receiving cisplatin to prevent kidney damage. A diuretic drug, called mannitol, may also given to decrease the risk of kidney damage. All urine output should be measured during the infusion. The child should be given a baseline hearing test before cisplatin is given and be monitored for possible hearing loss.

Common side effects:
- Nausea and vomiting
- Low blood counts, which may increase risk of infection or bleeding and cause weakness, fatigue, and paleness
- Loss of appetite
- Taste distortion
- Hearing loss
- Ringing in the ears
- Abnormalities of sodium, potassium, calcium, and magnesium
- Kidney damage
- Tingling and weakness in the hands and feet
- Hair loss that is not permanent

Infrequent side effects:
- Low blood pressure
- Allergic reactions
- Rapid or slow heart rate

- Damage to the liver

- Dizziness, agitation, paranoia

- Temporary blindness, color blindness, or blurred vision

> *Missy's protocol required her to have both cisplatin as well as carboplatin (for her stem cell transplant). Both of these drugs, over the course of her treatment, damaged her high-pitch frequency hearing so much that her speech development took a turn for the worse. She needed hearing aids to help correct the problem.*

· · · · ·

> *Molly had a pineoblastoma, had surgery, then was placed on a clinical trial for infants with medulloblastoma. She was too young for radiation. She had vincristine and cisplatin, Cytoxan®, thiotepa, carboplatin, and a few others. She had a good bit of muscle wasting from the vincristine, but did really well with the "platins" with no hearing loss. Molly is 3 years old now, and is doing physical therapy twice a week just for muscle strength issues from the vincristine and being in the hospital for so long.*

Hints for parents: Administering IV fluids at home for several days after receiving cisplatin can help eliminate the drug from your child's system. Because elimination of this drug is much slower than many other agents, make sure that you have adequate antinausea medication on hand at home. Promptly report any hearing or neurological symptoms to your child's doctor or nurse.

Cyclophosphamide (sye-kloe-FOSS-fa-mide)

How given: Intravenous (IV) injection

How it works: Cyclophosphamide is an alkylating agent that disrupts DNA in cancer cells, preventing reproduction.

Precaution: The child should drink lots of water or be given large amounts of IV fluids while taking cyclophosphamide to prevent bladder damage. A drug called Mesna® may be given to prevent bladder irritation. Antinausea drugs should be given before and for several hours after this drug is administered.

Common side effects:
- Low blood counts, which may increase risk of infection or bleeding and cause weakness, fatigue, and paleness

- Nausea, vomiting, and diarrhea

- Loss of appetite

- Hair loss that is not permanent
- Mouth sores

Infrequent side effects:

- Bleeding from the bladder
- Cough or shortness of breath
- Skin rash, dryness, and darkening of the skin
- Metallic taste during injection of the drug
- Blurred vision
- Irregular or absent menstrual periods in postpubertal girls (temporary)
- Permanent sterility in postpubertal boys (rare at routine doses, more common at doses given for high-risk or relapse treatment or for transplants)

> *Erica just could not tolerate the Cytoxan®. She had continuous vomiting. At one point she had lost more than one third of her body weight. Our HMO (health maintenance organization) wouldn't authorize using ondansetron (a very effective antinausea drug) because it was so expensive.*

> • • • • •

> *Christine breezed through the Cytoxan® infusions. She would go to Children's in the afternoon, they would give her lots of IV fluids, and then ondansetron a half hour before the Cytoxan®. She would sleep through the night with absolutely no nausea, because they were so good about giving her the ondansetron all night and the next morning. It was hard on me because I had to wake up every 2 hours to change her diaper so that the nurse could weigh it to make sure she was passing enough urine.*

Dacarbazine (da-KAR-ba-zeen)

How given: Intravenous (IV)

How it works: Dacarbazine is an alkylating agent that prevents cancer cell reproduction.

Precautions: The child should be given an antinausea drug prior to infusion. Dacarbazine causes severe skin reactions if it leaks outside the IV.

Common side effects:

- Low blood counts, which may increase risk of infection or bleeding and cause weakness, fatigue, and paleness
- Nausea, vomiting, and diarrhea

- Hair loss that is not permanent

- Sun sensitivity

- Loss of appetite

- Mouth sores

- Flu-like symptoms, including low fever and body aches

Infrequent side effects:

- Pain on injection if the drug is given through a peripheral vein

- Clotting in blood vessels in the liver

- Allergic reactions

- Confusion, blurred vision, and seizures

Hints for parents: Make sure to have an adequate supply of antinausea medication at home during treatment with this drug. Ibuprofen or Tylenol® will help relieve flu-like symptoms if your child develops these. Promptly report any neurological or visual symptoms to your child's doctor or nurse. Avoid prolonged sun exposure and use SPF 30 sunscreen liberally when your child is outside.

Dexamethasone (dex-a-METH-a-zone)

See **Prednisone**

Etoposide (e-TOE-poe-side)

How given: Intravenous (IV) injection or infusion; pills by mouth (PO)

How it works: Etoposide prevents DNA from reproducing and causes cells to die.

Precautions: No live vaccines should be given while taking etoposide. It also interacts with several common drugs and herbs, such as aspirin, cyclosporine, glucosomide, and St. John's wort. Etoposide may cause birth defects if taken during pregnancy. It can also irritate the vein where it is injected or damage nearby tissue if it leaks out of the vein.

Common side effects:

- Low blood counts, which may increase risk of infection or bleeding and cause weakness, fatigue, and paleness

- Loss of appetite

- Nausea and vomiting
- Hair loss that is not permanent
- Temporary changes in menstrual cycle in girls

Infrequent side effects:
- Low blood pressure
- Shortness of breath
- Numbing of fingers and toes
- Fever with or without chills

Gemtuzumab (jem-TOO-zah-mab)

How given: Intravenous (IV)

How it works: Gemtuzumab is a monoclonal antibody that binds to and enters cancer cells, then delivers a substance that causes the cells' DNA to break, thus inhibiting growth. It is a targeted therapy that only affects cancer cells.

Precautions: Although few side effects have been reported, in very rare cases, patients suffer from veno-occlusive disease (VOD), in which the small veins in the liver become blocked. This condition is a medical emergency. The signs of VOD include swelling or tenderness of the liver and increased bilirubin levels in the blood.

Common side effects:
- Low blood counts, which may increase risk of infection or bleeding and cause weakness, fatigue, and paleness
- Fever
- Chills

Infrequent side effects:
- Liver toxicity
- Mouth sores
- Rashes
- Cold sores or fever blisters

Ifosfamide (eye-FOSS-fah-mide)

How given: Intravenous (IV)

How it works: Ifosfamide is an alkylating agent that disrupts DNA in cancer cells, preventing reproduction.

Precautions: The child should be given extra fluids by mouth or intravenously during infusion. Mesna®, a drug that protects the bladder, should also be given. Your child must urinate every 1 to 2 hours during the treatment, and her urine will be tested for blood.

Common side effects:

- Hair loss that is not permanent
- Low blood counts, which may increase risk of infection or bleeding and cause weakness, fatigue, and paleness
- Nausea and vomiting
- Dizziness
- Excessive sleepiness and mental confusion

Infrequent side effects:

- Kidney damage that may be permanent
- Bladder irritation and bleeding
- Liver damage
- Irritation to veins used for administration

Hints for parents: Have your child drink plenty of fluid, if possible, prior to treatment. This drug is usually given over 3 to 5 consecutive days, so make sure you have an adequate supply of antinausea medicine at home for your child. This drug may cause the kidneys to lose important substances, such as calcium and phosphorus, and it may be necessary for your child to take oral supplements.

Interferon-alpha (in-ter-FEAR-on-AL-fah)

How given: Subcutaneous (SQ), intramuscular (IM), or intravenous (IV) injection

How it works: Interferon-alpha boosts the body's immune system, enabling it to fight cancer cells. It may also directly interfere with the growth of malignant cells.

Precautions: In very rare cases, interferon-alpha can cause permanent vision loss or congestive heart failure. Patients using interferon should have regular thyroid tests. The drug interacts with theophylline, a drug used to treat respiratory diseases.

Common side effects:

- Fatigue
- Flu-like symptoms
- Low blood counts, which may increase risk of infection or bleeding and cause weakness, fatigue, and paleness

Infrequent side effects:

- Dizziness or confusion
- Depression, anxiety, or irritation
- Swelling or irritation at the injection site
- Insomnia
- Abdominal pain, nausea, vomiting, and diarrhea
- Temporary hair loss
- Rashes, sweats, dry skin, or itching
- Allergic reaction
- Tingling in hands and feet
- Swelling of feet and ankles
- Changes in taste or smell
- Dry mouth
- Temporary liver or kidney toxicity
- Chest pain or irregular heartbeat

Irinotecan (eye-rin-oh-TEE-can)

How given: Intravenous (IV)

How it works: Irinotecan is a plant alkaloid that disrupts the structure of DNA, preventing cell reproduction.

Common side effects:

- Loss of appetite
- Low blood counts, which may increase risk of infection or bleeding and cause weakness, fatigue, and paleness
- Nausea and vomiting
- Abdominal cramping and diarrhea
- Excessive sweating, salivation, and facial flushing during administration
- Hair loss that is not permanent
- Fatigue

Infrequent side effects:

- Mouth sores (stomatitis)
- Muscle cramps
- Temporary damage to the liver
- Skin rash
- Sugar in the urine
- Dizziness
- Numbness and tingling of hands and feet

Hints for parents: Many of the side effects that occur while or immediately after your child receives this drug may be controlled by the administration of a drug called atropine.

> *The big side effect that comes along with irinotecan like a shadow is diarrhea. There are two forms: early and late. Early diarrhea could happen even during the infusion (we had this problem during the second dose). Late diarrhea is every bit as much irinotecan's fault but might not be so obvious, because it can take 4 to 11 days post-infusion to show up. I guess I should say that there are really two other forms: the kind you can tolerate as a mild inconvenience and the more potent kind. Most doctors suggest that Imodium A-D® (over the counter) be given per label instructions, and if that doesn't control the diarrhea, you should call them for something more.*

Our second-line drug was Lomotil® by prescription (we gave that AND Imodium® and still had no luck). Use common sense with any diarrhea. Call in if it seems out of line, and hydrate, hydrate, hydrate to replace the fluids.

Seizure medications may affect the metabolism of irinotecan, and families should check with their medical team about interaction of seizure medications with other chemotherapy drugs as well.

Lomustine (low-MUS-teen)

How given: Capsules by mouth (PO)

How it works: Lomustine is an alkylating agent that interferes with DNA and RNA replication, resulting in cell death.

Precautions: Your child will probably have baseline pulmonary function tests performed, and these will be repeated at specified intervals throughout treatment with this drug.

Common side effects:

• Low blood counts, which may increase risk of infection or bleeding and cause weakness, fatigue, and paleness

• Nausea and vomiting

• Loss of appetite

• Hair loss that is not permanent

Infrequent side effects:

• Mouth sores

• Kidney damage

• Permanent lung damage

• Disorientation and confusion

• Menstrual cycle irregularities

• Second cancer (cancer that occurs as a result of treatment)

Hints for parents: Give your child her dose of this drug at bedtime to decrease the possibility of nausea and vomiting. Promptly report any shortness of breath or dry, nonproductive cough to your child's doctor.

Methotrexate (meth-o-TREX-ate)

How given: Intravenous (IV) infusion

How it works: Methotrexate is an antimetabolite that replaces nutrients in the cancer cells, causing cell death.

Precautions: Children should not be given extra folic acid in vitamins or the methotrexate will not be effective. Several drugs can cause methotrexate to stay in the system too long or worsen its side effects. Some of these drugs include aspirin, non-steroidal anti-inflammatory drugs, penicillin, bactrim, septra, and several anti-seizure drugs. Children taking methotrexate are very sensitive to the sun and should always wear protective clothing and sunscreen.

Common side effects:

- Low blood counts, which may increase risk of infection or bleeding and cause weakness, fatigue, and paleness
- Extreme sun sensitivity, including allergic reactions
- Diarrhea
- Skin rashes

Infrequent side effects:

- Mouth sores
- Temporary hair loss
- Nausea and vomiting
- Loss of appetite
- Fever, with or without chills
- Liver damage (temporary)
- Kidney damage (temporary)
- Shortness of breath and dry cough
- Nervous system damage (can be temporary or permanent)
- Neurotoxicity that can cause learning disabilities
- Redness at the site of previous radiation ("radiation recall")

Hints for parents: Most of the common side effects of this drug are temporary and reversible. Mouth sores can be quite painful, and your child may not eat or drink well when she has them. Always remember to have your child use sunscreen when playing outside (SPF 30 or higher). Minor skin rashes can be treated effectively with over-the-counter cortisone cream. When given as high-dose therapy, methotrexate requires administration of a reversing agent (antidote) called leucovorin. It is critical that your child begin the leucovorin at the correct time to prevent serious, possibly irreversible, side effects.

> Carl was on an experimental IV high-dose methotrexate protocol funded through the National Institutes of Health. Side effects ranged from nausea and vomiting to diarrhea, sore bones, mood swings, and disorientation.

Prednisone (PRED-ni-zone)
Dexamethasone (dex-a-METH-a-zone)

These two steroids are grouped together because they are closely related chemically and have similar action and side effects. The biggest difference in side effects appears to be the increased risk of avascular necrosis (death of bone due to decreased blood supply) from dexamethasone.

Dexamethasone is given in high doses as a chemotherapy drug and in low doses to prevent nausea. To see the side effects of dexamethasone when it is used as an antinausea drug, look under "Drugs given to prevent nausea" later in the chapter.

How given: Pills or liquid by mouth (PO), intravenous (IV), or intramuscular (IM) injection

How they work: These drugs are hormones that kill lymphocytes.

Precautions: Every parent interviewed described problems that their child had while on prednisone or dexamethasone. The side effects ranged from mild to severe, but were universal. At high doses, steroids create major behavioral problems in children, which gradually subside after the drug is stopped.

Common side effects:

- Mood changes, from extreme irritability to rage
- Increased appetite and food obsessions
- Increased thirst
- Indigestion
- Weight gain
- Fluid retention
- Round face and protruding belly

- Sleeplessness

- Nightmares

- Nervousness, restlessness, hyperactivity

- Loss of potassium

- Loss of bone mass

- Hypersensitivity to lights, sound, and motion

Infrequent side effects:

- Decreased or blurred vision

- Seeing halos around lights

- Increased sweating

- Weakness with loss of muscle mass

- Muscle cramps or pain

- Swelling of feet or lower legs

- High blood pressure

- High blood sugar

- Hallucinations

Rachel had a dual personality on steroids. She would be fine one minute and then fly into a rage. One time, she literally had an argument with herself. She asked to watch a tape, and then for 20 minutes she argued with herself over whether she should watch the tape. It was painful to watch.

• • • • •

Steroids were the worst drugs for Katy. She hallucinated horrible things. She'd scream that boys were chasing her or that her heart had stopped beating. She'd sob that I was melting and would disappear. She'd dig her fingers into my arm begging me to help her. She sometimes did this all night, and nothing consoled her. She slept very little while taking steroids. She spent day after day and night after night in my arms while I rocked her in the rocking chair, only leaving my arms to eat huge amounts of food. She would eat an entire loaf of bread, and always asked to have "butter spread on it like icing on a cake." She has never once said that since ending treatment.

• • • • •

When you add steroids to a teen boy's already hyped up emotional level, you get ignition. It helped to talk to him about how it would change how he feels and thinks. After a while, he could describe how he was becoming more agitated and wanted to stay in his room alone. He really didn't like being crabby and angry and would voluntarily isolate himself. I suggested ways for him to control his environment while on the steroids so things wouldn't irritate him as much. He also knew that rules of behavior did not change just because he was on steroids.

Procarbazine (pro-KAR-ba-zeen)

How given: Pills by mouth (PO)

How it works: Procarbazine is an alkylating agent that prevents cancer cell reproduction.

Precautions: This drug is best taken at bedtime, and it is often helpful to take antinausea medicine 30 minutes before taking the drug. Adverse effects, such as headache, tremor, excitation, heart arrhythmias, and visual problems, may occur if the drug is taken with foods rich in tyramine such as fermented cheese, cured meat, and fava beans.

Common side effects:

- Low blood counts 2 to 3 weeks after taking the drug
- Nausea, vomiting, and diarrhea
- Mouth sores
- Skin rash and itching
- Sun sensitivity
- Light sensitivity, double vision
- Low blood pressure
- Rapid heart rate
- Flu-like symptoms, including low fever and body aches
- Tingling and weakness in hands and feet, dizziness, lethargy, nightmares, hallucinations, seizures

Infrequent side effects:

- Frequent urination
- Blood in the urine
- Drug interactions with ephedrine, epinephrine, tricyclic antidepressants, certain narcotic drugs (Demerol®), antihistamines, barbiturates, and certain high blood pressure medications
- Increased side effects if the drug is taken with tyramine-rich foods, such as those listed in the "Precautions" section above

Hints for parents: Make sure to have an adequate supply of antinausea medication at home during treatment with this drug. Give your child the antinausea medication about 30 minutes before giving this drug. Ibuprofen or Tylenol® will help relieve flu-like symptoms if your child develops these. Promptly report any neurological or visual symptoms to your child's doctor or nurse. Avoid prolonged sun exposure, and use SPF 30 sunscreen liberally if your child is outside. Be sure to tell the doctor if your child is taking any drugs that can enhance the side effects of this drug. Avoid tyramine-rich foods while your child is taking this drug.

Temozolamide (tem-oh-ZO-la-mide)

How given: Capsules by mouth (PO)

How it works: Temozolamide works as an alkylating agent to interfere with DNA replication, causing cell death.

Precautions: Capsules should not be broken open. If this inadvertently occurs, avoid inhaling the powder or directly touching it.

Common side effects:

- Low blood counts, which may increase risk of infection or bleeding and cause weakness, fatigue, and paleness

- Hair loss that is not permanent

- Nausea and vomiting

- Headache

- Constipation

- Fatigue

Infrequent side effects:

- Seizures

- Dizziness

- Poor coordination

- Weakness on one side of the body

- Infertility

- Second cancer (cancer that occurs as a result of treatment)

Hints for parents: Give your child this medication at bedtime to decrease nausea. Capsules should be swallowed whole and not chewed. The manufacturer states that mixing with applesauce or apple juice is acceptable for children who cannot swallow capsules.

> *I gave Nikki her Zofran® and Temodar® [temozolomide] every night for 42 nights on and 28 off. I let her eat dinner and dessert and do a time check. One hour after her last bite, she would take 4 mg Zofran and 1 hour following that, I'd give her the Temodar® [temozolomide].*

Thalidomide (tha-li-DO-mide)

How given: Capsules by mouth (PO)

How it works: Thalidomide is an anti-angiogenesis agent that may disrupt the blood supply to the tumor, resulting in death of tumor cells.

Precautions: Girls of childbearing age must not become pregnant while taking this drug because it can cause serious birth defects.

Common side effects:

- Drowsiness and excessive sleeping
- Tingling and weakness of the hands and feet
- Constipation
- Dizziness when sitting or standing up
- Low blood counts, which may increase risk of infection or bleeding and cause weakness, fatigue, and paleness

Infrequent side effects:

- Slow heart rate
- Allergic reactions
- Severe skin reactions (Stevens-Johnson syndrome)
- Severe birth defects

Hints for parents: Your child should take this drug at bedtime. Give your child a stool softener during therapy with this drug to prevent constipation.

Thiotepa (thigh-oh-TEE-pah)

How given: Intramuscular (IM), intrathecal (IT), intravenous (IV)

How it works: Thiotepa is an alkylating agent that disrupts DNA and inhibits protein synthesis.

Precautions: A small percentage of children have an allergic reaction to this drug.

Common side effects:

• Low blood counts, which may increase risk of infection or bleeding and cause weakness, fatigue, and paleness

• Nausea and vomiting

• Loss of appetite

• Headache and dizziness

• Weakness of the legs and tingling after intrathecal injection

Infrequent side effects:

• Hair loss that is not permanent

• Allergic reactions

• Severe mouth sores

• Bronzing, redness, peeling skin

• Confusion, cognitive impairment

• Impaired fertility

• Second cancer (cancer occurring as a result of treatment)

Hints for parents: Two to three showers per day are necessary to reduce the possibility of serious skin reactions. When skin peeling occurs, keeping the skin clean and dry is very important. Your child may become very confused for several days after receiving this drug and, depending on her age and developmental level, may require much patience and comforting.

Topotecan (toe-poe-TEE-can)

How given: Intravenous (IV)

How it works: Topotecan is a derivative of a plant alkaloid and interferes with an enzyme involved in maintaining the structure of DNA.

Precautions: Dose may need to be adjusted for children with kidney damage.

Common side effects:

- Low blood counts, which may increase risk of infection or bleeding and cause weakness, fatigue, and paleness
- Nausea and vomiting
- Diarrhea
- Loss of appetite
- Hair loss that is not permanent
- Headache during the infusion
- Dizziness and light-headedness during the infusion
- Fever
- Fatigue

Infrequent side effects:

- Mouth sores
- Skin rashes
- Kidney damage
- Elevated blood pressure and heart rate
- Blood in the urine

Hints for parents: Your child may have diarrhea during treatment with this drug that persists for several days after therapy is completed.

> Matthew tolerated the topotecan very well. He had the usual nausea and vomiting that he experienced with other chemotherapy drugs, though. He wouldn't eat much during the treatments, but within a day or two he was usually back to his old self again.

Vinblastine (vin-BLAS-teen)

How given: Intravenous (IV)

How it works: Vinblastine is an alkaloid derived from the periwinkle plant that causes cells to stop dividing.

Precautions: Care should be taken to prevent leakage of vinblastine from the IV site. The child should take medications to prevent constipation.

Common side effects:

- Low blood counts, which may increase risk of infection or bleeding and cause weakness, fatigue, and paleness
- Nausea and vomiting, usually mild
- Constipation
- Pain and a burn if the medicine leaks into the tissues

Infrequent side effects:

- Hair loss that is not permanent
- Mouth sores
- Headache
- Numbness or tingling in fingers and toes

Hints for parents: This drug is often given weekly for a number of weeks. Start a mild stool softener when your child begins taking this drug. If your child develops a burning sensation in the anus from the medication, promptly notify your child's doctor or nurse.

Vincristine (Vin-CRIS-teen)

How given: Intravenous (IV) injection or infusion

How it works: Vincristine is an alkyloid derived from the periwinkle plant. It causes cells to stop dividing.

Precautions: Care should be taken to prevent leakage of vincristine from the IV site because it will damage tissue. Before taking the first dose of vincristine, your child should be started on a program to prevent constipation. Vincristine interacts with several other chemotherapy drugs, so care should be taken in planning the dosing schedule. Grapefruit or grapefruit juice may affect the functioning of this drug, so parents should check with the doctor about whether their child should avoid these while taking vincristine. Children on vincristine should be tested frequently for kidney and liver toxicity.

Common side effects:

- Severe constipation

- Pain (may be severe) in jaw, face, back, joints, and/or bones

- Foot drop (child has trouble lifting front part of foot)

- Numbness, tingling, or pain (may be severe) in fingers and toes

- Extreme weakness and loss of muscle mass

- Drooping eyelids

- Hair loss that is not permanent

- Pain, blisters, and skin loss if drug leaks during administration

Infrequent side effects:

- Headaches

- Dizziness and light-headedness

- Seizures

- Paralysis

Hints for parents: This drug is given weekly for a number of weeks and then monthly. Start your child on a stool softener at the beginning of treatment with this drug and give it consistently. Jaw pain is an early and temporary side effect, but it is often severe enough to warrant an oral narcotic. Watch your child's gait and strength, especially going up and down stairs and performing fine-motor activities, such as coloring, writing, or buttoning clothes. Report problems in these areas to your doctor promptly so your child's dose can be altered. Sometimes medications (e.g., Neurontin®) and physical therapy are necessary to counteract the neurological effects of this drug.

> *Erica (diagnosed at age 1) once had a vincristine burn on her arm at the IV site. It was red when we went home from the clinic, but by the second day it was badly burned. She developed a blister as big as a half dollar, which left a bad scar. It hurt and was sensitive for a long time. She also developed severe foot drop (she could not lift up the front part of her foot) and fell a lot.*

· · · · ·

Preston (diagnosed age 10) had an awful time from vincristine. He would develop cramping in his lower legs, and would just curl up in bed, in great pain. It would start a couple of days after he received the vincristine, and would last a week. I would massage his legs, use hot packs, and give him Tylenol®. I would have to carry him into the clinic, because he couldn't walk. I did some research and discovered that when the bilirubin is high, the child can't excrete the vincristine and therefore the toxicity is increased. We lowered his vincristine dose and got him into physical therapy.

· · · · ·

Soon after diagnosis at age 5½, Robby became so weak in the hospital that he stopped walking. He did not walk for at least a week, maybe more. When Robby did walk, he was up on his toes. I kept asking the doctors about it, and they poohpoohed it, saying it was just the vincristine. Finally, I took Robby to the pediatrician, who was horrified at how bad his feet had gotten. We immediately started daily physical therapy and major exercises and got traction boots to wear at night.

Prophylactic antibiotics

Children and teens on chemotherapy take antibiotics 2 to 3 days each week to prevent pneumocystis pneumonia (PCP). They usually continue taking the antibiotics for a few months to a year after treatment ends. The antibiotic of choice for PCP prevention is a combination drug containing sulfamethoxazole and trimethoprim; it is sold under the brand names Bactrim® and Septra®. This antibiotic can cause gastrointestinal upset, skin rashes, sun sensitivity, and low blood counts. If a substitute is needed, one of the following is used:

• Pentamidine, administered as an aerosol or through a nebulizer (can be difficult for children because it takes 20 minutes to administer and it smells and tastes bad), or by IV once a month.

• Dapsone®, pills given orally every day.

> *We just started the Dapsone® because Katie was starting to buck the nebulizer treatment. (It smells and tastes horrible.) The Bactrim® costs about $3/month, the dapsone about $7/month, and the pentamidine nebulizer treatment is about $300/month!*

Colony-stimulating factors

Colony-stimulating factors (CSFs) are often used for children with brain tumors or for those who have had stem cell transplants. High-dose chemotherapy reduces the number of white blood cells used by the body to fight infections. The administration of CSFs, such as granulocyte colony-stimulating factor (G-CSF) and granulocyte-macrophage colony-stimulating factor (GM-CSF), can reduce the severity and duration of low white blood counts, lessening the chance of infection. G-CSF may be administered by IV or by subcutaneous injection. GM-CSF must be administered by subcutaneous injection.

> Kenny was only 2 years old when he was receiving G-CSF, so he was too young to understand why he needed the shots. He would cry and beg us not to hurt him—that he was sorry. My heart would break, but I would have to give him the shot. We finally developed a really good system. Right before being discharged after a round of chemo, we would put EMLA® on Kenny's arm and then have the nurse place an insulflon. It was a small catheter that Kenny didn't even notice was in his arm. It was good for 7 to 10 days, which was the duration of his G-CSF for the entire month. We would draw up the amount needed for injection, then place it in the insulflon and inject it very slowly. Kenny never felt it and no longer begged us not to do the G-CSF. Oh, how I wished we had done this from the beginning! Kenny's counts would usually start to decline about 4 days after his chemo. At about Day 10 the G-CSF would kick in, and his counts would skyrocket.

· · · · ·

> Katie had no side effects from Neupogen® that I can recall. The worst thing about it for us was giving the shots at home. They're subcutaneous, so the needle is short, but Katie still said they hurt, even with EMLA®.

Antinausea drugs used during chemotherapy

Antinausea drugs, also referred to as antiemetics, make chemotherapy treatments more bearable, but they sometimes cause side effects. The following section lists some commonly used antinausea drugs.

There are many drugs used to prevent nausea that are not described here, including Marinol®, Reglan®, scopolamine patch, and Atarax®.

Antinausea drug list

As with chemotherapy drugs, several different names can be used to refer to each antinausea drug. The list below will help you find detailed information about each drug on the following pages.

Drug Names	Brand Name(s)
Aprepitant	Emend®
Diphenhydramine	Benadryl®
Granisetron	Granisol®, Kytril®, Sancuso®
Lorazepam	Ativan®
Ondansetron	Zofran®
Prochlorperazine	Compazine®
Promethazine	Phenergan®

Aprepitant (a-PREP-it-ant)

How given: Capsule by mouth or intravenous (IV) infusion

When given: Capsule is taken 1 hour before chemotherapy. IV infusion is given over a 15-minute span, starting 30 minutes before chemotherapy.

Precaution: This drug interacts with many drugs, so make sure the pharmacist knows about every drug your child takes.

Common side effects:

- Fatigue
- Dizziness
- Constipation
- Diarrhea
- Hiccups
- Heartburn
- Itchiness
- Loss of appetite

Diphenhydramine (die-fen-HIGH-dra-meen)

How given: Liquid, pills, or capsules by mouth, or intravenous (IV) injection

When given: Usually given every 6 to 8 hours.

Common side effects:

- Drowsiness
- Dizziness
- Impaired coordination
- Dry mouth
- Excitability (in young children)
- Low blood pressure

Granisetron (gran-ISS-eh-tron)

How given: Intravenous (IV) injection, pills by mouth (PO), or a patch on the skin (called Sancuso®)

When given: Granisetron is usually given 30 minutes prior to the start of chemotherapy infusion. Doses may be repeated every 12 to 24 hours.

Common side effects:

- Headaches
- Diarrhea
- Constipation

Infrequent side effects

- High blood pressure
- Fatigue
- Fever
- Allergic reaction
- Abnormal heart rhythms

Sarah got Zofran® at first, then the clinic switched to liquid Kytril®. Sarah usually hates liquid meds (she much prefers pills), but she loves Kytril®. She thinks it's really yummy. And it works, too!

· · · · ·

Kytril® is an antinausea pill. It is incredibly expensive but brilliant in treating chemo-related sickness. It sometimes takes a bit of juggling to get the timing right; Michael used to take it an hour before taking the CCNU, which he then took at bedtime and slept right through with no ill effects. None of the other antiemetics worked for him nearly as well.

Lorazepam (lor-AZ-a-pam)

How given: Pills or liquid by mouth (PO), sublingually (pill dissolved under the tongue), or subcutaneous (Sub-Q), intravenous (IV), or intramuscular (IM) injection

When given: This tranquilizer is generally given in combination with other antinausea drugs.

Precaution: This drug interacts with several other drugs, so parents should tell the doctor about everything else their child is taking, including over-the-counter drugs.

Common side effects:
- Drowsiness and sleepiness
- Poor short-term memory
- Impaired coordination
- Low blood pressure
- Excitability (in young children)

Ondansetron (on-DAN-se-tron)

How given: Intravenous (IV) injection, liquid by mouth, pills by mouth (PO), or sublingual (pill dissolved under the tongue)

When given: Usually given 30 minutes prior to chemotherapy drugs, then every 4 to 8 hours until nausea ends or in a higher dose once a day.

Note: Ondansetron comes in flavored oral solutions; 1 teaspoon = 4 mg. You can mix the dose in a small amount of a drink your child likes.

Common side effects:

• Headache with rapid IV administration

• Diarrhea

• Constipation

Infrequent side effects:

• Serious allergic reaction

• Abnormal heart rhythm

> *After Jeremy had his first inpatient treatment, he was allowed to go on an outpatient basis, wearing a cad pump at home. He felt fine, but every couple hours he would vomit for no reason. The next morning, when his oncologist asked him how it had gone, Jeremy was hesitant to tell him about the vomiting. When he did, the doctor asked us if the Zofran® hadn't helped. I gave him a confused look and asked him what a Zofran® was. I can laugh about it now, but it was an oversight. Everyone thought someone else had taken care of it! We rarely had any problems with nausea after that.*

· · · · ·

> *The absolute best for me were the Zofran® lozenges: simply dissolve on or under the tongue for instant relief. The prescription must state lozenges. You'll love those "melty pills."*

· · · · ·

> *Ondansetron works great for Ethan. He does have late nausea after chemo, so he takes it once a day for 10 days afterwards, and hasn't vomited or felt nauseated.*

Prochlorperazine (pro-chlor-PAIR-a-zeen)

How given: Pills, long-acting capsule, or liquid by mouth; rectal suppository; or intramuscular (IM) or intravenous (IV) injection

When given: Used alone if only mild nausea is expected.

Common side effects:

• Drowsiness

• Low blood pressure

• Nervousness and restlessness

• Uncontrollable muscle spasms, especially of jaw, face, and hands

• Blurred vision

Promethazine (pro-METH-ah-zeen)

How given: Pills or liquid by mouth (PO), rectal suppository, or intramuscular (IM) or intravenous (IV) injection

When given: Usually given every 4 to 6 hours.

Common side effects:

- Drowsiness

- Dizziness

- Impaired coordination

- Fatigue

- Blurred vision

- Euphoria

- Insomnia

Drugs used to relieve pain

As with other medicines, drugs used for pain relief can be given by various methods and can cause side effects. The following section lists some drugs commonly used to relieve pain. Many other medications are used to relieve pain in children, including acetaminophen, nalbuphine, fentanyl, hydrocodone, and others.

Pain medication list

Several different names can be used to refer to each of the pain medications. You may hear the same drug referred to by its generic name, an abbreviation, or one of several brand names, depending on which doctor, nurse, or pharmacist you talk to. The following list provides the generic name of several commonly used pain medications and some of the most common brand names.

Drug Names	Brand Name(s)
Codeine	Codrix®
Dexamethasone	Decadron®
Hydromorphone	Dilaudid®

Drug Names	Brand Name(s)
Meperidine	Demerol®, Mepergan®
Methadone	Methadose®, Dolophine®
Morphine	Astramorph PF®, Avinza®, Duramorph®, Infumorph®, Kadian®, MS Contin®, Oramorph SR®, Roxanol®
Oxycodone	Percocet®, Percodan®, Oxycontin®, Roxicet®, Roxilox®, Roxycodone®, M-Oxy®, Oxyfast®, OxyIR®, ETH-Oxydose®, Tylox®

Codeine

How given: Intramuscular (IM) injection, intravenous (IV) injection or infusion, sub-cutaneous injection (Sub-Q), or pills or liquid by mouth (PO)

How it works: Codeine is an opiate that reduces pain.

Note: Codeine is added to numerous other non-narcotic pain relievers.

Common side effects:

- Light-headedness
- Dizziness
- Sedation
- Euphoria
- Constipation

Infrequent side effects:

- Nausea
- Vomiting
- Allergic reaction
- Slowed heart rate

Dexamethasone

How given: Intravenous (IV) injection or pill by mouth (PO)

Note: At low doses, this drug is used to treat headaches associated with increased intracranial pressure.

Common side effects:

- Euphoria
- Restlessness
- Confusion

Hydromorphone

How given: Intravenous (IV) injection or infusion, pill by mouth (PO), rectal suppository, or subcutaneous (Sub-Q) injection

How it works: Hydromorphone is a narcotic pain reliever.

Precautions: Hydromorphone can cause slowed breathing.

Common side effects:

- Dizziness and light-headedness
- Sedation
- Nausea and vomiting
- Excessive sweating
- Euphoria and other mood alterations
- Headaches
- Constipation
- Slowed breathing

Infrequent side effects:

- Hallucination and disorientation
- Diminished circulation
- Shock
- Cardiac arrest

Meperidine

How given: Intravenous (IV), intramuscular (IM), or subcutaneous (Sub-Q) injection; or liquid or pill by mouth (PO). It is not as effective if taken by mouth.

How it works: Meperidine is a narcotic that works similarly to morphine.

Common side effects:

- Sedation
- Constipation
- Dizziness
- Nausea and vomiting
- Dry mouth
- Flushing or sweating

Infrequent side effects:

- Respiratory depression (slowed breathing)
- Decreased blood pressure
- Seizures
- Headaches
- Visual disturbances
- Mood changes
- Slowed heart rate

Methadone

How given: Intravenous (IV), intramuscular (IM), or subcutaneous (Sub-Q) injection; or liquid or pill by mouth (PO)

How it works: Methadone is a narcotic pain reliever.

Common side effects:

- Light-headedness and dizziness
- Sedation
- Nausea and vomiting

- Excessive sweating
- Euphoria
- Constipation
- Loss of appetite

Infrequent side effects:
- Respiratory depression (slowed breathing)
- Decreased circulation
- Depression or euphoria
- Confusion
- Shock

Morphine

How given: Intravenous (IV) injection or infusion, pill by mouth (long-acting or short-acting), liquid by mouth, or suppository

How it works: Morphine is a narcotic derived from the opium plant.

Common side effects:
- Euphoria
- Nausea and vomiting
- Sedation
- Dry mouth
- Headaches
- Drowsiness
- Constipation

Infrequent side effects:
- Reduction in body temperature
- Respiratory depression (slowed breathing)
- Allergic reactions, including hives
- Seizures

Zachary's first surgery was fairly easy to recover from. His second, however, had a horrible 3-week recovery period, involving painful bladder spasms, extreme diarrhea, an infection in his Hickman® line, and massive weight loss. It took a lot of morphine to help him feel comfortable.

Oxycodone

How given: Pills or liquid by mouth (PO)

How it works: Oxycodone is a narcotic derived from opium.

Common side effects:

- Light-headedness
- Dizziness
- Sedation
- Constipation
- Nausea and vomiting

Infrequent side effects:

- Respiratory depression (slowed breathing)
- Skin rash
- Mood changes
- Headaches
- Insomnia
- Low blood pressure
- Slowed heart rate
- Delayed digestion
- Allergic reactions

Topical anesthetics to prevent pain

Several products are commonly used to prevent pain from injections, finger pricks, IV insertions, and spinal taps. Most of these drugs fall into two categories, which are described below. Use of these drugs is also discussed in Chapter 6, *Coping with Procedures*.

Topical anesthetizing creams

Examples: EMLA®, ELA-Max®, and many other brand names

How given: Each product has slightly different instructions. In general, they are applied to the skin between 30 to 90 minutes before a procedure. Some must be covered with an airtight dressing.

How they work: These are creams that contain the topical anesthetic lidocaine. ELA-Max® uses lidocaine alone; EMLA® uses lidocaine in combination with prilocaine.

Note: It may take longer than an hour to achieve effective anesthesia in dark-skinned children. When using EMLA®, sometimes the blood vessels constrict, making it harder to find a vein. To prevent this problem, it helps to apply a warm damp cloth immediately before the injection. For more information about use of these products, see Chapter 6, *Coping with Procedures*.

> We use EMLA® for everything: finger pokes, accessing port, shots, spinal tap. I even let her sister use it for shots because it lets her get a bit of attention, too. Both of my children have sensitive skin that turns red when they pull off tape, so I cover the EMLA® with plastic wrap held in place with paper tape. I also fold back the edge of each piece of tape to make a pull tab so the kids don't have to peel each edge back from their skin.

Vapocoolant sprays

Examples: Fluori-Methane Spray® and Fast Freeze®

How given: This aerosol spray is applied to the sterilized target area immediately before the procedure. It can also be applied by spraying the solution into a medicine cup for 10 seconds, then dipping a cotton ball into the solution and holding it on the site for 15 seconds immediately before the procedure.

How they work: Most vapocoolant sprays use the refrigerant ethyl chloride to numb the area before an injection or infusion.

Note: If the spray is applied too long, it can cause frostbite. Spray just until skin begins to turn white (3 to 10 seconds). The spray can should be held between 3 and 9 inches away from the skin.

Complementary treatments

In recent years, increasing research has been done on mind-body medicine and its effect on coping with the side effects of illness. Complementary (also called adjunctive) therapies are those that can be expected to add something beneficial to the treatment. For example, imagery and hypnosis are widely used to help children and teens prepare for or cope with medical procedures. Other helpful complementary therapies are relaxation, biofeedback, massage, visualization, acupuncture, meditation, music therapy, aromatherapy, Reiki, and prayer.

> *Christine was terrified of needles, and it was a nightmare every time we went in to get her port accessed or blood drawn. We went to a psychologist who specialized in methods to cope with pain. She taught my daughter visualization. They made an audiotape of an underwater snorkeling trip. It included watching all of the colorful fish and feeling the soothing warm water. She would listen to it in the clinic, or visualize the trip without the tape. It really helped her develop a technique to cope with accessing the port.*

Alternative treatments

Alternative treatments can be defined as either treatments that are used in place of conventional medical treatments or treatments that may have unknown or adverse effects when used in addition to conventional treatments. Sometimes alternative treatments are illegal or unavailable in the United States or Canada, and patients travel to other countries to obtain them.

Alternative treatments are usually based on word-of-mouth endorsements, called anecdotal evidence. Medical therapy is based on scientific studies using data collected from large groups of patients. In treating cancer, these large clinical trials have resulted in increases in survival rates over the past 3 decades.

Many alternative treatments can help parents and children feel they are aiding the healing process. Even with a good prognosis for your child, it is difficult to ignore the advice of friends and relatives extolling the virtues of various alternative treatments. Parents just want to help their children in every way possible; they often feel helpless and agonize over the pain their child endures for many months or years while on conventional therapy.

However, it is extremely important that any alternative therapy that involves ingestion or injection into the body (e.g., herbs, vitamins, special diets, enemas) only be given with the neuro-oncologist's knowledge. The neuro-oncologist's involvement is necessary to prevent you from giving something to your child that could lessen the effectiveness of the conventional chemotherapy or cause additional toxicity. For instance, folic acid (a type of B vitamin) replaces methotrexate in cells and reduces or eliminates its effectiveness, allowing cancer cells to flourish. The neuro-oncologist will be much more knowledgeable about these potential conflicts than a parent, herbalist, or health food store salesperson.

If you want to evaluate claims made about alternative treatments, here are several ways to collect information:

- Check the National Institutes of Health's National Center for Complementary and Alternative Medicine to see if any scientific evidence or warnings exist about the treatment that interests you. This information is available online at *http://nccam.nih.gov.*

- Contact your local American Cancer Society or Canadian Cancer Society's division office and ask for information about the therapy you are considering. These organizations have compiled information about many therapies describing the treatment, its known risks, side effects, opinions of the medical establishment, and any lawsuits that have been filed in relation to the therapy. The American Cancer Society has an online database at *www.cancer.org/treatment/treatmentsandsideeffects/ complementaryandalternativemedicine/index* with information about many alternative treatments.

- Collect and study all available objective literature about the treatment. Ask the alternative treatment providers if they have treated other children with cancer, what results have been achieved, how these results have been documented, and where they have reported their results. Ask for the reports so your child's doctor can review them.

- Talk with other people who have gone through the treatment. Inquire about the training and experience of the person administering the treatment. Be sure to find out how much the therapy costs, because your insurance company may not pay for alternative treatments.

- Beware of any practitioner who will give your child the alternative therapy only if you stop taking the child in for conventional treatments.

- Never inject any alternative product into a central line. Children have developed life-threatening infections and have died from this.

Take all the information you gather to your child's neuro-oncologist to discuss any positive or negative impacts the alternative treatment may have on your child's current medical treatment. Do not give any alternative treatment or over-the-counter drugs to your child in secret. Some treatments prevent chemotherapy from killing cancer cells, and other substances, such as those containing aspirin or related compounds, can cause uncontrollable bleeding in children with low platelet counts.

> At one point, we decided to try some alternative therapies with our son. Our plan was to use it in conjunction with his conventional treatment. I scheduled a meeting with his oncologist and discussed the alternatives with him. I wouldn't dare attempt to start anything, not even vitamin supplements, without first talking it over with the doctor, because I was scared that I would cause my child more harm than good. I was grateful that the oncologist was willing to listen to what I had to say and offer his opinion.

> We both agreed that the alternative therapy we had in mind wouldn't do any damage or interfere with the chemotherapy my son was receiving. Two months later, we decided that it was doing absolutely nothing for him, so we stopped. I figured the money would be better spent at the toy store than on a useless therapy. I learned a valuable lesson from that experience. I'm much more skeptical now than I used to be. My new motto is "show me the proof."

• • • • •

> I gave my son echinacea when he received chemotherapy. I checked with his doctor first. He didn't think it would hurt but didn't think it would help, either. Still, all the nurses in emergency swore by the stuff. We got good results, too. We started the echinacea after lots of treatment, and it was the first time that he didn't have to be readmitted 3 days after chemo for febrile neutropenia. I'm convinced that it helped him during the recovery period when his counts would bottom out.

If, after thorough investigation, you feel strongly in favor of using an alternative treatment in addition to conventional treatment and your child's neuro-oncologist opposes it, listen to her reasons. If you disagree, get a second opinion from another oncology specialist. Remember, your child's health should be everyone's priority.

> When Zack (age 6) was treated, he always developed a fever after chemotherapy. I could tell when his counts were dropping because the fever would start off low and go up to around 102°. When his fever went over 101°, the doctor would put him on IV antibiotics and draw blood cultures every day. His fevers usually started about 7 days after the first day of chemo. His counts would drop real fast. For us, it became normal. He'd also always need platelet and red blood cell transfusions after chemotherapy. It was a scary time but we became used to it.

> I thank God daily for sustaining Zack this long. Yesterday was just a horrible day. But today I arose with positive thoughts. I will take care of my son and live life for we have been blessed to be his parents.

Chapter 12

Common Side Effects of Chemotherapy

In the depth of winter, I finally learned that within me there lay an invincible summer.

— Albert Camus

CHEMOTHERAPY DRUGS INTERFERE with tumor cells' ability to grow and reproduce. Because tumor cells divide frequently, they are more susceptible to chemotherapy drugs than most normal cells. Unfortunately, normal, healthy cells that multiply rapidly can also be damaged by chemotherapy. These normal cells include those of the brain, bone marrow, mouth, stomach, intestines, hair follicles, and skin.

This chapter explains the most common side effects of chemotherapy drugs and explores ways to deal with them effectively. It also covers questions about owning pets when your child is receiving chemotherapy. Chemotherapy side effects that prevent good nutrition are discussed in Chapter 20, *Nutrition*. Side effects are listed in alphabetical order below.

Bed wetting

Bed wetting can be a very upsetting side effect of cancer treatment. Some drugs increase thirst and others disrupt normal sleep patterns, both of which make bed wetting more likely. Receiving intravenous (IV) fluids at night can also cause bed wetting. When the bed wetting is caused by drugs or IVs, time will cure the problem. Once the drugs or extra fluids are no longer needed, the bed wetting will stop.

There are also psychological reasons for bed wetting during treatment. The trauma of treatment for brain and spinal cord tumors causes many children to regress to earlier behaviors such as thumb sucking, baby talk, temper tantrums, and bed wetting.

Punishment for these behaviors only adds to the child's distress and rarely solves the problem. Following are parents' suggestions:

- Adopt an attitude that lets your child know bed wetting is "no big deal." There should be no shaming or punishment.

- For younger children, you can use disposable, absorbent underwear.

- Put down a plastic liner covered by fitted and flat sheets, then put another plastic liner with a fitted and flat sheet on top. During the night, simply pull off the wet top sheets and plastic and there are fresh sheets below.

- Keep a pile of extra-large or beach towels next to the bed. Cover the wet spot with towels and save the bed change for the morning.

- Give the last drink 2 hours before bedtime so your child can go to the bathroom right before bed.

- If your child is extremely distressed by bed wetting, ask if he wants you to set the alarm for the middle of the night so he can get up and go to the bathroom.

- Change sleeping arrangements.

> *During treatment, my daughter had nightmares and frequent bed wetting. I felt if she could sleep through the night, the bed wetting might stop. I told her she could sleep with me during that round of chemo, but that after that she would move back into her own bed. It calmed her to sleep with me. The nightmares and bed wetting decreased, and she moved back into her own bed without complaint when the time came.*

- Give extra love and reassurance.

> *My teenaged son wet the bed whenever he was given antinausea medicine prior to high doses of chemotherapy. He was so embarrassed. I stayed with him every night at the hospital. He was so groggy that even if he woke up in time, I had to help him out of bed and support him while he stood, half asleep, to use the urinal.*

· · · · ·

> *When my daughter started bed wetting, I didn't think it was the drugs. I thought long and hard about any additional worries that she might have, and I realized that because her dad had emotionally withdrawn from her during her illness, she might be worried that I would do the same. So I told her one night, "You know, I just real-ized that every day I tell you how much I love you. But I've never told you that no matter how hard life gets and no matter how mad we get at each other, I will always love you. I love you now as a child, I will love you as a teenager, and I will love you when you are all grown up." She started to sob and hugged and hugged me. She has never wet the bed again.*

Changes in taste and smell

Chemotherapy can cause changes in the taste buds, altering the brain's perception of how food tastes. Meats often taste bitter and sweets can taste unpleasant. Even foods that children crave can taste bad. The sense of smell is also affected by chemotherapy, heightening smells that other family members do not notice and sometimes causing nausea in the child on chemotherapy.

Both the senses of smell and taste can take months to return to normal after chemotherapy ends. During chemotherapy and radiation treatment, it is best to avoid favorite foods that do not taste the same, so that when treatment ends they can be enjoyed once again.

> *Once Katy begged me to make her my special double chocolate sour cream cake. Surprisingly, it smelled really good to her as it baked. She took a big bite, spit it out all over the table, and ran back to her room sobbing. She cried for a long time. She told me later that it had tasted "bitter and horrible."*

Constipation

Constipation means a decrease in a child's normal number of bowel movements or dry, hard stool that is painful to pass. Some drugs, such as vincristine, slow the movement of stool through the intestines, resulting in constipation. Pain medication, decreased activity, decreased eating and drinking, and vomiting can all affect the normal rhythm of the intestines.

Following are parents' suggestions for preventing and coping with constipation:

• Encourage your child to be as physically active as possible.

• Encourage your child to drink plenty of liquids every day. Prune juice is especially helpful.

• Serve high-fiber foods such as raw vegetables, beans, bran, graham crackers, whole-wheat breads, whole-grain cereals, dried fruits (especially prunes, dates, and raisins), and nuts.

• Check with the doctor before using any medications for constipation. He may recommend a stool softener such as Colace®. If the doctor suggests liquid Docusate®, be aware that many children don't like the taste. Senokot®, another frequently prescribed stool softener, comes in a tablet, chocolate-flavored liquid, and granules that can be mixed into yogurt or ice cream. Metamucil® and Citrucel® increase the volume of the stool, which stimulates the intestines. Milk of Magnesia®, magnesium citrate, and MiraLax® help the stool retain fluid and remain soft.

Vincristine constipation resulted in horrible screaming, bottom itching, and constant trips to the bathroom with no luck, for days at a time. It is absolutely frustrating! We now have a preventative routine so that never happens again. Beginning the morning of a vincristine injection, I give one Peri-Colace® (stool softener plus laxative) each morning and evening until things improve—which is usually after about a week or so. Then, I taper down to one a day until things seem to be getting on the too soft side, then stop. The Peri-Colace® is manufactured in a brown "soft-gel" thing, and the liquid inside it tastes horrible. If at any time during our Peri-Colace® phase there are 2 consecutive days with no bowel movements, I give bisacodyl in the evening of the second day, and things usually get straightened out the next morning. Unfortunately, if it's a school day, I have to keep him home until mid-morning, as the prednisone diet and laxatives lead to a very busy morning in the bathroom.

- Do not give enemas or rectal suppositories. These can cause anal tears that can be dangerous for a child with a weakened immune system.

- When your child feels the need to have a bowel movement, sipping a warm drink can help the feces come out.

My 4-year-old daughter either had diarrhea or severe constipation for months. When constipated, she would just sob and try to hold it in. This made her stool even harder and more painful. One time she cried, "Why is my anus round and my poop square?" We ended up just putting her in a bathtub full of warm water, gave her warm drinks, and let her go in the bathtub.

Dental problems

Both cranial radiation and chemotherapy can cause changes in the mouth, teeth, and ability to salivate. Awareness of the potential problems, coupled with good preventive care, can help maintain oral health during treatment. Ask your dentist to refer to the current issue of the *Pediatric Dentistry Reference Manual* to formulate a dental plan.

During treatment, plaque can build up rapidly on your child's teeth, increasing the likelihood of cavities and gum infections. Take your child to the dentist for a cleaning and check-up every 3 to 4 months, as long as her blood counts are high (an ANC of more than 1,000 and platelets of more than 100,000). Children with a central venous catheter should be given antibiotics before and after each visit to the dentist.

When Kevin (diagnosed with posterior fossa ependymoma) turned 2, I asked our oncologists if they thought he should see a dentist, that I was worried about his teeth. They tried to take a peek at his teeth, but Kevin was like Fort Knox. They both said that he shouldn't have any problems because of his illness and that we could bring him to our regular dentist when he turned 3. When Kevin was a little over 2½, I suspected that he had a few cavities. I brought him to a local pediatric dentist.

After a horrible exam of three people holding him down, the dentist said he had four cavities. He wanted to fill them all without putting Kevin under anesthesia.

After talking to our pediatrician, she said, "Why don't you go to a Children's Hospital dentist?" So we did, and the exam was much better. Anyway, they thought he had more than four cavities and that two of his teeth would have to be removed. They wouldn't know for sure until they did an x-ray during surgery. He was put under for his surgery and they removed two teeth and filled five cavities. We were told that the cavities were probably due to radiation. He also had a right paralyzed vocal cord and right facial paralysis. He always chewed his food on the left side of his mouth. But the cavities were on both sides. And he hated to have his teeth brushed! After his cavities were filled, the Children's dentist wanted to see him every 3 months for a cleaning and checkup.

Ask your child's oncologist and dentist for advice about tooth care when counts are very low. Often parents are advised to use a sponge or damp gauze to gently wipe off their child's teeth after meals instead of brushing.

My daughter had problems with thick yellow saliva during the entire time she was treated. It coated her teeth and formed a lot of plaque. I brought her to an excellent pediatric dentist every 3 months to have the plaque removed. She took antibiotics half an hour before treatment and then again 6 hours afterward. He also put sealants on all of her molars and, even though there were many weeks when her teeth could not be brushed, she never got a cavity.

Some parents report delays in the arrival of their child's permanent teeth. Children who receive chemotherapy or cranial radiation therapy may also have poorly developed or absent permanent teeth and blunted tooth roots.

Diarrhea

Because chemotherapy destroys cells that are produced at a rapid rate, such as those that line the mouth, stomach, and intestines, it can cause diarrhea, ranging from mild (frequent, soft stools) to severe (abundant quantities of liquid stool). Diarrhea during chemotherapy can also be caused by some antinausea drugs, antibiotics, and intestinal infections. After chemotherapy ends and immune function returns to normal, the lining of the digestive tract heals and the diarrhea ends.

The following suggestions for coping with diarrhea come from parents:

- Do not give any over-the-counter drug to your child without approval from the oncologist. She might want to test your child's stool for infection prior to treating the diarrhea. Frequently recommended drugs for diarrhea are Kaopectate®, Lomotil®, and Immodium®.

- It is very important that your child drink plenty of liquids. The liquids will not increase the diarrhea, but they will replace the lost fluids.

> My 3-year-old daughter had stopped drinking from bottles long before her diagnosis. When she first began her intensive chemotherapy, she had uncontrollable, frequent diarrhea. Liquid would just gush out without warning. It was hard for her to drink from a cup, so one night she said in a small voice, "Mommy, would it be okay if I drank from a bottle again?" I said, "Of course, honey." It was a great comfort to her, and she took in a lot more fluids that way.

- Hot or cold liquids can increase intestinal contractions, so give your child lots of room-temperature clear liquids or mild juices such as water, Gatorade®, ginger ale, peach juice, or apricot nectar.

- Diarrhea depletes the body's supply of potassium, so give your child foods high in potassium, such as bananas, orange juice, baked or mashed potatoes without the skin, leafy greens, fish, tomato juice, and milk or yogurt (if tolerated).

- Low potassium can cause irregular heartbeats and leg cramps. If these occur, call the doctor.

- Do not serve greasy, fatty, spicy, or sweet foods.

- Do not serve foods high in fiber, such as bran, fruits (dried or fresh), nuts, beans, or raw vegetables.

- Serve bland, low-fiber foods such as bananas, white rice, plain noodles, applesauce, unbuttered white toast, creamed cereals, cottage cheese, fish, and chicken or turkey without the skin.

> During treatment, my son had severe diarrhea for a week. He had large amounts of liquid stool 20 times a day. I felt so sorry for him. The doctor cultured a stool specimen, but they never identified a cause. It cleared up after a week of the BRAT diet (bananas, rice, applesauce, toast).

- Keep a record of the number of bowel movements and their volume to keep the doctor informed. Call the doctor if you notice any blood in the stool, or if your child has any signs of dehydration such as dry skin, dry mouth, sunken eyes, decreased urination, or dizziness.

- Keep the area around the anus clean and dry. Wash with warm water and mild soap after every bowel movement, then gently pat the area dry.

- If your child's anus is sore, check with the doctor before using any non-prescription medicine. She may recommend using Desitin®, A&D ointment®, or Bag Balm® after each bowel movement.

During treatment, my daughter had a terribly sore rectum, which was a big problem. It hurt to have bowel movements, she'd cry and have to squeeze our hands to go, then the urine would run back and burn. She was very itchy. We carried around bags with Q-tips® and every known brand of rectal ointment—A&D®, Preparation H®, Desitin®, and Benadryl®.

• Call the doctor if your child has significant pain with bowel movements, especially if your child has low blood counts.

Fatigue and weakness

Fatigue, a feeling of weariness, is an almost universal side effect of treatment for cancer. General weakness, although different from fatigue, is caused by many of the same things and is treated the same way. Fatigue and weakness may be constant throughout therapy or intermittent. They can be minor annoyances or totally debilitating. Fatigue and weakness are usually caused by one, or a combination, of the following things:

• Cranial radiation

• Your child's body working overtime to heal tissues damaged by treatment and to rid itself of dead and dying tumor cells

• Medications to treat nausea or pain

• Mineral imbalances caused by chemotherapy, diarrhea, or vomiting

• Malnutrition caused by nausea, vomiting, loss of appetite, or taste aversions

• Anemia (low red blood cell count)

• Infections

• Emotional factors such as anxiety, fear, sadness, depression, or frustration

• Disruption of normal sleep patterns (common when hospitalized or when taking some drugs)

Following are suggestions from parents:

• Make sure your child gets plenty of rest. Naps or quiet times spaced throughout the day help.

Erica took a 2 ½ hour nap every afternoon throughout therapy. She's 4 now and off treatment, but her endurance is low and she still tires easily.

• Limit visitors if your child is weak or fatigued.

While in the hospital, my daughter was very weak. She had too many visitors, yet didn't want to hurt anyone's feelings. We worked out a signal that solved the problem. When she was too tired to continue a visit, she would place a damp washcloth on her forehead. I would then politely end the visit.

- Serve your child well-balanced meals and snacks, but don't get upset if he doesn't eat them (see next point about stress).

- Parents and children should try to avoid physical and emotional stress.

- Encourage your child to pursue hobbies or interests, if able. For example, if your child is too weak to play on an athletic team, let her go to cheer the team on.

   My eighth-grade daughter was a fabulous athlete prior to her diagnosis. When she went back to school after missing a year, she wasn't very competitive, but she managed the softball team and dressed for basketball. So she was still part of the social scene and was able to do things with the teams.

- Help your child make a prioritized list of activities. If he feels strongly that he wants to attend a certain event and you think he may run out of energy, throw a wheelchair or stroller into the car and go.

- Encourage your child to attend a kid or teen support group, and go to the parent group yourself. Seeing that others have the same problems and talking about how you are feeling can lighten the load.

Some children go through treatment without fatigue or weakness, but other children are not so lucky. The following stories describe two common experiences.

   Before Brent was diagnosed at age 6, he was exceptionally well coordinated and a very fast runner. During treatment, he slowed down to about average. He played soccer and T-ball throughout, and was very competitive.

· · · · ·

   Jeremy has had some major, persistent problems with weakness and loss of coordination. When he was 9 years old, a year off therapy, he still could not catch a ball. When he ran, he was like a robot, and the trunk of his body stayed straight. Some kids made fun of him, and he got very frustrated with himself. He had lots of physical therapy, and now, 3 years off treatment, his skills have improved, but he still has to work harder than the other kids. We put him into martial arts in hopes of further increasing his motor skills and his confidence.

Hair loss

Because hair follicle cells reproduce quickly, chemotherapy causes some or all body hair to fall out. The hair on the scalp, eyebrows, eyelashes, underarms, and pubic area may slowly thin out or fall out in big clumps.

Hair regrowth usually starts 1 to 3 months after chemotherapy ends. The color and texture may be different from the original hair. Straight hair may regrow curly; blond hair may become brown. If your child had cranial radiation for treatment of a brain tumor, some or all of the hair follicles may be permanently damaged, and your child may only experience partial or patchy regrowth in the area that was radiated.

The following suggestions for dealing with hair loss come from parents:

- When hair is thin or breaking, use a brush with very soft bristles.

- Avoid bleaches, curlers, blow dryers, and hair gels, as these may cause additional damage.

- If hair is thin, use a mild shampoo specifically designed for overtreated or damaged hair.

- A flannel blanket placed on the pillow at night will help collect hair that falls out.

- Once hair loss begins, consider a very short hair cut to ease the transition to complete hair loss.

- Recognize that coping with hair loss is difficult for almost all children, but it is especially hard on teenagers.

- Emphasize to your child that the hair loss is temporary and that it will grow back.

> During the first year after Belle was diagnosed (and lost her hair), her brother and I found some Barbie® hats/bandanas with wigs attached at the local dollar store. So the Barbies® whose heads were shaved had something to wear while their hair grew out! Belle also made numerous outfits for "chemo Barbie®" out of supplies at the hospital: napkins, masks, various kinds of tape. She even made furniture out of straws and stuff!

- Try to have your child meet children off therapy so she can see for herself that hair will regrow soon.

- Allow your child to choose a collection of hats, scarves, or cotton turbans to wear. These are tax-deductible medical expenses and may be covered by insurance.

- To order several styles of reversible, all-cotton headwear for girls and teens, contact Just in Time Soft Hats® at (215) 247-8777 or online at *www.softhats.com*. Another company called Hip Hats with Hair® sells hats with human hair, which are soft, comfortable, and fun to wear. Visit its website at *www.hatswithhair.com*.

- If your child expresses an interest in wearing a wig, take pictures of her hairstyle prior to hair loss. Also, cut snippets of hair to take in to allow a good match of original color and texture. The cost of the wig may be covered by insurance if the doctor writes a prescription for a "wig prosthesis" and includes the medical reason for the wig, such as "alopecia due to cancer chemotherapy."

- To find a wig retailer, look in the phone book's yellow pages under "Hair Replacements, Goods, and Supplies" or do an online search. The American Cancer Society, (800) ACS-2345, and some local cancer service organizations offer free wigs in some areas.

- Advocate that school-aged children be permitted to wear hats or other head coverings in school. Use a 504 Plan, described in Chapter 18, *School,* if necessary.

- Separate your feelings about baldness from your child's feelings. Many parents rush out to buy wigs and hats without discussing with their child how he or she wants to deal with baldness. Allow your child to choose whether to wear head coverings or not. Let it be okay to be bald. An oncologist comments:

  > Consider whether hair loss bothers your child. If it bothers him, then you should pursue things to hide or resolve the problem. If it bothers you but not him, then focus your efforts on trying to deal with your concern and anxiety. Think of this as an opportunity to teach him that it is what is on the inside that counts. In today's culture that places so much emphasis on outward appearance and conformity, this is a valuable lesson. It has been my experience that kids who have visible late effects after cancer treatment can adjust quite well to external differences if they are given a lot of support at home. As a parent, if you let him know he is a great kid, he will believe it.

The amount of hair loss varies among children being treated for brain or spinal cord tumors. Some children lose part of their hair, some have hair that thins out, and some quickly lose every hair on their head.

> Preston never completely lost his hair, but it became extremely thin and wispy. When he was first diagnosed, a friend bought him a fly-fishing tying kit, and he became very good at tying flies. He even began selling them at a local fishing shop. When his hair began to fall out, we would gather it up and put it in a plastic bag. He started tying flies out of his hair, and they were displayed in the shop window as "Preston's Human Hair Flies." He was only 11, but the shop owner hired him to help around the shop. He became very popular with the clientele, because everyone wanted to meet the boy who tied flies from his own hair. He really turned losing his hair into something positive.

Three-year-old Christine's hair started to fall out within 3 weeks of starting chemo. She had beautiful curly hair, but she never talked about losing it, and I thought it didn't bother her. Occasionally she would wear a hat or the hood of a sweatshirt, but most of the time she went bald. One day, I learned how she really felt. We were talking about the different colors of hair in our family, and she began shouting, "I don't have brown hair! I'm bald, just like a baby."

• • • • •

My daughter, Katie (age 11), cut and dyed her hair bright fuchsia as soon as she realized she had cancer. It made her hair seem less hers than something to play with. Then, when she started receiving chemo, she asked that it be cut and shaved really short like some of her boy friends in her class. Our local coach came over and shaved it for her. It was only about a quarter of an inch long at that point. Then when it fell out a week later, it was no big deal for her, because she had already taken it off. That was her way of controlling the situation.

Now we celebrate her baldness by painting henna designs on her head and using face paints to paint fancy designs whenever we go somewhere special, or visit the hospital. On July 4th, we painted stars and rockets in red, white, and blue. On our last visit to the hospital, we painted a floral vine with flowers and lightning bolts above her ears to show she's hot stuff. She even had her sisters add two eyes at the back of her head—to watch the doctors and nurses when her back is turned. Everyone loves to check out her head when she comes in the hospital, and she receives tons of attention as a result of it. Also, now she's beginning to play with rub-on tattoos and is placing them where the doctors like to inspect, just to surprise them when they pull up her shirt.

She also loves to dress up her head with funny wigs and masks. Last week she was dancing in the front yard with a black/blue fright wig, monster ears, a Grateful Deadhead shirt and black platform heels. She literally stopped traffic! It was a riot. She absolutely refuses to talk to most of her doctors and nurses, and is extremely shy, but this is her silly way of poking fun at them and the whole situation with her cancer.

Low blood cell counts

Bone marrow—the spongy material that fills the inside of the bones—produces red cells, white cells, and platelets. Chemotherapy drugs damage or destroy the cells inside the bone marrow and can dramatically lower the number of cells circulating in the blood. Frequent blood tests are crucial in determining whether your child needs transfusions. Many children treated for brain or spinal cord tumors require transfusions of red cells and sometimes platelets. When the number of infection-fighting white cells is low, your child is in danger of developing serious infections.

Absolute neutrophil count (ANC)

The activities of families of children with cancer revolve around the sick child's white blood cell (WBC) count, and, specifically the absolute neutrophil count (ANC). The ANC provides an indication of the child's ability to fight infection.

When a child has blood drawn for a complete blood count (CBC), one section of the lab report will state the total WBC count and a "differential." This means each type of WBC will be listed as a percentage of the total. For example, if the total WBC count is 1500 mm^3, the differential might appear as follows:

White Blood Cell Type	Percentage of Total WBC
Segmented neutrophils (also called polys or segs)	49%
Band neutrophils (also called bands)	1%
Basophils (also called basos)	1%
Eosinophils (also called eos)	1%
Lymphocytes (also called lymphs)	38%
Monocytes (also called monos)	10%

To calculate the ANC, add the percentages of segmented and band neutrophils, then multiply by the total WBC. Using the example above, the ANC is 49% + 1% = 50%; 50% of 1,500 (.50 x 1500) = 750; so the ANC is 750.

> Erica ran a fever whenever her counts were low, but nothing ever grew in her cultures. They would hospitalize her for 48 hours as a precaution. She was never on a full dose of medicine because of her chronically low counts. She's 2 years off treatment now and doing great.

How to protect a child with a low ANC

Generally, an ANC of 500 to 1,000 provides children with enough protective neutrophils to fight off exposure to infection due to bacteria and viruses. With an ANC this high, you can usually allow your child to attend all normal functions such as school, athletic events, and parties. However, it is wise to keep close track of the pattern of the rise and fall of your child's ANC. If you know the ANC is 1,000, but is on the way down, it will affect what activities are appropriate for your child. Each hospital has different guidelines concerning activities for children with low ANCs.

Following are parents' suggestions for ways to prevent and detect infections:

- Insist on frequent, lengthy (at least 1 to 2 minutes), and thorough hand washing for every member of the family. Use plenty of soap and warm water, lather well, and rub all portions of the hands, including between all the fingers and under the fingernails. Children and parents need to wash before preparing meals, before eating, after playing outdoors, and after using the bathroom.

We always had antibacterial baby wipes in our car. We washed Justin's hands, and our own, after going to any public places such as parks, museums, or restaurants. They can also be used to wipe off tables or high chairs at restaurants.

- Make sure all medical personnel at the hospital or doctor's office thoroughly wash their hands before touching your child.

- Keep your young child's diaper area and skin creases clean and dry.

- Whenever your child needs a needle stick, make sure the technician cleans your child's skin thoroughly with both betadine and alcohol.

- If your child gets a small cut, wash it with soap and water, rinse it with hydrogen peroxide, and cover it with a small bandage.

- When your child is ill, take his temperature every 2 to 3 hours. Call the doctor if your child's temperature is 101° F (38.5° C) or above.

- Do not permit anyone to take your child's temperature rectally (in the anus) or use rectal suppositories, as these may cause anal tears and increase the risk of infection and bleeding.

Believe it or not, we once stopped the nursing assistant from doing a rectal temp during an inpatient admission. When we had a room on the pediatric oncology side, this never happened. But for that admission those rooms were full, and we were on the other side of the floor.

- Do not use a humidifier, as the stagnant water can become a reservoir for contamination.

- Apply sunscreen whenever your child plays outdoors. The skin of children taking certain chemotherapy drugs or who have recently received cranial radiation therapy is sun sensitive, and a bad sunburn can easily become infected.

- Your child should not receive routine immunizations while on chemotherapy. Your child's doctor or nurse can complete medical exemption forms for your child's school.

- Siblings should not be vaccinated with the live polio virus (OPV); they should get the killed polio virus (IPV). Verify that your pediatrician is using the appropriate vaccine for the siblings.

Katy was diagnosed just a week after her younger sister, Alison, had been given the live polio vaccine. Because there was a small risk that Alison could infect any immunosuppressed child with polio, she was not allowed to visit the oncology floor of the hospital.

- If your child's ANC is low, an infected site may not become red or painful.

> *My daughter kept getting ear infections while on chemotherapy. They would find them during routine exams. I felt guilty because she never told me her ears were hurting. I told her doctor that I was worried because she didn't complain of pain, and he reassured me by telling me that she probably felt no pain because she didn't have enough white cells to cause swelling inside her ear.*

> • • • • •

> *Shawn had continual ear infections while on treatment. He had two sets of tubes surgically implanted while on chemotherapy.*

- Never give aspirin for fever, because aspirin and drugs containing aspirin interfere with blood clotting. Aspirin is not recommended for children in general. Ibuprofen may be given if approved by your child's oncologist. If your child has a fever, call the doctor before giving any medication.

- Ask your child's oncologist about using a stool softener if your child has problems with constipation. Stool softeners can help prevent anal tears.

- Call the doctor if any of the following symptoms appear: fever above 101° F (38.5° C), chills, cough, shortness of breath, sore throat, severe diarrhea, bloody urine or stool, and pain or burning while urinating. Bring your child immediately to the hospital if there is a fever and you know that your child is neutropenic (low ANC) because if not treated immediately, this could be a life-threatening situation.

> *Some people choose to keep their kids away from everything and everyone during treatment, while others restrict their activities when they're neutropenic or receiving a particularly heavy dose of chemo. You will learn how to trust your instincts and your doctor's advice, and also learn how to take your cues from your child. For us, we try to walk a fine line between keeping Hunter's life as normal and stimulating as possible, while not taking any foolish risks with his health. When he's neutropenic (ANC below 500), when he's in a particularly heavy round of chemo, or when there's chicken pox going around we keep him at home. When he's doing well then we take him out a bit more, but sensibly: no shopping malls on Saturdays, no contact with anyone who's sick, and limited contact with other kids. During the week, I will take him with me to the grocery store, or to see his grandparents or cousins, provided everyone is healthy. When he's feeling well, we also go to the park, ride our bikes, and do normal kid stuff. I carry around antibacterial hand wipes with me so I can keep him clean after playgrounds.*

Mouth and throat sores

The mouth, throat, and intestines are lined with cells that divide rapidly and can be severely damaged by chemotherapy drugs. This damage is more common for children on very intensive protocols and for those having stem cell transplants. The sores that result in the mouth, throat, and intestines are extremely painful and can prevent eating and drinking. Check your child's mouth periodically for sores, and if any are present ask the neuro-oncologist for advice. Following are some suggestions from parents:

- To prevent infection, the mouth needs to be kept as clean and free of bacteria as possible. After eating, have your child gently brush teeth, gums, and tongue with a soft, clean toothbrush.

- If your child is old enough, the doctor may recommend a rinse to decrease the amount of bacteria in your child's mouth, which helps prevent mouth sores.

> When David was told to use Peridex®, I asked the doctor if we could substitute 0.63 percent stannous fluoride rinse. He said yes. As a dentist, I knew Peridex® kills bacteria and lasts up to 8 hours, but it tastes terrible and stains teeth. Children do not like using it. The 0.63 percent stannous fluoride has the same bacteria-killing properties and also lasts up to 8 hours, but has a better taste and does not stain as badly. The fluoride also helps prevent cavities and makes the teeth less sensitive. It comes in a variety of flavors like mint, tropical, and cinnamon. It is a prescription drug that a lot of dentists dispense.

> Mix ⅛ ounce of concentrate with warm water, making 1 ounce. A measuring cup comes with the bottle. I have David swish with half the mixture for 1 minute. (Time it, because it's longer than you think!) This can only be used by kids who are old enough not to accidentally swallow it. Six-year-old David has no problem taking this once a day before he goes to bed. If and when he starts developing mouth sores, he will take it morning and evening. It's important not to eat or drink for 30 minutes after rinsing. That is why David rinses before bedtime, after he has taken his meds and brushed his teeth.

- Serve bland food, baby food, or meals put through the blender.
- Use a straw with drinks or blender-processed foods.

> Preston got bad mouth sores every time he was on high-dose metho-trexate. He could not swallow, but we were supposed to be forcing fluids to flush the drugs out. The only thing that felt good on his throat was guava nectar. It was very expensive and hard to find, and he would drink several quarts a day through a straw. Unfortunately, my daughter and husband both developed a liking for it, too. At one point, we cornered the market on guava nectar at three grocery stores in our neighborhood.

- There are several prescription products available to treat mouth sores. One common product is called "magic mouthwash," which contains an antibiotic, an antihistimine, an antifungal, and an antacid. Some formulations add dexamethasone. More information about this product is available at *www.mayoclinic.com/health/magic-mouthwash/AN02024*. If your child has painful mouth sores, ask the neuro-oncologist for a prescription. Because large amounts of lidocaine can numb the back of the throat and cause difficulty swallowing, this medication should be used at a dose recommended by the neuro-oncologist.

- Glutamine, a nutritional supplement available at most drug and health food stores, may help prevent or minimize mouth sores in some children. If your child is receiving chemotherapy with a high probability of causing mouth sores, you may want to try glutamine as a preventive measure. The powder can be mixed in juice and should be started 1 or 2 days before your child receives a cycle of chemotherapy. Be sure to get your neuro-oncologist's approval before giving glutamine.

> *Roger just began his second round of chemo. He is on lomustine, procarbazine, and some intravenous chemo. He seemed to be tolerating it fairly well until he started breaking out in terrible sores all through his mouth and under his tongue, very painful to him. He couldn't even eat. I decided to get him to gargle and swish 100% pure aloe vera juice all through his mouth. He held the aloe vera in his mouth for 5 minutes before swallowing it that night before he went to bed and then 3 or 4 times a day for the next few days until he felt better. Strangely enough, the sores were almost all gone by morning. Roger woke up the next morning and said, "Wow that stuff works fast!"*

Nausea and vomiting

The effects of anticancer drugs vary from person to person and dose to dose. A drug that makes some children violently ill often has no effect on other children. Some drugs produce no nausea until several doses have been given, but others cause nausea after a single dose. Because the effects of chemotherapy are so variable, each child's treatment for nausea must be tailored to her individual needs.

There is no relationship between the amount of nausea and the effectiveness of the medicine. The development of newer antinausea medications has made a significant impact on the amount of nausea and vomiting associated with chemotherapy. Many children eat normally and never exhibit any signs of nausea while on chemotherapy because of the effectiveness of the antinausea medications.

Following is a list of suggestions for helping children and teenagers cope with nausea and vomiting:

- Give your child antiemetic (antinausea) medications as prescribed. Nausea is easier to keep under control than to get control of, so never miss a dose.

- Ask your doctor whether a drug that blocks gastric secretions, such as Pepcid® or Zantac®, would be helpful.

- Have your child wear loose clothing, because it is both more comfortable and easier to remove if soiled.

- Try to have at least one change of clothes for your child in the car.

- Keep large zip-lock plastic bags in the car. They are an easy-to-use and highly effective container if your child gets sick. They can be sealed and disposed of quickly and neatly, ridding the car of unpleasant odors that could make your child's nausea worse.

- Carry a bucket, towels, and baby wipes in the car in case of vomiting.

- Try to keep your child in a quiet, well-ventilated room after chemotherapy.

- Try not to cook in the house when your child feels nauseated. If possible, open windows to provide plenty of fresh air. Smells can trigger nausea.

- Use a covered cup with a straw for liquids if your child is nauseated by smells.

- Do not serve hot foods if the odor aggravates your child's nausea.

- Serve dry foods such as toast, pretzels, cereal, or crackers in the morning or whenever your child is feeling nauseated.

- Serve several small meals rather than three large ones.

- Have your child keep his head elevated after eating. Lying flat can induce nausea.

- Provide plenty of clear liquids such as water, juice, Gatorade®, and ginger ale.

- Avoid serving sweet, fried, or very spicy food. Instead, stick with bland foods such as potatoes, cottage cheese, soup, bananas, applesauce, rice, or toast when your child feels nauseated.

- Watch for any signs of dehydration, including loose or dry skin, dry mouth, sunken eyes, dizziness, and decreased urination. Call the doctor if your child appears dehydrated.

- Use distractions such as TV, videos, music, games, or reading aloud to divert attention from nausea.

- Have your child rinse her mouth with water or a mixture of water and lemon juice after she vomits to help remove the taste.

- Let your child chew gum or suck on Popsicles® if he develops a metallic taste in his mouth; it may help alleviate the taste of metal.

- Consider trying acupuncture, aromatherapy, or meditation to help alleviate symptoms.

> *A friend whose wife had undergone radiation for breast cancer recommended acupuncture to us as being good for energy and mood and lessening nausea. We were*

certainly worried about his regimen, which for medulloblastoma is 13 sessions of radiation to the full cranium and spine and then 18 sessions to the tumor bed—that's an awful lot of radiation. So, Ezra went to the acupuncturist every week while he did radiation and the doctors were impressed with his energy level. The fact that he managed to pull off his bar mitzvah on the last day of 6 weeks of radiation speaks well of his stamina.

Another reason we liked the acupuncture was this: because cancer treatment is so grueling, it seems everything we do for the kids harms them in some overt way. They never saw the cancer, and in our case, did not experience any significant harm prior to diagnosis, but since then, Ezra's life has been a series of painful, damaging, exhausting, and nauseating treatments. Acupuncture was something that was only there to make him feel better, no bad effects. He likes the warm room, the soft table, the soothing music. There is a trickling fountain in the room which he loves. Because it's hard to fit this treatment into a school week, he didn't go to the acupuncturist during the 6-week rest period or the first 6-week round of chemotherapy, but at that point he was so miserable, had been vomiting every morning and basically had no good days for 6 weeks, we sent him back to the acupuncturist and he went weekly during the second 6-week round. Maybe it was a coincidence, but his mood has been wonderful and the nausea almost nonexistent over this period. He likes and looks forward to his sessions.

If antinausea medications do not work well for your child, investigate the Food and Drug Administration (FDA)-approved Relief Band®. This wrist band gives an electrical stimulation (too faint to feel) to an acupuncture point on the wrist that affects the portion of the brain that controls nausea. Information about one type of band is available online at *http://neurowavemedical.com/products/motionsickness*.

Kytril® is an antinausea pill. It is incredibly expensive but brilliant in treating chemo-related sickness. It sometimes takes a bit of juggling to get the timing right; Michael used to take it an hour before taking the CCNU, which he then took at bedtime and slept right through with no ill effects. None of the other antiemetics worked for him nearly as well.

· · · · ·

Liquid promethazine worked fine for controlling nausea, but James' preschool teacher mentioned how drowsy he was at school, so we asked for something else.

· · · · ·

During Megan's treatment for anaplastic ependymoma, nausea was a big problem at first. I made a point to work with the staff to address this, and this is the plan we came up with: Megan would be given the maximum tolerated dose of Zofran® the first time chemo was administered, then 4 hours later she'd get the regular dose, then we would give the regular dose every 6 hours.

Seizures

Seizures can be compared to an electrical storm in the brain. They can happen anytime, but most commonly occur during the year following surgery and during treatment. Seizure activity may happen just once, occasionally, or regularly, depending on the individual nature of your child's disease and treatment.

Around 40 types of seizures or seizure disorders have been identified. The three main kinds experienced by children with brain or spinal cord tumors are:

- **Absence seizure (also known as petit mal seizure).** During an absence seizure, children lose awareness for less than a minute and may blink repeatedly. Adults often think the child is "zoning out" rather than having a seizure.

- **Partial seizure.** Children lose awareness for longer periods of time, but don't lose consciousness. They sometimes have strange sensations and make involuntary grunts or noises.

- **Tonic clonic seizure (also called grand mal seizure).** These seizures include loss of consciousness and visible arm/leg tremors or whole body convulsions.

For more information about local and national support organizations and about seizure management at school and home, contact the Epilepsy Foundation at (800) 332-1000 or see its website at: *www.epilepsyfoundation.org.*

Serious illnesses

Two illnesses that are especially dangerous for children during treatment are pneumonia and chicken pox.

Pneumonia

Pneumonia is inflammation of the lungs caused by bacteria, viruses, or other organisms. The symptoms of pneumonia are rapid breathing, trouble getting a breath, chills, fever, chest pain, cough, and bloody sputum. Children with low blood counts can rapidly develop a fatal infection and must be treated quickly and aggressively. Most cancer centers recommend an annual influenza (flu) shot to help prevent pneumonia.

> *My son received chemotherapy just days before he was scheduled to go to the camp for kids with cancer. His ANC was 1,200 and he looked so sick, but he begged to go and I let him. It was early in his treatment, and I didn't realize the pattern of his blood counts. They called me from camp on Friday to say he had a temperature of 103° and needed to go to the hospital. He was very weak and feverish; his WBC was 140, and his ANC was 0. Both lungs were full of pneumonia. I was furious at the*

doctor for giving him permission to go to camp and at myself for not paying closer attention to how quickly his counts dropped. I'm sure he had the pneumonia before he even went to camp. They started him on five different antibiotics, and his fever went up to 106° that night. We didn't know if he would live or die. He started to improve the next morning and was completely recovered in a week.

· · · · ·

Erica complained that her back hurt for 2 days. Then she woke up in the night crying, and she couldn't move because it hurt her too badly. She was blazing with fever, and screamed if I touched her. Her x-ray showed that her left lung was half full of fluid. They put her on antibiotics, and within 24 hours she was on the mend.

If your child has received carmustine (BCNU), lomustine (CCNU), or bleomycin, she may be at greater risk for respiratory infections. Children taking steroids (e.g., prednisone, dexamethasone) are at increased risk for contracting serious and potentially life-threatening lung infections from an organism called *Pneumocystis jirovecii*. In most cases, the infection can be prevented by taking trimethoprim-sulfamethoxazole (brand names Septra®, Bactrim®) 2 or 3 days per week.

Chicken pox

Chicken pox is a common childhood disease (although less so than it used to be because of the vaccine) caused by a virus called varicella zoster. The symptoms are headache, fever, and tiredness, followed by eruptions of pimple-like red bumps that typically start on the stomach, chest, or back. The bumps rapidly develop into blister-like sores that break open, then scab over in 3 to 5 days. Any contact with the sores can spread the disease. Children are contagious up to 48 hours before breaking out.

Chicken pox can be fatal for immunosuppressed children, so extreme care must be taken to prevent exposure. You will need to educate all teachers and friends so they will vigilantly report any outbreaks. Your child should not go to school or preschool until an outbreak is over.

Chicken pox can be transmitted through the air or by touch. Exposure is considered to have occurred if a child is in direct contact or in a room for as little as 10 minutes with an infected person. If an immunosuppressed child is exposed to chicken pox, call the neuro-oncologist immediately. If the child gets a shot called VZIG (varicella zoster immune globulin) within 72 hours of exposure, it may prevent the disease from occurring or minimize its effects.

We knew when Jeremy was exposed, so he was able to get VZIG. He did get chicken pox, but only developed a few spots. He didn't get sick; he got bored. He spent 2 weeks in the hospital in isolation. We asked for a pass, and we were able to go outside for some fresh air between doses of acyclovir.

If a child develops chicken pox while on chemotherapy, the current treatment is hospitalization or, if possible, home therapy for IV administration of acyclovir, a potent antiviral medication that has dramatically lowered the complication rate of chicken pox.

> Kristin broke out with chicken pox on the Fourth of July weekend. Our hospital room was the best seat in the house for watching the city fireworks. She did get covered with pox, though, from the soles of her feet to the very top of her scalp. We'd just give her gauze pads soaked in calamine lotion and let her hermetically seal herself. They kept her in the hospital for 6 days of IV acyclovir; then she was at home on the pump (a small computerized machine that will administer the drug in small amounts for several hours) for 4 more days of acyclovir. She had no complications.

A child who has already had chicken pox may develop herpes zoster (shingles). If your child develops eruptions of sores similar to chicken pox that are in lines (along nerves), call the doctor. The treatment for shingles is identical to that for chicken pox.

> Kristin also got a herpes zoster infection, this time on Thanksgiving. It looked like a mild case of chicken pox, limited to her upper right arm, her upper right chest, and her right leg. They kept her overnight on IV acyclovir and then let her go home for 9 more days on the pump.

Untreated chicken pox or shingles can result in life-threatening complications including pneumonia, hepatitis, and encephalitis. Parents must make every effort to prevent exposure and watch for signs of these diseases while their child is on treatment.

Skin and nail problems

Minor skin problems are frequent while on chemotherapy. The most common problems are rashes, redness, itching, peeling, dryness, and acne. Following are suggestions for preventing and treating skin problems:

- Avoid hot showers or baths, as these can dry the skin.

- Use moisturizing soap.

- Apply a water-based moisturizer after bathing, and once or twice daily, depending on the level of skin dryness.

- Avoid scratchy materials such as wool. Your child may feel more comfortable in loose, cotton clothing.

- Have your child use sunscreen with a sun protection factor of at least SPF 30. This is especially important for areas that have been irradiated.

- Insist on head coverings or sunscreen every time your child goes outdoors if she is bald, especially if she had cranial radiation.

- Buy your child lip gloss with sunscreen.

> *Matthew's lips would get very dry and eventually start to peel. It irritated him, and he developed a habit of biting on his lips. To minimize the problem I learned that wiping a cool, wet cloth over his mouth many times a day worked well. I would then apply a light coating of Vaseline® to his lips to keep them moist.*

- Rub cornstarch on itchy skin to help sooth it.

If your child has chemotherapy drugs injected into the veins (rather than a central venous catheter), you may notice a darkening along the veins; this will fade after treatment ends. However, skin and underlying tissues can be damaged or destroyed by drugs that leak out of a vein. If your child feels a stinging or burning sensation, or if you notice swelling at the IV site, call a nurse immediately.

Call the doctor anytime your child gets a severe rash or is very itchy. Scratching rashes can cause infections, so you need to get medications to control the itching.

Chemotherapy also affects the growing portion of nails located under the cuticle. After chemotherapy, you may notice a white band or ridge across the nail as it grows out. These brittle bands are sometimes elevated and feel bumpy. As the white ridge grows out toward the end of the finger, the nail may break.

Steroid problems

Some children with brain or spinal cord tumors require therapy with steroid medications at intervals throughout treatment. Prednisone, dexamethasone, hydrocortisone, and others in this category can cause many unpleasant side effects, including fluid retention, high blood pressure, elevated blood sugar, sleep disturbances, muscle weakness, cataracts, and bone weakening. Many children experience profound mood swings and are very emotional. If your child is having these kinds of problems, consult the neuro-oncologist to see whether the dose of steroid medication can be adjusted or whether a different type of steroid with fewer side effects is appropriate. For more information about steroids, see Chapter 11, *Chemotherapy*.

> *My 3-year-old niece was on Decadron® during treatment for a brainstem anaplastic astrocytoma. She had localized radiation, then later whole brain and spinal radiation, plus various chemos, but nothing whacked her out like Decadron®. She was on a high dose during radiation, and we were waiting to see her head turn all the way round or for her to start vomiting great gobs of green stuff. When the Decadron® was reduced, sanity returned to the household.*

Meagan is very emotionally labile after only two doses of prednisone. She is very frustrated, quick to anger, hits, screams. On those days we try to stay home, and this helps to decrease the stimulation. We plot it out on the calendar in advance so that we can plan accordingly. I think the kids deserve some tender, loving care while taking prednisone. Of course, I don't allow the hitting, but I do try hard not to aggravate the situation when she is on prednisone. I can see how she is uncomfortable being out of control, but she just can't help it.

Can pets transmit diseases?

Some oncologists recommend that parents rehome pets while their child is being treated for cancer. Although it is very unlikely that your child will be harmed from living with a household pet, several common-sense precautions are needed to protect a child with a low ANC from disease, worms, or infection:

- Make sure your pet is vaccinated against all possible diseases.

- Have pets checked for worms as soon as possible after your child is diagnosed, and then every year thereafter (more often for puppies). Give preventative treatments to your pets as directed by your veterinarian.

- Do not let pets eat off plates or lick your child's face.

- Keep children away from the cat litter box and any animal feces outdoors.

- Have all of your children wash their hands after playing with the pet.

- Make sure your pet has no ticks or fleas.

- If you have a pet that bites or scratches, consider finding another home for it. But if you have a gentle, well-loved pet, it may be a source of great comfort.

> *I think parents should know that you should not automatically get rid of your dog because your child has a low ANC. We went through a small crisis trying to decide whether to give away our large but beloved mongrel. The doctors wouldn't really give us a straight answer, but a parent in the support group said, "DO NOT get rid of your dog. Your son will need that dog's love and company in the years ahead." She was right. The dog was a tremendous comfort to our son.*

If at all possible, try to delay getting a new pet until your child has finished treatment. If your child wants a pet while undergoing cancer treatment and the family is in a position to take care of it, follow these guidelines:

- Do not get a puppy. All puppies bite while teething, increasing the chance that your child may contract an infection.

- Do not get a parrot or parakeet, as these species can transmit an infection called psittacosis to humans.

- Do not get a turtle or other reptile (e.g., snake, iguana) as they sometimes carry salmonella.

- Get an animal that is unlikely to bite or scratch.

> We bought Sarah an older puppy. We were very selective about the breeder and the breed. The dog has given my little girl back to me. After she got the dog, she started to want to walk again. She started to laugh. She had reason to think beyond herself and how terrible this illness is. She had someone who needed her. Someone who was delighted to see her and made her feel special in a way no human can. It literally transformed my child.

> The dog's name is Libbe, and after having Libbe for about a week, Sarah started asking when Libbe was going to die. She knew Libbe was just a puppy, but she really was asking about herself. We were able to tell her that Libbe will be around when she is a teenager and she can take Libbe with her on those big-girl sleepovers. Heck, she could take Libbe in the car for a ride, if she wanted. She beamed. It put the death and dying issue to rest.

If you have any concerns or questions about pets you already own or are thinking about purchasing, ask your neuro-oncologist and veterinarian for advice.

> There were times during my son's protocol that I felt he suffered more from the side effects of treatment than from the disease. It was emotionally painful for me to watch him go through so much. I think one of the hardest moments for me was the day he lost all his hair. Up until that point I had been living in a semi-state of denial. His bald head was more proof of our reality—he really did have cancer.

> I had to learn how to accept our situation, because I needed to be strong for my child. To get through, I reminded myself every day that the treatments were necessary, and that without them he would die. It was a struggle, but the unpleasant side effects soon passed, and he was able to resume his normal activities. I was constantly amazed at his resilience.

Chapter 13

Radiation Therapy

Nothing is so strong as gentleness,
and nothing is so gentle as true strength.

— St. Francis de Sales

RADIATION THERAPY IS ONE of the oldest and most effective therapies for many brain and spinal cord tumors. It can be used to shrink a tumor, delay tumor growth, prevent a tumor from returning, or treat symptoms associated with tumor growth, such as pain.

Radiation therapy can cause acute short-term side effects and permanent damage that may not be evident until months or years after treatment. Children who are younger than age 5 when they receive radiation are at much higher risk for developing serious permanent side effects. For this reason, radiation treatment is sometimes postponed for very young children, and the benefits and risks of treatment with radiation must be carefully weighed by both doctors and parents.

This chapter explains what radiation is, when and how it is used, and its potential side effects. It clearly explains what you and your child can expect from radiation treatment.

Parts of the body where radiation is used

Radiation can be directed at tumors, as well as at parts of the body that may be harboring tumor cells. The most common locations in the body that receive radiation to treat childhood brain or spinal cord tumors are:

- The entire tumor and a small amount of healthy tissue around the tumor (called "margins").

- The primary tumor site. After a tumor is surgically removed, the area where the tumor grew is irradiated (e.g., the posterior fossa in children with ependymoma) to prevent the tumor from returning.

- The entire brain and spinal cord. For example, children with medulloblastoma receive a high dose of radiation to the primary tumor site and a lower dose to the entire brain and spinal cord to kill any cancer cells that may have spread.

Types of radiation therapy

Radiation therapy directs high-energy x-rays at targeted areas of the body to destroy tumor cells or interfere with their ability to grow. Because tumor cells often remain after surgery, radiation is used to destroy them after a biopsy or after total or partial surgical removal of a tumor. Radiation is also used to relieve symptoms, such as pain. When used for pain relief, the treatment is called palliative radiation.

Radiation can be given internally or externally. This section describes the types of radiation that are used to treat children with brain and spinal cord tumors.

External radiation

External radiation uses high-energy x-rays called photons or protons to kill tumor cells. For photon radiation therapy, a large machine called a linear accelerator directs x-rays to the precise portion of the brain or spinal cord where the tumor is located. The treatment is usually given in doses measured in units called gray (Gy).

Radiation oncologists create an individualized treatment plan for each child using computers that combine images from MRIs and CT scans of the tumor and surrounding areas of the brain and spine. This plan allows the radiation oncologist to aim the radiation directly at the tumor or surgical cavity and a small margin around it; this way normal brain tissue can be spared as much as possible.

Radiation is usually given every day for a specific number of days, excluding weekends. This process is called standard or conventional fractionation, and it is the most common way brain and/or spinal cord radiation is given. Radiation given more than once a day is called accelerated fractionation, or hyperfractionation. It uses smaller amounts of radiation for each treatment. Hyperfractionation may reduce long-term side effects, but short-term side effects are sometimes more pronounced.

Specific types of external radiation therapy are:

- **3D conformal radiation therapy.** This type of therapy delivers high-dose radiation tailored to the precise area of the tumor, while delivering a lower dose to the normal tissue surrounding the tumor. It uses 3D images from CT, MRI, and PET scans to identify the margins of the tumor and their relationship to normal brain structures. Multiple radiation beams are delivered from several different directions so that they overlap at the tumor. By using this technology, the tumor receives the high-dose radiation and the normal tissues surrounding it receive a lower dose.

- **Intensity modulated radiation therapy (IMRT).** This type of 3D conformal therapy can spare adjacent critical structures by varying the intensity of one beam of radiation.

IMRT is the most advanced form of photon radiation available. A disadvantage of this type of radiation is that a lower dose of radiation is given to a larger amount of normal brain tissue.

- **Stereotactic radiosurgery.** This sophisticated 3D technique directs radiation to small tumors that cannot be surgically removed because of their location deep within the brain. Using highly specialized computer-assisted equipment, it delivers radiation via multiple independent beams directed to the single target. Stereotactic radiosurgery is delivered as a single treatment (radiosurgery) or as fractionated treatment (stereotactic radiotherapy). This innovative treatment requires precise planning and the combined efforts of multiple specialists. A neurosurgeon works in collaboration with the radiation oncologist to deliver the treatment.

> *My daughter Stacia's inoperable tumor (a GBM) located in the basal ganglia was treated with stereotactic radiosurgery by way of focused radiation beams. She had to put on the bird cage, she thought the screws in her head were annoying, and the anesthetic shots in the scalp were a nuisance, but otherwise she was fine. Two months after this treatment, her basal ganglia tumor was completely dark, and she clinically was terrific. Two months after that, recurrence on the edges of the cavity had begun. But in my opinion this treatment was effective in increasing both the quantity and quality of her life.*

- **Proton beam radiation.** Proton therapy delivers high doses of radiation to the tumor while limiting damage to surrounding healthy tissue. This advanced technique generally results in fewer short- and long-term side effects than does conventional radiation therapy. Proton beam therapy is only available at a few specialized centers, but it will soon be available at some major pediatric centers.

> *Our daughter Megan (age 8) received proton beam therapy for her optic glioma. She was so full of spunk she would run down the hall with her pink blanket dragging behind her and jump on the table. Megan lay on a table where they placed pliable plastic mesh over her face first to get a mold, then the mask was bolted to a board during treatment. The radiation took about a minute per location, and there were three locations. She had this treatment for 6 weeks; there was no sickness, no skin burning. After proton treatment, the tumor did not grow for about 7 years.*

Children do not become radioactive from these types of radiation treatments, and no specific precautions or activity restrictions are necessary.

> *I was very proud of my 6-year-old son for handling his radiation treatments so well. He never required sedation and was always cooperative. I'm convinced that it was partly because of his personality, and partly because of how the staff treated him. Every day that he received radiation, his favorite stuffed toy, Mr. Bear, was radiated, too.*

For a listing of facilities that offer specific kinds of radiation treatment, contact the American Brain Tumor Association, listed in Appendix B, *Resource Organizations*.

Internal radiation

Internal radiation—also called brachytherapy, implant therapy, or interstitial therapy— is not commonly used to treat childhood brain and spinal cord tumors. Internal radiation uses radioactive materials (called seeds or implants) placed directly into the tumor (interstitial implants) or applied to the surface of the tumor (plaques). It differs from external radiation because it provides a continuous low dose of radiation to the tumor, rather than intermittent bursts one or two times per day.

The radioactive seeds or implants are delivered through a catheter that is placed surgically with CT scan guidance. The catheter remains in place for a specific number of days (usually 2 to 5 days), until the required amount of radiation has been given, and is then removed.

Your child will become radioactive from internal radiation. He will need to stay in a special isolation room with a private bathroom during treatment. The room has plastic covers on all fixtures, and disposable serving plates and utensils are used. Parents are allowed to spend a limited amount of time with their child, typically several hours a day. The rest of the time you can sit outside your child's room to talk or read to him. Children and pregnant women cannot visit when your child is radioactive.

Although experience with internal radiation in children is limited, efforts are ongoing to evaluate various types of internal radiation in children with recurrent brain and spinal cord tumors.

> Megan had an anaplastic ependymoma in the left occipital/parietal region of her brain. She had a gross total resection of the tumor. While all of her MRIs were clear following the initial surgery, we all know that you can't get every cell in surgery and we don't know how well chemo works on these brain tumors. So, we went with the aggressive approach and (2½ years ago now) Megan had a second surgery to implant brachytherapy seeds.
>
> The doctor had 150 seeds ready to be implanted in the tumor bed. Our doctor called us from the operating room, happy and amazed that there were no visible traces of tumor. Five biopsies were done while Megan was in surgery, only one showed traces of tumor. The doctor then removed some tissue in the area where the traces of tumor were and then did five more biopsies in that area. Those five biopsies came back clear. As there was only one area that had any active tumor cells, that is the only area where the seeds were implanted and they only used 34 seeds.

Megan had no side effects, either at the time of surgery or since, from this type of radiation. Her MRIs are still clear and do not show any signs of radiation damage to the area where the seeds were implanted. We do know that some of the seeds have since fallen out of place and rest at the bottom of her spine. The doctors aren't concerned about this and they don't affect her.

Experimental treatments used with radiation

In some clinical trials, radioimmunotherapy and chemical modifiers are used in conjunction with radiation to treat children with brain and spinal cord tumors.

Radioimmunotherapy uses radiolabeled antibodies as radiation carriers. The antibodies are attached (labeled) to a radioactive material and then injected into the body through a venous catheter or IV. Once injected, the antibodies begin a "seek and destroy" mission, searching for specific tumor cells. Radiolabeled antibodies lessen the chance of radiation damage to normal cells. Experience with this method of radiation in children is limited.

Chemical modifiers are compounds used at the same time as radiation therapy. Two classes of compounds are currently under study in children: radiation sensitizers and radioprotectors (drugs that are administered with the radiation treatments). Radiation sensitizers increase delivery of oxygen to tumor cells, thereby rendering them more sensitive to the effects of radiation. Radioprotectors are designed to shield normal cells from radiation damage by using substances absorbed by healthy normal cells but not by tumor cells. Studies using these compounds are ongoing or under development in the Children's Oncology Group and may provide important new ways to treat children with brain and spinal cord tumors.

Who needs radiation treatment?

Your child's doctor will recommend radiation treatment based on your child's type and location of tumor. Radiation is used for slow-growing tumors that cannot be reduced in size by surgery because of their location and for tumors that continue to grow despite chemotherapy. Fast-growing tumors usually need radiation in conjunction with surgery and chemotherapy.

Childhood brain and spinal cord tumors that usually respond to radiation include high-grade gliomas, medulloblastomas, ependymomas, germinomas, and some low-grade astrocytomas. Although radiation to the brain or spinal cord can cause long-term complications, it is an important part of successful treatment for many types of brain and spinal cord tumors. Because of the greater risk of long-term complications in younger children, radiation treatments are delayed until the child reaches the age of 3 by using surgery or chemotherapy whenever possible.

> *My daughter Ayla had maximum craniospinal radiation the day after she turned 3. Prior to that she had a 50% resection of a brainstem PNET and the highest dose of chemo. While taking chemo, her cancer spread to several locations throughout her midbrain. We were told that she had a 10% chance to live. We chose radiation as a last recourse and it is my belief that this was what "zapped" that cancer! She is doing great now and even attended school full time a few weeks after completing the radiation. I know that every kid is different but there are many successes from radiation, so it should not be discounted. I also know that in the future she may have some cognitive problems, but at least we have her.*

Questions to ask about radiation treatment

If radiation has been recommended as a treatment for your child, some questions you can ask the radiation oncologist include:

- Why does my child need radiation?

- What type of radiation does she need?

- What type of radiation treatments do other facilities offer?

- What part of his brain or spinal cord will be treated with radiation?

- What is the total dose of radiation that she will receive?

- How many treatments of radiation will he get?

- How much experience does this institution have in administering this type of radiation to children?

- How will she be positioned on the table?

- Will any restraints be used?

- Will anesthesia or sedation be needed?

- How long will each treatment take?

- What are the possible short-term and long-term side effects?

- Could this type and dosage of radiation cause cancer later?

- What are the alternatives to radiation?

- Are there any precautionary procedures to be done prior to spinal radiation therapy?

My daughter Rachel (age 14) had medulloblastoma. She had one of her ovaries moved to protect it from the field of spinal radiation. It's not a guarantee, but it does seem to be the standard procedure.

Where should your child go for radiation treatment?

To have optimal treatment, children should receive radiation therapy only at major medical centers with extensive experience treating children with brain and spinal cord tumors. Doctors who are experienced in pediatric radiation oncology should supervise all treatments. State-of-the-art equipment, expert personnel, and vast experience with many types of childhood tumors are what you should look for when choosing a center. Pediatric anesthesiologists should administer sedation or general anesthesia during radiation.

Radiation oncologist

A radiation oncologist is a medical doctor with years of specialized training in using radiation to treat cancer. In partnership with the other members of the treatment team, the radiation oncologist develops a treatment plan specifically tailored for your child.

The radiation oncologist will explain to you and your child what radiation is, how it will be administered, and any possible side effects. She will also answer all your questions regarding the proposed treatment. You will be given a consent form to review prior to the first treatment. Take the consent form home if you need extra time to read it. Parents should not sign the consent form until they thoroughly understand all benefits, risks, and possible side effects of the radiation. The radiation oncologist will meet at least weekly with you and your child to discuss how the treatment is going and to address concerns or answer questions.

Radiation therapist

Radiation therapists are specially trained technologists who operate the machine that delivers the dose of radiation prescribed by the radiation oncologist. This member of the medical team will give your child a tour of the radiation room, explain the equipment, and position your child for treatment. The technologist will operate the x-ray machine and will monitor your child via closed-circuit TV and a two-way intercom.

*When 3-year-old Katy was being given the tour of the radiation room by her tech-
nologist, Brian, he was just wonderful with her. He gave her a white, stuffed bear
that he used to demonstrate the machine. He immobilized the bear on the table using
Katy's mask (device to hold the head still during treatment), then moved the machine
all around it so that she could hear the sounds made by the equipment. He then
took a Polaroid picture of the bear on the table, in the mask, for Katy to take home
with her.*

Immobilization devices

Different institutions use a variety of devices to immobilize children or teens to ensure
that the radiation beam is directed with precision. Custom fitting the devices on a
child who has already undergone numerous procedures requires skill and patience.
This is especially true for children being fitted for a mask in preparation for radiation
to the head or spine. Great care should be taken to ensure that making the mask is not
traumatic. This can often be accomplished by using play therapy to demonstrate the
procedure.

Masks are made from a lightweight, porous, mesh material. First, the technologist
should explain and demonstrate the entire mask-making process to the child. The child
then lies down on a table. The technologist places a sheet of the mask material in warm
water to soften it. This warm mesh sheet is placed over the child's face and quickly
molded to his features. The child can breathe the entire time through the mesh material, but must hold still for several minutes as the mask hardens. The mask is lifted off
the child's face, and the technologist cuts holes in it for the eyes, nostrils, and mouth.

*The cancer center staff had scheduled 2 hours to make a mask for my 3-year-old
daughter. I asked them to very quietly explain every step in the process. I told her
that I would be holding her hand, and I promised that it would not hurt, but it would
feel warm. I asked her to choose a story for me to recite as they molded the warm
material to her face to make the time go faster. She picked "Curious George Goes to
the Hospital." She held perfectly still; I recited the story; the staff were gentle and
quick; and the entire procedure took less than 20 minutes.*

For children having radiation to the spine, immobilization devices can be as simple as
Velcro straps to hold the body in place. Some children will have special foam or plaster
molds made to allow greater accuracy when directing the radiation.

*My 4-year-old son needed 6 weeks of radiation scheduled to begin just weeks after
his stem cell transplant. His immune system was still so low, although he was starting to recover from the month-long ordeal. The technicians thought he would lay face*

down quietly in a tub of warm plaster so that they could make his mold. I don't think so! He was scared, and kicked and screamed, so we went home. We came back the next day, they sedated him with propofol, and then it took just a few minutes to make the mold and prepare him for radiation.

Immobilization devices can be fitted on well-prepared, calm children or sedated children. The following are parent suggestions for preparing a child for the fitting of an immobilization device:

• Give the child a tour of the room where the fitting will take place.

• Explain each step of the process in clear language.

• Be honest in describing any discomfort the child may experience.

• For small children, fit the device onto a mannequin or stuffed animal to demonstrate the process.

• For older children or teenagers, show a video or read a booklet describing the procedure.

> *Seventeen-month-old Rachel was fitted with two immobilization devices. They made a mask to hold her head in position, as well as a body mold from her neck to her thighs.*

Spending ample time on preparation generally means less time will be needed to fit a device. If the fitting goes well, it establishes trust and good feelings that will help make the actual radiation treatments proceed smoothly.

Sedation

All infants, most preschoolers, and some school-age children require sedation or a short-acting anesthesia (most commonly propofol given intravenously) to ensure they remain perfectly still during radiation therapy. The radiation facility should give parents written instructions concerning pediatric anesthesia, including guidelines about when to stop eating and drinking before sedation or anesthesia. Children can eat and drink after treatment, as soon as they are alert enough to swallow.

> *About 1 month after he was diagnosed with ependymoma, Sam started a course of 30 daily radiation treatments. In some ways, this was the easiest part. Each day we woke up at the same time we always had, got dressed and went directly to the hospital. Because of Sam's young age, he received anesthesia so that he would lie still for the radiation session. He had a Hickman® catheter in his chest, so that made getting the anesthesia into him a quick process. The anesthesia acted very quickly, and the*

technicians and nurse would place him in position and the treatment would start. Each session lasted about 15 minutes. He'd then be moved into a recovery area where I'd wait while he awoke. He usually came out of it happy, but hungry. I learned to pack lots of easy snacks, like cheerios, crackers, and juice boxes. Once he was fully awake, I'd wheel him to the car in the baby stroller. Most days we were home by 9:30 am. One of the blessings of daily radiation is seeing nurses and technicians every day. I was very touched by the caring and comfort of the staff in the radiation department. Another benefit of the daily radiation was being able to change the dressing on Sam's Hickman® while he was under anesthesia.

Anesthesia is given through a mask or through the child's catheter or intravenous line (IV). Sometimes the parent can hold or comfort the child while anesthesia is administered, but the parent must leave the room once radiation treatment begins. Once your child is easily aroused and can swallow, you can take her home. The entire procedure generally takes from 30 to 90 minutes. Nausea and vomiting are occasional side effects of anesthesia, but they are usually well controlled by anti-nausea drugs such as ondansetron (Zofran®). Over time, your child may become comfortable with the treatment and not require anesthesia.

Each time my young son came in for radiation, part of the routine was to place the hard plastic mesh mask over his face while he was awake, just for an instant, to get him used to the idea of trying to wear it for treatments without sedation. No pressure was ever put on him about it, it was just mentioned as a possibility of something he could try, something that would let him keep eating and drinking all through the day, instead of having to fast for a few hours before each sedation, which was very hard for such a small boy who was getting sedation twice a day.

They left the mask on him for a tiny bit longer each time, until he was tolerating it for several seconds, and by the end of the third week, close to a minute. His fifth birthday was at the exact middle of treatment, and he decided that since he was such a big boy now, he would try to do it without sedation. I know he was trying to please and impress all these kind people. He worked it out quietly with a favorite technician, asked the "sleepy medicine doctor" to wait outside the treatment room, let them screw the mask down to the table and did the whole thing awake.

I've never been more proud in my life. Everyone cheered and hugged him. He finished the last three weeks of treatments without sedation, sometimes eating and drinking on his way in the door just to show off that he could!

What is a radiation treatment like?

Radiation treatments can be very stressful for both children and parents, but knowledge and preparation can make the entire process much easier. This section describes radiation simulation and the various types of radiation therapy.

Radiation simulation

Prior to receiving any external radiation therapy, measurements and technical x-rays are taken to map the precise area to be treated. This preparation for therapy is called the "simulation." The simulation will take longer than any other appointment—from 30 minutes to 2 hours. Because simulation does not involve any high-energy radiation, parents may be allowed to remain in the treatment room to help and comfort their child. Some children require sedation for the simulation.

During simulation, the radiation oncologist and technologist use a specialized x-ray machine or a CT scanner to outline the treatment area. They will adjust the table that the child lies on, the angle of the machine, and the width of the x-ray beam needed to give the exact dosage in the proper place. Ink marks or permanent tattoos are placed on the skin or the immobilization device to ensure accuracy of treatment. After the simulation is completed, the child can leave while the radiation oncologist carefully evaluates the developed x-ray film and measurements to design the treatment field.

External radiation treatment

To receive external radiation, children are given appointments to visit the radiation clinic for a specific number of days, usually the same time each day. Standard radiation treatment for many brain and spinal cord tumors is given 5 days a week for 5 to 7 weeks (weekends off). At some institutions and for some protocols, children go more than once a day to receive hyperfractionated dosing.

When the parent and child arrive, they must check in at the front desk. The technologist or nurse comes out to take the child into the treatment room. Often, parents accompany young children into the room. If the child requires anesthesia, it is usually given in the treatment room.

> I desperately wanted my 3 year old to be able to receive the radiation without anesthesia. I asked the center staff what I could do to make her comfortable. They said, "Anything, as long as you leave the room during the treatment." So I explained to my daughter that we had to find ways for her to hold very still for a short time. I said, "It's such a short time, that if I played your Snow White tape, the treatment

would be over before Snow White met the dwarves." Katy agreed that was a short time, and asked that I bring the tape for her to listen to. She also wanted a sticker (a different one every day) stuck on the machine for her to look at. I brought her pink blanket to wrap her in because the table was hard and the room cold. Each day, she chose a different comfort animal or doll to hold during treatment. So we'd arrive every day with tapes, blanket, stickers, and animals. She felt safe, and all treatments went extremely well.

The technologist will secure children or teens in place with an immobilization device. Measurements are taken to verify that the child's body is perfectly positioned. Frequently, the technologist will shine a light on the area to be irradiated to ensure that the machine is properly aligned. The technologist and parents leave the room, closing the door behind them.

At some institutions, parents are allowed to stay and watch the TV monitor and talk to their child via the speaker system. If this is the case, the parent should be careful not to distract the technologist as he administers the radiation. At other institutions, parents are asked to wait in the waiting room. It's important that parents understand the department's policies; they should ask the radiation therapist if anything is unclear.

The treatment takes only a few minutes and can be stopped at any time if the child experiences any difficulty. When the treatment is finished, the technologist turns off the machine, removes the immobilization device, and parents and child can go home. There is no pain at all when receiving x-ray treatment.

There was something about the radiation or the anesthesia that frightened Shawn terribly. He would scream in the car all the way to the hospital. It was a scream as if he was in pain. He had nightmares while he was undergoing radiation and every night after it was over. We decided a month after radiation ended to bring a box of candy to the staff who had been so nice. Shawn asked, "Do I have to go in that room?" When I explained that it was over and he didn't need to go in the room anymore, he asked if he could go in to look at it once more. He stood for a long time and just looked and looked at the equipment. Somehow he made his peace with it, because he never had any more nightmares.

Internal radiation treatment

Children are admitted to the hospital to receive internal radiation. Certain hospital rooms are specially designed for children undergoing this type of treatment. The walls may contain lead, and often items such as sheets and eating utensils are disposable. This is because the child and everything he touches will become radioactive during therapy.

Internal radiation may be given in the child's hospital room after catheters have been placed in the radiology department or in the operating room. The child is then transported to the special room, where he will remain until he is no longer radioactive. The interstitial implants will generally remain in place for several days. Once they are removed, your child may resume normal activities and will no longer require isolation.

Children and pregnant women cannot visit while a child is receiving internal radiation. Parents and nursing staff can spend a limited amount of time in the child's room. This may be distressing for very small children who are unable to understand why people must maintain a safe distance. It may be possible to keep the door to your child's hospital room open. In these instances, you can sit in the hall and talk to your child to help alleviate any fears or feelings of boredom. Parents should talk with the nursing staff and the child life specialist and ask if they have suggestions about how to make the child as comfortable as possible.

> Our son was 5 years old when he was admitted for his internal radiation. The biggest issue we had to deal with was boredom. It was hard for him to understand that I wasn't allowed to spend all my time at his bedside. The door to his room was open at all times, so I moved a reclining chair into the hall, and that was where I stayed for 4 days. I would read him stories, stopping from time to time to hold up the book so he could see the pictures. He had a Nintendo® machine and a VCR in his room, and that helped to keep him entertained. The nurses even thought of clever games to play. They would inflate rubber gloves and bat them into his room as they passed by his door. After a while they became more and more creative, taking time to draw faces and hair onto the rubber gloves.

Possible short-term side effects

Generally, radiation therapy given to children with brain and spinal cord tumors takes place over 4 to 6 weeks. If side effects occur, it is often hard to differentiate those caused by radiation from those caused by the chemotherapy, which is sometimes given at the same time. The severity of the side effects depends upon the sensitivity and size of the area being irradiated. The radiation oncologist is familiar with all possible side effects and is responsible for their treatment.

> The side effects Sam experienced from the radiation were typical: hair loss, sunburned skin in the radiated area, irritability, and headaches. Eventually, he started on Decadron® to reduce the internal brain swelling. The side effects of this were markedly increased appetite, mood swings, and irritability. A 3 year old on Decadron® is no picnic! There were many days that all I did was prepare and serve food! On those days I was too worn out to worry.

Possible short-term side effects include the following:

- Loss of appetite

    Calories are most important; nutrition can come after treatment. We use whole milk, and put butter on everything: Ethan would eat any time, anything. When Ethan completely lost his appetite during radiation, we used Megase®, a prescription appetite stimulant. It has fairly few side effects and did seem to work for him.

- Nausea and vomiting

    About a month after radiation was over for my residual pilocytic astrocytoma, I started experiencing all my side effects. I started having problems with my stomach, and was vomiting every morning. I also had balance problems, headaches, cold chills, and had problems with my shunt. I am still experiencing side effects 6 months later. Radiation did stop the growth of my brain tumor.

- Ear, nose, or throat problems
- Mouth and throat sores

    There are several concoctions that radiation oncologists prescribe, sometimes called "Miracle Mouthwash," that often work wonders for mouth and throat sores.

- Fatigue
- Reddened, itchy, or peeling skin

    Where the beams entered at two places, his scalp was burned like a sunburn, and aloe vera gel helped to keep that soft.

· · · · ·

    During radiation I was told to use baby shampoo, not to use a hair dryer, and was given samples of a cream for my scalp called Aquaphor®.

- Hair loss (sometimes permanent)

    My son, Dan, experienced really no side effects for the first 3 weeks of radiation to treat anaplastic astrocytoma. Then, at the beginning of the fourth week, his hair began to fall out in quite big clumps. By the end of radiation, he had no hair on his head except for a small ball-shaped spot on top, and a sharp line between his ears and below to his neck. Now, 14 months later, he has all of his hair back except in two places, the two spots where the beams entered his head. The exit spots have all filled in nicely, just the two entrance spots remain. One is very bald while the other has a thin fine film of hair. The rest is long and black and curly again. The docs have told Dan that if the hair hasn't come back by now, it probably won't. But Dan is handling it. Hats are still cool. And he doesn't really care what people think.

- Low blood counts
- Changes in taste and smell (sometimes occurring during treatment sessions)
- Increased or decreased saliva or dry mouth (ask your physician about saliva substitutes such as Moi-Stir® or Salivant®)

> My daughter Mandy (age 4) had a problem with thick saliva while she was being treated. We started to give her about 200 ml of extra water each day through her G-tube. This seemed to help although she would still have the problem some days, just not as much.

For additional methods of coping with many of the above side effects, see Chapter 12, *Common Side Effects of Chemotherapy*.

Somnolence syndrome is uniquely associated with cranial radiation and is characterized by drowsiness, prolonged periods of sleep (up to 20 hours a day), low-grade fever, headaches, nausea, vomiting, irritability, difficulty swallowing, and difficulty speaking. It may occur during radiation or as late as 12 weeks after radiation treatment ends; it can last from a few days to several weeks.

> Nine weeks after ending her cranial radiation, my daughter started complaining of severe headaches. She would hold her head and just sob with pain. She also vomited several times. Then she became very sleepy, and dozed on the couch most of the day. She developed a low fever and choked when she tried to swallow liquids or solid food. This lasted for about a week.

· · · · ·

> Stephan (8 years old) had no side effects from the cranial and spinal radiation other than sleepiness, but he was very affected by it. First, he just started taking naps and generally slowing down. Then the naps got longer, and he was awake less. Finally, he only woke up to eat. Luckily, that part coincided with Christmas vacation so he didn't miss much school. Altogether, it lasted about 6 weeks.

Possible long-term side effects

Short-term effects appear quickly and then subside, but long-term side effects may not become apparent for months or years after treatment ends. Specific late effects depend on the age of the child when radiation was given, the dose of radiation, and what part of the brain was irradiated.

The effects of radiation on cognitive functioning, bone growth, soft tissue growth, teeth and sinuses, puberty, and fertility, range from none to severe and life-long impacts. Brain tumor survivors can develop seizure disorders, gait and balance problems, hand/eye coordination problems, personality changes, and learning disabilities. Vision problems and cataracts can develop after radiation, and second tumors in the radiation field are a rare but possible long-term side effect. Detailed information about possible late effects are described in *Childhood Cancer Survivors: A Practical Guide to Your Future, 3rd edition* by Nancy Keene, Wendy Hobbie, and Kathy Ruccione (see *www.childhoodcancerguides. org/survivors*).

Cognitive problems

Injury to the brain can result from a multitude of factors, including tumor extension, surgical procedures, radiation, and chemotherapy. Children with brain and spinal cord tumors often develop mild to severe learning disabilities that can start immediately or develop later. Whole brain radiation can result in problems with mathematics, understanding visual/spatial relationships, problem solving, attention span, memory, and concentration skills.

> My daughter received 1.8 Gy of cranial radiation when she was 17 months old. She is now 9 years old and in third grade. She has many learning challenges, including slower processing speed, attentional difficulties, and difficulty with short-term memory and multi-step processing. She benefits from additional help in school. In the past she has needed additional drilling in phonics, math fact repetition, and refocusing on multi-step directions, as well as additional time to complete testing. It is challenging for her to maintain her focus throughout the day.

> After much observation, I am convinced that these kids have a quirky organizational system. My husband and I both realize that school is a struggle for her. We have sought help through the special education system, and our daughter is now classified as traumatically brain injured. Her self-esteem is high, and she is a very bright, verbal child with a lot of strengths. We are working diligently with all of her teachers and all of the resources available to ensure that she gets the best education possible.

Children at greatest risk for significant cognitive problems are those treated with radiation when younger than 5 years of age, with those younger than 2 at the highest risk. Children treated with radiation after age 5 or into adolescence are also at risk for developing early or late cognitive difficulties. Chapter 18, *School*, discusses in great detail the types of educational problems some children face and methods to deal with the problems.

Endocrine function

The endocrine system is composed of glands that secrete hormones into the blood. The endocrine glands that can be damaged by brain or spinal cord radiation include the pituitary gland, thyroid gland, ovaries, and adrenal glands. Problems with these glands may develop years after treatment, so long-term follow-up by experts in the late effects after childhood cancer is essential. Long-term followup should include careful monitoring by an endocrinologist, a doctor who specializes in hormonal issues.

Growth

The brain contains the hypothalamus and the pituitary gland, which control many body processes, including growth and reproduction. Effects on growth usually begin to be seen in children who receive 2.4 Gy or more of radiation to these two glands. If your child receives radiation therapy to the brain and/or spine, her growth will require close observation, and she should be measured (sitting and standing) at every follow-up visit. Your child's growth chart should be kept up to date so that it will be easier to quickly observe subtle changes that may indicate early plateauing of your child's growth.

If your child is one of the rare individuals who experience precocious puberty (before the age of 8 for girls and 10 for boys), growth may also be affected. An early growth spurt with early sexual maturation results in short stature because bones stop growing when sexual maturity is reached. When this happens at a young age, the child loses 2 to 3 years of additional growth. After treatment for a brain or spinal cord tumor, growth hormone injections are sometimes given to support your child's growth until he reaches his final height.

> Mandy (age 16) is a tad short-waisted, but grew 7 inches on growth hormone treatment! The doctors closely monitor wingspan (that is, outstretched arms fingertip to fingertip), to make sure it correlates to height. Otherwise they may have longer arms and be out of balance. The growth hormone adds energy and good spirits as well.

Early or delayed puberty

Some young children who receive radiation to the brain do not experience puberty at the appropriate age. As mentioned earlier, a very small percentage of children develop precocious puberty, which means puberty begins several years earlier than normal. This is most common in children who also have impaired growth. Conversely, puberty is significantly delayed in some children who have received cranial radiation.

A pediatric endocrinologist with extensive experience treating children and adolescents who had cancer should evaluate girls and boys who show signs of early or delayed puberty.

Vision

Problems with vision may occur as a result of tumor location, tumor spread, surgery, or radiation therapy. If such problems are present, the early involvement of a pediatric ophthalmologist and serial evaluations are important. Your child may need special glasses, selective seating in the classroom, or a reading machine. If your child has significant visual impairment or is considered legally blind, she is probably eligible for a variety of services, including Talking Books, a free library service (*www.nlstalkingbooks. org*). It is important that you keep a copy of all reports of your child's vision testing for your records. Such reports are very useful when dealing with your child's teachers and school administrators.

Teeth

Although newer conformal treatments have reduced the late effects of radiation on teeth, cranial radiation given in previous decades often resulted in disrupted tooth development and in the blunting of roots of children's permanent teeth. This resulted in some children missing certain permanent teeth or in early tooth loss because of shortened roots. Even with newer treatments, the involvement of a pedodontist (children's dentist) is important.

Any child who received cranial or spinal radiation is at additional risk for dental decay because of diminished function of the salivary glands. Appropriate dental evaluations and treatment with fluoride preparations may be necessary. You should ask your radiation oncologist for a summary of the dose to the teeth and to let you know whether the dose is enough to be concerned about future dental problems.

Secondary cancers

Children who receive radiation to the brain have an increased risk of developing another tumor years after treatment. The risk is reported to range from 1 to 5 percent.

Despite the possibility of these short- and long-term effects, radiation therapy remains an important treatment for children with brain and spinal cord tumors. Technological advances have allowed for more targeted treatments intended to cure the child while minimizing or avoiding these complications.

As I carried my unconscious son back to the waiting room after radiation treatment, a woman there stared intently. On impulse, I took the seat next to her. As I arranged Ben into a bear hug with my arms wrapped around him, she whispered to me, "I'm so jealous." I was taken aback by the heat in her voice. She told me she was making these daily treks with her son, too. Only, he was 21 years old, and wouldn't let her hold him or hug him. It broke her heart to see Ben and I wrapped up in ourselves in that unique mom-child world of clinging hugs, multiple kisses, and rubby-faces. Her son was brave, a valiant independent young man, and she was proud of him. But what she really wanted to do was wrap herself around him, tuck his head under her chin, and make everything all better like she used to.

Chapter 14

Peripheral Blood
Stem Cell Transplantation

*The courage of life is often a less dramatic spectacle
than the courage of the final moment; but it is no less
a magnificent mixture of triumph and tragedy.*

— John Fitzgerald Kennedy
Profiles in Courage

PERIPHERAL BLOOD STEM CELL TRANSPLANTATION (PBSCT) is a complicated procedure used to treat some cancers and blood diseases that were once considered incurable. In this procedure, stem cells in the blood are collected and then children are given high-dose chemotherapy. After the chemotherapy, the stem cells that were collected earlier are infused into the child's veins. The stem cells migrate to the cavities inside the bones where new, healthy blood cells are then produced.

Stem cell transplants are expensive, technically complex, and potentially life-threatening. Understanding the procedure and its ramifications at a time of crisis can be tremendously difficult. This chapter explains the type of PBSCT currently used to treat a small number of children with brain and spinal cord tumors, and it shares the experiences of several families.

What is a peripheral blood stem cell transplant?

Bone marrow is the spongy material inside bones. It is full of the youngest type of blood cells—called stem cells—from which all other blood cell types develop (white blood cells, red blood cells, and platelets). Stem cells are also found in circulating (also called peripheral) blood, although in a much less concentrated form.

At present, some types of brain and spinal cord tumors cannot be cured with conventional doses of chemotherapy or radiation. For some of these tumors, the very high doses of chemotherapy needed to kill tumor cells also permanently destroy the normal stem cells in the bone marrow.

There are different types of stem cell transplants. When peripheral blood is used as a source of stem cells for a transplant, it is called a peripheral blood stem cell transplant or PBSCT. If the child does not have cancer cells in the bone marrow, as is the case for children with brain and spinal cord tumors, the child usually is able to donate his own stem cells for a transplant. This type of transplant is called an autologous PBSCT, and this chapter deals specifically with this type of stem cell transplant.

In an autologous PBSCT, the child's own stem cells are harvested in a procedure called apheresis. After collection and storage of the stem cells, children are given high-dose chemotherapy, followed by an infusion of their own stem cells. See the section entitled "Stem cell harvest and storage" later in this chapter for a description of the collection and storage process.

This process can be done one or more times, allowing doctors to expose the tumor cells to high doses of chemotherapy while limiting toxicity and the risk of life-threatening infections. When this process is done more than once, it is called tandem PBSCT, serial PBSCT, or sequential PBSCT.

When are transplants necessary?

Some clinical trials use tandem PBSCTs as front-line treatment for some primitive neuroectodermal tumors, high-risk embryonal tumors, germ cell tumors, and malignant tumors diagnosed in very young children. Although preliminary data from some of these studies are encouraging, tandem transplants are still considered experimental in most, but not all, situations.

If a PBSCT has been recommended for your child or teenager, you may want to get a second opinion before proceeding. In addition, you may want to ask the neuro-oncologist some or all of the following questions:

- What are all the treatment options for my child's tumor?
- For my child's type of tumor, history, and physical condition, what chance for survival does she have with a transplant? What are her chances with other treatments?
- What are the risks? Explain the statistical chance of each risk.
- What are the benefits of this type of transplant?
- What will be my child's likely short-term and long-term quality of life after the transplant?
- Where would my child receive this type of transplant?
- What portion of the procedure will be outpatient versus inpatient?

- What is the average length of stay in the hospital for children undergoing this procedure?

- What are the anticipated and rare complications of this type of transplant?

- Will my child have to take medicines after the transplant? For how long?

- What are the side effects of these medicines?

- Is this transplant considered to be experimental, or is it the current standard of care?

Choosing a transplant center

If the institution where you child is treated is also an accredited transplant center, you will not need to travel for this part of your child's treatment. However, if you need to choose a transplant center, it is an important and often difficult decision. Institutions may just be starting a stem cell transplant program, or they may have vast experience. Some centers may be excellent for adults, but have limited pediatric experience. Some may allow you to stay overnight with your child; others may restrict access.

The center closest to your home may not provide the best medical care available for your child or allow the necessary quality of life (rooming in, social workers, etc.) that you need. In addition, your insurance plan may require your child to have the PBSCT at a specific center. To see a list of transplant centers, visit *www.bmtinfonet.org/before/ choosingtransplantcenter.* Asking the following questions can help you learn about the policies of different transplant centers:

- Is your center accredited by the Foundation for Accreditation of Cellular Therapy (*http://factwebsite.org/AboutFACT/*)? This agency inspects transplant programs and certifies programs that provide high-quality care.

- What are your program's 1-, 2-, and 5-year survival rates? (Remember that some institutions accept very-high-risk patients, and their statistics would not compare to a center that performs less risky transplants.)

- What is the nurse-to-patient ratio? Do all staff members have pediatric training and experience?

- What support staff is available (educators, social workers, child life specialists, clergy, support groups, volunteers, etc.)?

- Will my child be on a pediatric or combined adult–pediatric unit?

- What are the institution's rules about parents staying in the child's hospital room?

- Are children allowed to visit?

- What kinds of temporary and long-term housing are available near the center? What are the costs for this housing?

- What infection control measures does this center use for transplant patients? Isolation? Gown and gloves? Washing hands?

- What kinds of activities are available for children during their hospital stay?

- Describe the transplant procedure in detail, including anticipated complications.

- Explain the risks and benefits of this procedure.

- What is the average length of time before a child leaves the hospital? For a child who has been discharged from the hospital but whose home is far away, how long before he can leave the area to go home?

- What are the long-term side effects of this type of transplant?

- What long-term follow-up is available? Does the center have post-transplant clinics that focus on late effects?

- How does the center stay in contact with the child's primary doctor?

- Explain the waiting list requirements.

- How much will this procedure cost? How much will my insurance cover?

Many transplant centers have videos and booklets for patients and their families that explain services and describe what to expect before, during, and after transplant. Call any transplant center that you are considering and ask them to send you all available materials.

> *The head of oncology from a major transplant center comes to our city every 2 months to follow up with the kids who have been treated there. It was a big draw for us to have post-transplant follow-up at home, rather than having to travel a great distance to get back to the center. The other thing was that children are not put in laminar air flow, and families weren't required to cap and gown, only scrub their hands. Since I'm allergic to those hospital gloves, this allowed me to stay with my daughter throughout. We did, however, call around to several centers to compare facilities, costs, and insurance coverage.*

Making an informed consent is a serious decision when considering a life-threatening procedure such as a PBSCT. It is very important to work closely with your child's neuro-oncologist and treatment team when making this decision. Do not hesitate to keep asking questions until you fully understand what is being proposed. Ask the doctor to use plain English if she has lapsed into medical jargon. Tape the conversation to review later, or take along a family member or friend to take notes. Many centers require the assent of children ages 7 to 17, in addition to parental consent. Do not sign the consent form until you feel comfortable that you understand the procedure and have had every question answered.

Paying for the transplant

PBSCTs are expensive. Some transplants are considered the standard of care, so insurers cover the procedure without problems. However, you will need to research carefully whether your insurance company considers the type of transplant proposed for your child to be experimental and therefore not covered. Most insurance plans have a lifetime cap, and many only pay 80 percent of the costs of the transplant up to the cap. Often, transplant centers will not perform the procedure without all of the money guaranteed. With time being of the essence, this can cause great anguish for families who struggle to raise funds or need to take out a second mortgage to pay for a PBSCT.

Most insurance companies will assign your child's care to a transplant coordinator or case manager who is responsible for making arrangements with the transplant center and handling financial issues. Getting to know your coordinator and letting that person know your needs and concerns may provide an additional valuable resource for you during this stressful time.

> *Our first quote from the transplant center was $350,000, but we were able to negotiate a lower price.*

· · · · ·

> *My son died soon after the transplant. I hate to talk about the money, because I don't want people to think I begrudge spending it. I know that I would feel differently if the transplant had been successful, but I honestly think that we were misled about the real chance of success for his type of disease. We spent the equity on our house, plus took out a second mortgage. We will be paying it off for the rest of our lives.*

If you are having difficulty getting your insurance company to pay for the transplant or coverage has been denied, BMT InfoNet provides a free referral service to attorneys and not-for-profit organizations that might be able to help you. To get this help, fill in the form at *www.bmtinfonet.org/services/insurancehelp* or phone (888) 597-7674.

If you do not have health insurance, check *www.healthcare.gov* to see if you are eligible for government-sponsored insurance plans. The National Cancer Institute (*http://bethesdatrials.cancer.gov*) offers transplants free of charge to patients who qualify for one of its research studies.

In Canada, each province and territory has a provincial health plan that usually covers the medical costs of transplantation. However, there are still expenses that will need to be covered by the family. Children will often have to travel long distances to facilities that can perform a transplant. Travel, accommodations, and related costs have to be paid by the parents.

Stem cell harvest and storage

Stem cells are collected through a process called apheresis. The stem cells are collected ("harvested") at your children's hospital or at the transplant center as your child's bone marrow recovers from an intensive cycle of chemotherapy. A medication called granulocyte colony stimulating factor (G-CSF) is given to your child after the chemotherapy to further increase the number of stem cells in the blood.

When your child's peripheral blood counts rise, blood is removed through a central venous catheter (specially equipped for apheresis) or a temporary catheter placed in a vein. For older children with large veins, the arms may be used, but usually the temporary catheter is placed in the neck or groin. This surgical procedure requires anesthesia. One side of the catheter collects blood, which then goes into a machine that filters out the stem cells. The filtered blood is returned to the body through the other side of the catheter. Each apheresis procedure takes 4 to 6 hours.

The number of sessions required is variable. Infants may need only one session, but older children usually need two or three sessions. In rare cases, it is impossible to get enough stem cells from the blood of children who have recently undergone extensive chemotherapy and/or radiation. In these rare instances, stem cells from the bone marrow are used.

> Six-year-old Ethan had a stem cell harvest after his recovery from the first Cytoxan® doses he got. He was on Neupogen® (G-CSF), which was a piece of cake for him. Once he had enough of the stem cells in his bloodstream, he had a femoral PICC line placed because they needed a larger catheter to do this. The only down side was that he had to lay completely flat for about 6 hours, and collection took 2 days, so he had limited movement the night between collections. Plan a lot of quiet activities! Videos, books on tape, handheld games, cards. He hated the no bathroom privileges and refused to use a urinal at all.

Possible complications of peripheral blood stem cell apheresis include:

- **Hypocalcemia (low calcium in the blood).** Your child may experience muscle cramps, chills, tremors, tingling of the fingers and toes, dizziness, and occasionally chest pain. He will be closely monitored during the procedure, and IV or oral calcium supplements will be given to prevent this problem.

- **Thrombocytopenia (low platelets).** Sometimes platelets stick to the inside of the apheresis machine. Your child's platelet count will be checked before and after the apheresis, and a platelet transfusion will be given if needed.

- **Hypovolemia (low blood volume).** This can occur at any time during the procedure and is more common in small children. Symptoms can include low blood pressure, rapid heart rate, lightheadedness, and sweating. To prevent this problem, the apheresis machine is generally "primed" with a unit of blood (from a blood donor) prior to the procedure.

- **Infection.** If your child develops fever, chills, or low blood pressure, blood cultures will be obtained and IV antibiotics given.

After collection, the child's stem cells are treated and stored until they are used. Various compounds (e.g., dimethyl sulfoxide [DMSO]) are used to protect the stem cells during storage.

Most apheresis procedures are safely performed on an outpatient or short-stay basis, so you and your child can go home each evening. Some transplant centers, however, do require hospitalization throughout the procedure.

The transplant

Prior to the transplant, the child's bone marrow is suppressed using high-dose chemotherapy (radiation is generally not used to prepare a child with a brain or spinal cord tumor for a PBSCT). This portion of treatment, called conditioning, kills tumor cells and makes room in the bone marrow for new stem cells. The child in the following story had conditioning for a single transplant that included the chemotherapy drug thiotepa. Children who receive thiotepa before tandem transplant do not usually have such severe symptoms.

> Our 2-year-old daughter had high-dose chemo and then a stem cell transplant to treat her medulloblastoma. The transplant was terribly hard. The thiotepa made her skin peel off, and she was wrapped in gauze like a mummy. Her mucous membranes sloughed off in her mouth and down her esophagus and she needed a morphine drip for pain. Her counts went to zero and it was very scary. There was certainly a lot that could go wrong. However, she recovered quickly and was back in preschool 2 months later. She is 6 now, and has mostly happy memories of those days. Our family sort of took over the room. We brought in a radio and we all danced. I'd take her out of bed and put her on the floor on a blanket and we'd picnic. We sang a lot. Now, she can't wait to go for her checkups.

Conditioning regimens vary according to institution and protocol and also depend on the medical condition and history of the child. For tandem transplants, the chemotherapy is given for 2 to 6 days; in many cases all or part of the therapy is given in the outpatient setting. Your child may need IV fluids at night to provide proper hydration. It is important that you understand who to call and the number to use if problems occur at night.

If your child receives conditioning chemotherapy as an outpatient, she will need to go to the transplant unit no later than the evening before the procedure for hydration. The transplant itself consists of simply infusing the stem cells through a central venous catheter into the child, just like a blood transfusion. The stem cells travel through the blood vessels, eventually settling in the bone marrow.

DMSO, the most common compound used to protect stem cells during storage, has a strong odor that might be present during the infusion. This odor can be minimized by washing the stem cells during the thawing process, although the DMSO can often still be smelled even after washing.

> I cannot say enough good things about the transplant center. They were very family-oriented, allowed us in the room 24 hours a day. I was allowed to sleep in bed with her (I just told the nurses to make sure to poke her and not me). The nurses were wonderful, and I still think of them as family.

A transplant doctor will monitor your child during the infusion of stem cells. A variety of minor to major complications might occur, including:

- Abdominal cramps
- Difficulty breathing
- Slow heartbeat
- Tightness in the chest
- Chills
- Cough
- Diarrhea
- Skin rash
- Fever
- Flushing
- Headache
- Changes in blood pressure
- Nausea and vomiting
- Unpleasant taste (usually relieved by sucking on hard candies or flavored liquids)
- Kidney failure (seen less frequently if stem cells were washed)

Treatment was a long haul for Andrew. It was a time that we had absolutely no control over anything. You watch your child in the most horrible state. It was literally a time that we lived minute-by-minute and sometimes second-by-second. We're still dealing with the side effects. He doesn't have his energy or full strength. It's coming back, but it's a slow process. He missed about a year and a half of school during treatment for his brain tumor.

Stem cell transplant was almost like a rebirthing for Andrew. He went from being so angry about his diagnosis to a much wiser, much more confident child. His insight is wise beyond his years. Andrew's involved in quite a bit of public speaking. He's gone before elementary, middle school, and high school groups and DARE groups, talking about how important life is, and why it's important to enjoy life, and how it feels to almost lose your life.

Andrew (now 13 years old) adds:

Public speaking started with my teacher. He asked me if I'd speak to a high school class, and I said sure, if someone can learn from what I've been through, I'm all for it. I consider myself blessed with a tumor, not diagnosed with it. So many good things have come from it. Treatment feels like a never-ending battle, but it's not. You can't be afraid to die; thinking like that will bring you down as fast as anything. You need to have faith in something, I had faith in God, but you need to believe you're going to make it. Treatment is painful, but you have to think of the outcome and keep your eye on the goal. It's difficult, but not impossible.

Emotional responses

PBSCT can take a heavy emotional toll on the child, the siblings, and the parents. It can be a physically and mentally grueling procedure, with the possibility of months or years of late effects. Most transplant team members are extensively trained to meet the needs of the child and family during the transplant itself and the convalescence that follows. The team usually includes doctors, nurses, social workers, educators, nutritionists, and physical, occupational, speech, and child-life therapists.

Levi's transplant experience was like watching someone wake up from a deep sleep. For 2 weeks he was flat on his back, suffering greatly from mucositis and a tummy bug that caused diarrhea for days straight. It was a real horror. Then one evening he sat up and said, "What's all that stuff?" He was referring to all the gifts that had piled up in the corner of his room. He opened every toy, got down on the floor, and drew pictures of all the foods he was craving, and he never looked back. It was like an instant transformation. I think my own recovery was longer. I believe part of me froze in order to survive the transplant, and it took a long time to thaw.

What helped me the most were the decorations and having a positive attitude. My mom decorated the area outside the transplant room with balloons, cards, and posters. It was hard to take the medicine, so my mom made a huge poster to mark off how well I did. Every time I took my medicine, I got a sticker. When I got one hundred stickers, I got some roller blades.

Often so much time and energy is focused on the child who needs the transplant that the needs of the siblings are overlooked. Siblings need careful preparation for what is about to occur, and all their questions should be answered and their concerns addressed. For more information about siblings, read Chapter 15, *Siblings*.

Organizations that offer emotional support to families during the transplant are listed in Appendix B, *Resource Organizations*.

Complications after transplant

Some children have a smooth journey through the transplant process, while others bounce from one life-threatening complication to another. Some children live, and some children die. There is no way to predict which children or teens will develop problems, nor is there any way to anticipate whether the new development will be a mere inconvenience or a catastrophe.

The transplant center was very clear about all of the potential problems. That was good, for it prepared me. My attitude is watch for them, hope they don't happen, if they do, then live with them. She had an easy time with the transplant, she's a happy third grader, she's alive, and we feel so, so very lucky.

This section presents some of the major complications that can develop post-transplant (in alphabetical order) and the experiences of several families who coped with these problems.

Bleeding

Bleeding may occur in different ways throughout your child's post-transplant recovery phase, including:

- Bruising
- Bleeding from the gums, urinary, or gastrointestinal tract
- Nosebleeds

These common problems are generally managed with platelet transfusions. Serious bleeding can also occur in the lungs, stomach, intestines, or brain. Most transplant centers strive to keep children's platelet counts at a safe level until blood cell recovery has occurred. In general, platelets are the last type of blood cell to fully recover following PBSCT.

Eating difficulties

Almost all children undergoing PBSCT require intravenous (IV) nutrition during their convalescence. Some centers feed children using tubes inserted through the nose to the stomach or small intestine. This is a good choice if the child isn't experiencing nausea and vomiting. Other children require IV nutrition (see Chapter 20, *Nutrition*). Most transplant centers initiate IV or tube feeding promptly after transplant and continue until the child's appetite and ability to take in adequate calories by mouth have returned.

A variety of factors contribute to eating difficulties, including pre-existing nutritional problems, side effects of conditioning chemotherapy, anticipatory nausea and vomiting, mouth sores, and infections of the gastrointestinal tract.

Your child may require ulcer medications to coat the lining of the stomach or to decrease the amount of stomach acid produced. He may experience ongoing nausea, in spite of the fact that he is long past his conditioning chemotherapy. Ask to speak to the transplant unit dietician and keep accurate records of your child's eating. Your child's ability to eat and drink more normally is closely correlated with the recovery of blood counts.

Hemorrhagic cystitis

Hemorrhagic cystitis (bleeding from the bladder) may result from certain chemotherapy drugs used in your child's conditioning regimen. If your child receives a chemotherapy drug that has the potential to cause this problem, she will probably also receive the drug Mesna® to help coat the bladder lining. Occasionally, hemorrhagic cystitis is caused by a bacterial or viral bladder infection. Symptoms include blood in the urine (which may be obvious to the eye or microscopic), blood clots in the urine, pain when urinating, and bladder discomfort. If your child develops hemorrhagic cystitis or a urinary tract infection, she will receive antibiotics, IV fluids, and pain medication as needed.

Infections

The immune system of healthy children quickly destroys any foreign invaders; this is not the case for children who have undergone a transplant. The immune systems of children undergoing PBSCT have been temporarily impaired by chemotherapy. Until the new stem cells begin to produce large numbers of white cells (2 to 4 weeks after the transplant), children are in danger of developing serious infections.

To combat bacterial infections, children receive large doses of several kinds of antibiotics if they develop a fever any time during the first weeks after transplant when their white blood cell count is low. Fungal infections can also occur. Fortunately, bone marrow growth factors, such as Neupogen®, stimulate and accelerate white blood cell recovery. Your child will begin receiving this medication 1 to 2 days after the transplant. In addition, your child will be carefully evaluated each day for signs and symptoms of infection. Potential sites for problems include the skin, mouth, anus, and central venous catheter exit site. Report any new symptoms, such as cough, shortness of breath, abdominal pain, diarrhea, pain on urination, vaginal discharge, or mental confusion to the nurses promptly.

After the first month post-transplant, children are also susceptible to serious viral infections, most commonly herpes simplex virus, cytomegalovirus (CMV), and varicella zoster virus (causes chickenpox and shingles). These infections can occur up to 2 years after the transplant. Viral infections are notoriously hard to treat, so many centers use prophylactic acyclovir, granciclovir, or immunoglobulin to prevent them. The most common organisms that cause infections are CMV and pneumocystis carinii (a type of pneumonia). CMV is usually preventable if your child is CMV-negative and all transfused blood products are CMV-negative or filtered to remove white blood cells. The risk of pneumocystis carinii infection can be decreased by using prophylactic trimethoprim/sulfamethoxazole or IV pentamidine.

> Our daughter (age 9) had a peripheral blood stem cell transplant. It's been several months and her white blood cell count is still low, but we have come to the conclusion that we can't make her live in a bubble anymore. We are careful to avoid potential risks, though, such as being around large crowds of people.

During immune recovery, a patient must redevelop immunity to the common organisms that infect all children, which may require redoing the usual childhood immunizations. Children are tested 6 to 12 months following transplant for their immunity, and reimmunization is done (or not) based on the results of the testing.

Preventing infection is the best policy for those children who have had a stem cell transplant. The following are suggestions to minimize exposure to bacteria, viruses, and fungi:

- Medical staff and all family members must thoroughly wash their hands before touching the child.

- Keep your child away from crowds and people with infections.

- Do not let your child receive live virus inoculations until the immune system has fully recovered; your child's neuro-oncologist will determine the appropriate date for getting immunizations.

- Keep your child away from anyone who has recently been inoculated with a live virus (e.g., chicken pox, polio).

- Keep your child away from barnyard animals and all animal feces.

- Avoid remodeling your home while your child is recovering.

- Have all carpets shampooed prior to your child's return home from transplant.

- Family pets should be shampooed prior to your child's return home.

- Call the doctor at the first sign of a fever or infection.

> *After Hunter's double stem cell transplant, we had to follow many precautions. We had to be careful when we took him out, avoiding large crowds or public places (especially those indoors). He needed to wear a mask when we took him to his doctor's visits. We would take him to plenty of outdoor places for fun. I found the precautions easy to follow.*

Mucositis

Mucositis (inflammation of the mucous membranes lining the mouth and gastrointestinal tract) and stomatitis (mouth sores) are common complications following PBSCTs. Symptoms include reddened, discolored, or ulcerated membranes of the mouth, pain, difficulty swallowing, taste alterations, and difficulty speaking. The majority of children undergoing transplants experience this problem.

Your child will require frequent mouth care, modifications in diet, and pain medications. It is very important to try and coordinate your child's required mouth care with the administration of appropriate pain medications. Likewise, making sure your child receives pain medication prior to eating often helps. When white blood cells return, your child's mouth will heal.

> *High-dose chemo kills your taste buds, and I wanted to only eat sweet or spicy food, anything else tasted like cardboard. I'd eat ribs with BBQ sauce. KFC® masedh potatoes and gravy was great. Drinking was hard. I used to suck on ice cubes. It's gross when the lining of your mouth comes out. It just pulls out, it's white, it doesn't hurt. It comes out during bowel movements, too, but you don't realize it. But, you can't swallow because of the sores, so you have to spit a lot.*

Neurological complications

Children with brain or spinal cord tumors are at increased risk of developing neurological complications after transplant. Mental confusion, acute hearing loss, and expressive and receptive communication problems may occur. Fortunately, these are usually temporary. Your child may need assistance with communicating her needs and wants. In many cases, a communication or picture board is helpful until your child is able to communicate better. Speech therapy helps, and you should request this service if your treatment team does not suggest it. Patience and a supportive attitude are very important and will reassure your child should this complication occur.

Pulmonary edema

Pulmonary edema (collection of fluid in lung tissue) is sometimes seen in children who have had single or tandem PBSCTs. Symptoms include shortness of breath, cough, bloody sputum, fever, sweating, chest pain, and swelling of the hands and feet. Your child may require oxygen, diuretic medications, corticosteroids, and temporary fluid restriction until the problem resolves.

Veno-occlusive disease

Veno-occlusive disease (VOD) is a complication in which flow of blood through the liver becomes obstructed. Children who have had more than one transplant, previous liver problems, or past exposure to intensive chemotherapy are more at risk of developing VOD. It can occur gradually or very quickly. Symptoms of VOD include jaundice (yellowing of the skin), enlarged liver, pain in the upper right abdomen, fluid in the abdomen, unexplained weight gain, and poor response to platelet transfusions. Treatment includes fluid restriction, diuretics (such as Lasix®), anti-clotting medications, and removal of all but the most essential amino acids from IV nutrition.

Long-term side effects

Increasing numbers of children are being cured of their disease and surviving years after a single or tandem PBSCT. The intensity of the treatment prior to, during, and after transplant can cause major effects not apparent for months or years. This section describes a few of the common long-term side effects that sometimes develop after transplant.

Dental development

Certain chemotherapy drugs, administered in high doses prior to transplant, may result in improper tooth development and blunted or absent tooth roots in children who had a transplant when they were younger than 5 years of age. Your child should have a comprehensive dental examination prior to the transplant and a dental follow-up after recovery from the PBSCT.

Thyroid function

Children who receive only chemotherapy do not develop thyroid deficiency as a result of treatment. If, however, your child receives radiation therapy to the brain and spinal cord, either before or following recovery from a transplant, she should be monitored for thyroid deficiency. Tablets containing thyroid hormone are usually effective in treating the problem.

> Our 4-year-old son had focal point and cranial/spinal radiation for medulloblastoma and high-dose Cytoxan® for his stem cell transplant. It took about a year for his counts to normalize and he was sick a lot during that time. He takes growth hormone and thyroid replacement. He has severe high frequency hearing loss. But these are nothing compared to the learning difficulties.

Puberty and fertility

If your child receives cranial radiation, either before or following recovery from a transplant, delays in puberty and sexual development can occur. In addition, some of the drugs given in high doses during conditioning (e.g., cyclophosphamide, thiotepa) can cause changes in future fertility (the ability to become a biological parent). For this reason, boys who have gone through puberty should bank sperm before treatment begins. You may also be told about any experimental protocols that are attempting to preserve fertility in girls.

Any child or teen who had a transplant should be followed closely by a pediatric endocrinologist, who can prescribe hormones (testosterone for boys, estrogen and progesterone for girls) to assist in normal pubertal development and can assess fertility in older survivors.

Second cancers

Children who receive a PBSCT have a small risk of developing a second cancer. The risk depends on the chemotherapy drugs given during conditioning. Use of etopoide and cyclophosphamide increases the risk of second cancers.

Because transplants are relatively new treatments for children and teens with brain and spinal cord tumors, the overall impact and long-term effects are not yet clear. Your child's doctor can explain known risks given your child's disease and treatment.

The road of chemotherapy treatment was long and harsh, but transplant was a test of faith and patience. Knowing that Mia's immune system would be zapped to the point of no return was scary. However, it felt like the last step in killing off any sign of cancer in my little girl's body and a step closer to the end of this nightmare. Isolation was tough on both of us but once again the staff, the programs, the volunteers, and everyone in the hospital were amazing. Mia's room was personalized and decorated just for her. She only asked to leave the room the day before we left for good, day 38! The nurses and doctors did everything in their power to make the whole transplant process go as smoothly as possible for all of us. They kept us informed, called us on their days off, helped me clean Mia up when she was sick, and even played dress up to help get her out of bed and shower. We survived, and Mia was discharged on day 39. She walked out dressed like a princess.

We came home on December 10, 2010. Mia has not been admitted since then. What a blessing to be home in time for Christmas. We had spent every holiday in the hospital since Mother's Day. We were so happy to be home at last and for good! I put the tree up the very next day.

Chapter 15

Siblings

Why was his hair falling out? Why was he going to
the hospital all the time? What was happening?
Why was he getting so many presents?

— Chet Stevens
Straight from the Siblings:
Another Look at the Rainbow

CHILDHOOD CANCER TOUCHES all members of the family, with especially long-lasting effects on siblings. The diagnosis creates an array of conflicting emotions in siblings; not only are the siblings concerned about their ill brother or sister, but they usually resent the turmoil that the family has been thrown into. They feel jealous of the gifts and attention showered on the sick child, yet feel guilty for having these emotions. The days, months, and years after diagnosis can be extremely difficult for the sibling of a child with a brain or spinal cord tumor.

Ways to explain the diagnosis to siblings are discussed in Chapter 4, *Telling Your Child and Others*. This chapter discusses common emotions and behaviors of siblings and provides insights about how to cope from parents and siblings who have been through this experience.

Emotional responses of the siblings

Brothers and sisters are shaken to the very core by cancer in the family. Parents, the leaders of the family clan, sometimes have no time, and little energy, to focus on the siblings. During this major crisis, siblings sometimes feel they have no one to turn to for help. They may feel concerned, worried, fearful, guilty, angry, sad, abandoned, or other powerful emotions. If you recognize these ever-changing emotions as normal, you will be better able to help your children talk about and cope with their strong feelings.

Although the years of treatment are emotionally potent for every member of the family, research has shown that siblings have good psychological outcomes, particularly if they have been assured that they are valuable, contributing members of the family whose thoughts and feelings matter. Siblings frequently report the experience as life-changing in many positive ways. Following are descriptions and stories about the emotions felt by siblings.

Concern for sick brother or sister

Children really worry about their sick brother or sister. It is difficult for them to watch someone they love be hurt by needles and sickened by medicines. It is scary to see a brother or sister lose weight and go bald. It is hard to feel so healthy and energetic when the brother or sister has to stay indoors because of weakness or low blood counts. The siblings may be old enough to know that death is a possibility. There are plenty of reasons for concern.

> My 10-year-old son Travis has had two brain bleeds since treatment for his tumor. It's hard for Travis' little brother Gregory. Here he had a big brother who took care of him and nurtured him, and now his brother can't talk, can't walk, and is totally disabled. The other night, I found Gregory sitting on the stairs crying. I asked him what was wrong, and he said, "I want all of us to watch TV together. I miss my brother watching TV with me."

· · · · ·

> I'm the mother of three children. Logan was 19 months old when diagnosed. It was very hard on all of us. Kathryn (5½ at the time of diagnosis) felt that she had to take so much on herself. She was there with us the entire time Logan was in the hospital. She had a cot right next to Logan's bed, and only she and I were the ones who could take care of "our Logan."

> She used to love to visit the other kids on the hospital floor and entertain them. She hated to go home. She would get so involved with the other kids and didn't want to leave them. She actually got very close to two little girls that lost the battle, so here she was at 6, dealing with the loss of two friends.

Fear and worry

It is extremely common for young siblings of children with cancer to think that the disease is contagious—that they can "catch it." Many also worry that one or both parents may get cancer. The diagnosis of cancer changes children's view that the world is a safe place. They feel vulnerable, and they are afraid. Many siblings worry that their brother or sister may get sicker or may die.

Fears of things other than cancer may emerge: fear of being hit by a car, fear of dogs, fear of strangers. Many fears can be quieted by accurate and age-appropriate explanations from parents or medical staff.

My 3-year-old daughter vacillated between fear of catching cancer ("I don't ever want those pokes") to wishing she was ill so that she would get the gifts and attention ("I want to get sick and go to the hospital with Mommy"). She developed many fears and had frequent nightmares. We did lots of medical play, which seemed to help her. I let her direct the action, using puppets or dolls, and I discovered that she thought there was lots of violence during her sister's treatments. She continues to ask questions, and we are still explaining things to her, 4 years later.

• • • • •

It's almost midnight, which means that it will be exactly 36 hours before my sister Kylie goes for her first MRI after radiation. I don't know what to expect, but I would really love to hear some positive words coming from the oncologist's mouth when we meet up with him to receive the results. I can hardly sleep because, although I am always hoping for a miracle, I constantly worry, to the extent of having nightmares, about hearing something that I don't want to hear.

Jealousy

Despite feeling concern for the ill brother or sister, almost all siblings also feel jealous. Presents and cards flood in for the sick child, Mom and Dad stay at the hospital with the sick child, and most conversations revolve around the sick child. When the siblings go out to play, the neighbors ask about the sick child. At school, teachers are concerned about the sick child. Is it any wonder brothers and sisters feel jealous?

The siblings' lives are in turmoil and they sometimes feel a need to blame someone. It's natural for them to think that if their brother or sister didn't get sick, life would be back to normal. Some siblings develop symptoms of illness in an attempt to regain attention from the parents.

Our 9-year-old son seemed to be dealing with things so well until one evening as I was tucking him in, he confided that he had tried to break his leg at school by jumping out of the swing. He began to cry and told me he doesn't want his brother to be sick anymore; that he needs some attention, too. As parents, we were always so concerned with our sick child that we didn't realize how much our healthy child was suffering.

Guilt

Young children are egocentric; they are not yet able to see the world from any viewpoint but their own. Some children believe that they caused their brother or sister to get cancer. They may have said in anger, "I hope you get sick and die," and then their sister got sick. This notion should be dispelled right after diagnosis. Children need to be told, many times, that cancer just happens, and no one in the family caused it. They need to understand that no one can make something happen just by thinking or talking about it.

Many siblings feel guilt about their normal responses to cancer, such as anger and jealousy. They think, "How can I feel this way about my brother when he's so sick?" Assure them that the many conflicting feelings they are experiencing are normal and expected. As a parent, share some of your conflicting feelings (such as anger at the behavior of a child due to a treatment side effect, guilt about being angry).

It is also common for some children (and parents) to feel guilt about being healthy. It is important for parents to provide many opportunities to remind their healthy children that there is no connection between their health and their sibling's illness and that no one, including the sick brother or sister, wants them to feel bad about feeling good.

Abandonment

If parental attention revolves around the sick child, siblings may feel isolated and resentful. Even when parents make a conscious effort not to be so preoccupied with the ill child, siblings sometimes still perceive that they are not getting their fair share of attention and may feel rejected or abandoned.

> Jay had undergone many surgeries as a child, besides treatment for an anaplastic ependymoma. On a well-child visit, the doctor said he was concerned about his left eye turning in, and surgery for stabismus repair was recommended. This noncancer-related surgery unearthed memories. Jealous feelings from Jay's numerous surgeries, from the cancer days, resurfaced in our 15-year-old daughter, Vanessa. "It's not fair, when Jay has surgery, nobody does anything special for me." Her anger is wholly that of the 10-year-old girl she was when her brother suddenly developed a brain tumor.

Sometimes it is necessary to have the siblings stay with relatives, friends, or babysitters. Parents may have to miss activities, such as soccer games or school events, they would otherwise have attended. Vacation plans may be scrapped. The reasons may seem obvious to parents, but the siblings may interpret these changes as evidence that they are not as well-loved as the sick child. Parents should explain in detail the reasons for any alterations in routines, solicit feelings about the changes from the siblings, and try to find solutions that work for everyone in the family.

Sadness

Siblings have many very good reasons to be sad. They miss their parents and the time they used to spend with them. They miss the life they used to have—the one they were comfortable with. They miss their sick sibling. They worry that he or she may die. Some children show their sadness by crying often; others withdraw and become depressed. Sometimes children confide in relatives or friends that they think their parents don't love them anymore.

When Jeremy was very sick and hospitalized, we sent his older brother Jason to his grandparents for long periods of time. We thought that he understood the reasons, but a year after Jeremy finished treatment, Jason (9 years old) said, "Of course, I know that you love Jeremy more than me anyway. You were always sending me away so that you could spend time with him." It just broke my heart that every time he made that long drive over the mountains with his grandparents, he was thinking that he was being sent away.

Anger

Children's lives are disrupted by the diagnosis of a sister or brother with cancer, and siblings often feel very angry. Questions such as "Why did this happen to us?" or "Why can't things be the way they used to be?" are common. Children's anger may be directed at their sick sibling, their parents, relatives, friends, or doctors.

Children's anger may have a variety of causes. They may resent being left with babysitters so often or having additional responsibilities at home, or they may notice that the sick child isn't always held to the same standards of behavior as the other children. Because each member of the family may have frayed nerves, explosions of temper can occur.

As we were driving home from school one day, Annie was talking, and I was only half listening. All of a sudden I realized that she was yelling at me. She screamed, "See, this is what I mean. You never listen, your mind is always on Preston." I pulled the car over, stopped, and said, "You're right. I was thinking about Preston." I told her that from now on I would try to give her my full attention. I realized that I would really have to make an effort to focus on what she was saying and not be so distracted. This conversation helped to clear the air for a while. I tried to take her out frequently for coffee or ice cream to just sit, listen, and concentrate on what she was saying.

Worry about what happens at the hospital

Children have vivid imaginations, and when they are fueled by disrupted households and whispered conversations between teary parents, children can imagine truly horrible things. Seeing how their ill sibling looks upon returning from a hospital stay can reinforce their fears that awful things happen at the clinic or hospital. Or, the sibling may think they are missing some grand parties when they see their sister or brother and parent come home from the hospital with presents and balloons.

My son is only in kindergarten. He has separation anxiety worse than a 6 month old. He doesn't want to go to bed alone. The last time Karissa had the flu, I thought he was going to die from worrying so much. He cried himself to sleep every night and woke up crying. He was so worried. He hasn't gotten much better since she has started feeling better, either. He doesn't even want to go near the hospital with his sister.

Age-appropriate explanations can help children be more realistic about what they think happens at the hospital, but nothing is as powerful as a visit. Of course the effectiveness of a visit depends on your child's age and temperament, but many parents say that bringing the siblings along helps everyone. The sibling gains an accurate understanding of hospital procedures, the sick child is comforted by the presence of the sibling(s), and the parent gets to spend more time with all the children.

> *Alissa's older brother Nicholas is her best friend. We are at the hospital for appointments and therapy three nights a week, every week. Nicholas helps Alissa with "hospital homework" and he also helps with her therapy. Nicholas is doing great at school. We include him on everything.*

Another way to help a worried sibling is to read age-appropriate books together. Many children's hospitals have coloring books for preschoolers that explain hospital procedures with pictures and clear language. School-age children may benefit from reading books with a parent (see Appendix C, *Books and Websites*). Adolescents might be helped by watching videos, reading books, or joining a sibling support group.

Several parents suggested that another way to reduce siblings' worries is to allow even the youngest children to help the family in some way. As long as children have clear explanations about the situation and concrete jobs to do that will benefit the family, they tend to rise to the occasion. Make them feel they are a necessary and integral part of the family's effort to face cancer together.

> *My younger kids have never known 11-year-old Zach as normal. He had his first surgery at 5 years old; Emily was 3 and Sarah was barely 1. Emily helped Zach go through 3 months of inpatient rehabilitation, when he relearned how to walk, talk, chew, swallow, etc. Zach having a brain tumor is all they know.*
>
> *All Zach's life, they treated him normally. No one ever let him win at games or anything (although I tried to make them). When we found out about the relapse, something got back to Emily in third grade. She got off the bus one day and asked if Zach was dying. I was shocked! I told her that his tumor was back but we were taking him to the best brain tumor doctor and we would do everything we could so he wouldn't die. That seemed to totally satisfy her.*
>
> *There was only one time that I remember Emily's and Sarah's teachers both telling me at parent conferences that the girls had been chatting a lot and not listening much. At the time, we were going through more surgery with Zach, so I think that is why.*
>
> *Lauren is 4. This past summer, Zach took horseback riding for physical therapy. It was great! The girls would take turns coming to watch. Well, one day, Lauren was watching and she picked out this beautiful horse and said, "When I have my brain tumor, I'm going to ride that horse." Oh my gosh! Can you imagine? It's just so normal to them.*

As far as I can tell, none of them have issues with embarrassment over Zach or anything like that. Often they think he is lucky because he can ride in the wheelchair (and they have to walk) or he was lucky because he got to ride horses. They all have a deep faith and pray a lot for Zach and other kids with brain tumors.

They also seem to reach out more to others. The oldest two belong to Chemo Angels where they volunteer to send out small cards or packages twice a week to a child with cancer.

Concern about parents

Exhausted parents are sometimes not aware of the strong feelings of their healthy children. They may assume children understand they are loved, and that they would be getting the same attention if they were the one who had cancer. Siblings frequently do not share their powerful feelings of anger, jealousy, or worry because they love their parents and do not want to place additional burdens on them. It is all too common to hear siblings say, "I have to be the strong one. I don't want to cause my parents any more pain." But burdens are lighter if shared. Parents can help themselves and the siblings by acknowledging their own conflicting feelings and encouraging children to share their feelings, especially the difficult ones. Try to listen without becoming defensive and use those moments as an opportunity to grow together and strengthen each other.

Immediately post-surgery Ethan was mute and paralyzed on his right side. He had been sharing a room with his eldest brother, Jake, prior to his diagnosis but because Ethan needed help going to the bathroom and was so non-communicative, either my spouse or I slept in the room with Ethan. Ethan gradually improved over the first couple of months to the point where he was more independently mobile and Jake said he wanted to sleep in Ethan's room again so that my spouse and I could go back to sleeping together. Jake has always been calm, thoughtful, and responsible, and he really seemed to handle Ethan's illness the best of the boys. When he and I participated in a survey to evaluate Post Traumatic Stress Disorder (PTSD) in siblings, I found out that he was much more distressed than I had imagined. We took some time to talk about how the stress affected each of us, and I was really grateful that we had agreed to do the research project.

Sibling experiences

Simply understanding the pain and fears of your healthy children eases their journey. Being available to listen and say, "I hear how painful this is for you," or "You sound scared. I am, too," reminds siblings that they are still valued members of the family and that even though their brother or sister is absorbing the lion's share of their parents' time and care, they are still cherished. Siblings need to hear that what they feel matters, especially if parents do not have a lot of time to spend with them. If parents understand that these overwhelming emotions are normal, expected, and healthy, they can provide solace.

Brothers and sisters of children with cancer shared the following stories about some of the difficulties they face.

Silent hurting heart

Dayna E. wrote the following poem when she was 13 years old. Two of Dana's brothers had cancer—one lived and one died. This poem was published in *Bereavement* magazine and is reprinted with permission.

"Oh, nothing's wrong," she smiled,
grinning from ear to ear.
The frown that just was on her face
just seemed to disappear.

But deep down where secrets are kept,
the pain began to swell.
All the hurt inside of her
just seemed to stay and dwell.

All the pain in her heart
was too much for her to take.
Pretending everything's OK
is much too hard to fake.

She'd duck into the bathrooms
and hide inside the stalls.
Because no one could see her tears,
behind those dirty walls.

She was sick and tired of losing
and things never turning out right.
She had no hope left in her.
She was ready to give up the fight.

But she wiped away the teardrops,
put a smile back on her face,
pulled herself together, and
walked out of that place.

Life went on and things got better.
She thought that was a start.
But still, no one could see inside
her silent hurting heart.

Alana's story

Alana F. (11 years old) remembers how family life changed when her sister, Laura, had cancer.

My sister was in fifth grade and had been sick for the last week or so. Laura always seemed to be my hero. Although we got into arguments, all siblings get into fights, so I didn't worry. I didn't know what was about to happen, but neither did anyone else.

I don't quite remember how my parents told me she had cancer, but I do remember a lot of tears.

As time progressed, my life changed. I lived with my best friend and her parents, Catherine and Bill, but that changed too. Kelsie (my friend) and I got into a lot of arguments, but we still do. I don't know if that is why my grandmother and grandfather moved up to live in our house so that they could take care of me. Living with them was different. My grandmother had different expectations of me than my mother did.

My parents would each take turns staying at the hospital. Some nights I would live with my mom, grammy, and grandpy; and the next it would be with my dad and them.

Of course going through this dilemma I felt left out. Here I was living with my grandparents, and my sister got to live with our parents. She got lots of flowers, cards, and gifts, and all I got was the feeling of love from my relatives. I know that love is better than material things, but when you are 6 years old, you don't think so.

Things stayed the same for a long time. Then my sister went into remission and started living at home. I had to get used to my parents again and missed my grandparents.

My sister was spoiled at home, too. They bought her a waterbed, so she wouldn't get cold. What did I get? A heating blanket; a used heating blanket.

Having a sister with cancer

Alison L. (6 years old) describes the experience of having a sister with cancer:

I think having a sister with cancer is not fun. My mom paid more attention to Kathryn, my sister. I had to stay with Daddy. Mommy picked Kathryn up and not me. I wanted my sister's PJs. Guess what? I did not get them! Although my mommy wanted to stay with me, she did not want to leave my sister alone. Sometimes I felt like I was going to throw up. But now it has been 2 years since she has stopped having medicine, and she is completely better. To celebrate we are going to Disneyland®.

My brother's a legend

To Erin H. (18 years old), her brother has become a legend by surviving childhood cancer.

I'm really proud of my brother Judson for handling everything so well. During those years, there were times when I was jealous of him, not only for the attention he received, but for his courage as well. This little boy was going through so much, and I still cowered at getting my finger pricked. As I look back, I wonder if I would have been able to make it through, not only physically, but emotionally as well.

According to some people, a person needs to be dead in order to be a legend, or to have been famous, or well liked. A legend to me, though, is someone who has accomplished something incredible, enduring many hardships and pains, and still comes out of it smiling.

Judd is a legend to me because he didn't give up in a time that he might have. He is a legend because he survived an illness that many do not. Now I look at him after being in remission for almost 5 years, and I hope that someday if I am ever faced with a challenge like his, I will have the same strength and courage he had.

When my brother got cancer

Annie W. (15 years old) relates some ways she benefited from her brother's battle with childhood cancer.

One experience in my life that was in no way comfortable for my family or myself and caused me a lot of confusion and grief was when my brother had cancer. Along with the disruption of this event, it also caused me to grow tremendously as a person. The Thanksgiving of my third-grade year, Preston, my brother, became very ill and was diagnosed a few weeks later with having cancer.

This event helped me to grow to become a better person in many ways. When my brother had very little hair or was puffed out from certain drugs, I learned to respect people's differences and to stick up for them when they're made fun of. Also, when Preston was in the hospital, I was taught to deal with a great amount of jealousy that I had. He received many gifts, cards, flowers, candy, games, and so many other material things that I envied. Most of all though, he received all the attention and care of my mother, father, relatives, and friends. This is what I was jealous of the most. As I look back now, I can't believe that I was that insensitive and self-centered to be mad at my brother at a time like that.

The thing that made this a "graced" experience was the fact that it enabled me to be very close to my brother as we grew up. My brother and I are now good friends and are able to talk and share our experiences with each other. I don't think that we would have this same relationship if he never had cancer, and I think that has been a very positive outcome. Another thing that has been a positive outcome of this event is the people I've been able to meet. Through all the support groups, camps, and events for children with cancer and their siblings, I have met some people with more courage and more heart than anyone could imagine. In no way am I saying that I'm glad my brother had cancer, but I will say I'm very glad with some of the outcomes from it.

My sister had cancer

Eleven-year-old Jeff P. explains what happened when "My Sister Had Cancer." (Reprinted with permission from Candlelighters Childhood Cancer Foundation Canada's *CONTACT* newsletter.)

> My sister Jamie got cancer when she was 23 months old. I was 8, and my two other sisters were 6 and 4.
>
> My sisters and I were scared that Jamie was going to die. We weren't able to go to public places and also weren't allowed to have friends in our house. We missed a lot of school when there was chicken pox in our school. I got teased in school sometimes because my sister had no hair. Once an older kid called my sister a freak. My mom was sad most of the time. It was very hard.
>
> We are all pleased that Jamie is doing well, and our lives are getting back to normal. It was an experience I'll never forget, and I hope it has made me a stronger person.

From a sibling

Fifteen-year-old Sara M. won first prize in a Candlelighters Creative Arts Contest with her essay, "From a Sibling."

> Childhood cancer—a topic most teens don't think much about. I know I didn't until it invaded our home.
>
> Childhood cancer totally disrupts lives, not only of the patient, but also of those closest to him/her, including the siblings. First, I was numbed with unbelieving shock. "This can't be happening to me and my family." Along with this came a whole dictionary full of incomprehensible words and a total restructuring of our (up to that time) fairly normal lifestyle.
>
> One day in July 1988, I was waiting for my parents to pick me up from summer camp and anticipating the start of our family vacation to Canada. When they arrived, they informed me that my older brother Danny was very sick, and we wouldn't be taking that trip after all. The following day, the call came that confirmed the diagnosis. Instead of packing for vacation, we packed our bags and headed for Children's Hospital in Denver, 200 miles away, where Danny was scheduled for surgery and chemotherapy.

I developed my own disease (perhaps from fear I would "catch" what Danny had) with symptoms similar to my brother's:

Sympathy pains. *I asked, "Why him?" when he came home from the hospital, exhausted from throwing up a life-saving drug for three days.*

Fear. *"How much sicker is Danny going to get before he gets well? He is going to get well, isn't he?"*

Resentment. *My parents seemed so worried about him all the time. They didn't seem to have time for me anymore.*

Confusion. *Why couldn't Danny and I wrestle around like we used to? Why couldn't I slug him when he made me mad?*

Jealousy. *I felt insignificant when I was holding down the fort at home.*

The parts I hated the most were: not understanding what was being done to him, answering endless worried phone calls, and hearing the answers to my own questions when my parents talked to other people.

I was helped to sort out these feelings and identify with other siblings when I attended a program held just for teens who had siblings with cancer. We got together, tried to learn how to cross-country ski, and talked about our siblings and ourselves.

Perhaps you remember this story: "US [speed skating] star Dan Jansen, 22, carrying a winning time into the back straightaway of the 1,000 meter race, inexplicably fell. Two days earlier, after receiving word that his older sister, Jane, had died of leukemia, Dan crashed in the 500 meter" (Life Magazine). Having a sibling with cancer can immobilize even an Olympic athlete. Dan was expected to bring home two gold medals, but cancer in a sibling intervened. He became, instead, the most famous cancer sibling of all time. He shared his grief before a television audience of two billion people. Dan later went on to win the World Cup in Norway and Germany, and capture the gold at the Olympics. He is the first to tell you the real champions can be found in the oncology wards of children's hospitals across our nation, and the siblings who are fighting the battle right along beside them.

Siblings: Having our say

A group of siblings at a national conference gave advice to parents and siblings of children with cancer.

Twelve young people aged 7 to 29 met at the 25th Anniversary Candlelighters Conference to talk about what it is like having a sibling with cancer in the family. We talked about our families, our anger, jealousy, worries, and fears, and thought about what we wanted to tell others about our experiences. In fact, we made lists of things we wanted other people to know: one for parents, one for other children or young adults in our position, and one for the child who has been diagnosed with cancer.

Some parts of these lists reflect anger and bitterness, but that was not the overriding feeling in the session. I hope it isn't the only message you take away. If nothing else, the issues raised here may provide you with a good starting point for discussions in your own family.

To parents:

- *We know you are burdened and trying to be fair. But try harder.*
- *Give us equal time.*
- *Be tough on disciplining the child with cancer. No free rides.*
- *Put yourself in our shoes once in a while.*
- *If you are away from home a lot, at least call and tell us, "I love you."*
- *Tell us what is going on. Don't just sit us in front of a video (about cancer); talk with us about it.*
- *Keep special time with us like lunch once a week or something. Time for just us. And if you can't be with us, find someone who can.*
- *When you talk to family members, say how everyone is doing—what we are doing is important, too.*
- *Ask how we are feeling. Don't assume you know.*

To siblings of newly diagnosed kids:

- *Keep a diary if you don't want to talk to your parents.*
- *Expect to not get as much attention.*
- *Expect that your parents are going to be extra cautious about what your brother/ sister does, who he/she hangs out with, etc.*
- *Hang in there. You're all you've got for now.*
- *Don't feel like you have to think about the illness all the time.*
- *Be understanding of your parents and stay involved.*
- *Tell someone how you are feeling—don't bottle it up.*
- *Go to the hospital to visit when you can.*
- *Make as many friends as possible at school.*

To our siblings who struggled or are struggling with cancer:

- *The world does not revolve around you.*
- *Stop feeling sorry for yourself.*

- *Not everything is related to cancer. Stop using that as an excuse for everything.*

- *I'm jealous of you sometimes, but I'm not mad. I know it sometimes seems like I'm mad, but I'm not.*

- *Don't take advantage of all the extra attention you get.*

- *Tell mom and dad to pay attention to me sometimes, too.*

- *Now that you are feeling better, where's the gratitude for all those chores that I did?*

- *I really admire your strength and courage. I wouldn't have gotten through your illness without you.*

Helping siblings cope

The following are suggestions from several families about ways to help brothers and sisters cope.

- Make sure you explain the tumor and its treatment to the siblings in terms they understand. Create a climate of openness so they can ask questions and know they will get answers. If you don't know the answer to a question, write it on your list to ask the doctor at the next appointment, or ask your child if he would like to go to the appointment with you and ask the question himself.

- Make sure all the children clearly understand that cancer is not contagious. They cannot catch it, nor can their ill brother or sister give it to anyone else. Impress upon them that nothing the parents or brothers and sisters did caused the cancer.

- Bring home a picture of the brother or sister in the hospital, and encourage the children to talk on the phone or send emails or text messages when their sibling is hospitalized.

- It is extremely hard for mothers and babies or toddlers to be separated when the mothers need to be at the hospital with the sick child and the baby or toddler sibling must stay at home.

  My daughter was 18 months old when her 3-year-old sister was diagnosed. Each member of the family flew in to stay at the house for 2-week shifts, so she had a lot of caregivers. A friend of mine gave her a big key chain that held eight pictures. We put a picture of each member of the family (including pets) on her key chain, and she carried it around whenever we were away. It seemed to comfort her.

- Try to spend time individually with each sibling.

  We began a tradition during chemotherapy that really helped each member of our family. Every Saturday each parent would take one child for a 2-hour special time. We scheduled it ahead of time to allow excitement and anticipation to grow. Each child picked what to do on their special day—such as going to the park, eating lunch at a restaurant, riding bikes. We tried to put aside our worries, have fun, and really listen.

- If people only comment about the sick child, try to bring the conversation back to include the sibling. For example, if someone exclaims, "Oh look how good Lisa looks," you could say, "Yes, and Martha has a new haircut, too. Don't you think she looks great?"

- Share your feelings about the illness and its impact on the family. Say, "I'm sad that I have to bring your sister to the hospital a lot. I miss you when I'm gone." This allows the sibling an opportunity to tell you how she feels. Try to make the illness a family project by expressing how the family will stick together to beat it.

  I never kept my feelings secret from Shawn's two older brothers (5 and 7 years old). If I was scared, I talked about it. Once when we thought he was relapsing, my stomach was so knotted up that I could barely walk. Kevin said, "Mom, I'm really worried about Shawn." I told him that I was, too, and then we both just hugged and cried together. They really opened up when we didn't hide our feelings.

- Include siblings in decision-making, such as giving them choices about how extra chores will be divided up or devising a schedule for parent time with the healthy children.

  We always gave the boys choices about where they would stay when Shawn had to be in the hospital. I felt like it gave them a sense of control to choose babysitters. They usually stayed at a close neighbor's house where there were younger children. It allowed them to ride the same bus to school and play with their neighborhood friends. Their lives were not too disrupted. They also really pitched in and helped with the younger kids. I think it helped them to help others.

  • • • • •

  Sometimes I think that my mom does not treat us equally. For example, if I left my snack garbage on the floor I would not get a snack the next night but Zach would get a snack if he left his garbage on the floor. I know he cannot walk but he could ask someone to take it out for him or he could say, "I need to take my garbage out so can somebody help me walk out so I can throw my garbage away."

- Allow siblings to be involved in the medical aspects of their brother's or sister's illness, if they want to be. Often the reality of clinic visits and overnight stays is easier than what siblings imagine. Many siblings are a true comfort when they hold their brother or sister's hand during procedures.

Just yesterday, Spencer (who screamed and shrieked at the blood draw for the BMT [bone marrow transplant] typing, and didn't match) out of the blue said "Mom, I wish I could have donated my marrow to Travis." And he's 5! He also donated money to plant a tree in Israel today at Sunday school and asked us to write that it was "In honor of God and my brother, Travis." Oh man, we can never forget how this experience is seared in the memory of our children who don't have cancer. I am convinced that for Spencer, too, we will be seeing effects of this entire experience in many ways, long into the future.

• Give lots of hugs and kisses.

We assumed everything was fine with Erin because she had her grandma, who adored her, staying with her. We made a conscious decision to spend lots of time with her and include her in everything. But we realized later that she felt very left out. My advice is to give triple the affection that you think they need, including lots of physical affection such as hugs and kisses. For years, Erin felt jealous. She thought her brother got more of everything: material things, time with parents, opportunities to do things she was not allowed to do. She finally worked it out while she was in college.

• Be sure to alert teachers of siblings about the tremendous stress at home. Many children respond to the worries about cancer by developing behavior or academic problems at school. Teachers should be vigilant for the warning signals and provide extra support or tutoring for the stressed child or teen. Continue to communicate frequently with the teachers of the siblings to make sure you are aware of any developing problems.

Lindsey was in kindergarten when Jesse was first diagnosed with medulloblastoma. Because we heard nothing from the kindergarten teacher, we assumed that things were going well. At the end of the year, the teacher told us that Lindsey frequently spent part of each day hiding under her desk. When I asked why we had never been told, the teacher said she thought that we already had enough to worry about dealing with Jesse's illness and treatment. She was wrong to make decisions for us, but I wish we had been more attentive. Lindsey needed help.

• Expect your other children to have some behavior problems as part of living with cancer in the family. This is a normal response.

When my 4-year-old healthy child screams and sobs over a minor skinned knee, she gets as much sympathy as my child with cancer does when having her port accessed. I put a bandage on the knee, rock her, sing a song, and get her an ice pack. The injuries are not equal, but the needs of each child are. They both need to be loved and cared for; they both need to know that mom will help, regardless of the severity of the problem. I even let Alison use EMLA® for routine shots. My pediatrician laughs at me, but I just tell him, "Sibs need perks, too."

- The child with cancer receives many toys and gifts, which can result in hurt feelings or jealousy in the siblings. Provide gifts and tokens of appreciation to the siblings for helping out during hard times, and encourage your sick child to share.

  My daughter Jacqueline is 7 years old. We have three other children, ages 14, 8 ½, and 3. We found (through trial and error) that letting them know as much as they were able to handle, and making sure they felt comfortable asking any questions they might have, helped a great deal. We also made sure we called them two or three times a day from the hospital, and talked to them about how THEIR day was. We let them come to the hospital any time they wanted, after checking that it was okay with the docs. The second time around, we made sure that anyone coming to visit, or sending her something through the mail, either brought something small for the other three kids, or didn't bring anything at all. We also kept a small stock of wrapped presents for those who didn't remember our rule.

- Encourage a close relationship between an adult relative or neighbor and your other children. Having a "someone special" when the parents are frequently absent can help your child feel cared for and loved.

  We tried very hard to attend to the feelings of Ethan's siblings ourselves, but we realized early on that we were going to need help. We have a friend who is a children's librarian. She and her husband took the boys out every week and spent the evening with them. The kids picked out books at the library with her help and input, talked about the things they were doing at school, what was going on in their lives, got an ice cream, and were made to feel wanted and special. When Ethan had to go to the hospital for chemotherapy, the children's music teacher would have a sleep over for the boys at her house. She made them a favorite meal, rented a movie, made popcorn, and had a pajama party at her house so that they felt there was something special for them.

Take advantage of any workshops, support groups, or camps for siblings. These can be of tremendous value for siblings, providing fun and friendships with others who truly understand their feelings.

Positive outcomes for the siblings

After reading about all the difficult emotions your children might experience, it is important to note that many siblings exhibit great warmth and active caretaking while their brother or sister is being treated for a brain or spinal cord tumor. Their empathy and compassion seem to grow with the crisis.

Some brothers and sisters of children with cancer feel they have benefited from the stressful experience in many ways, such as: increased knowledge about disease, increased empathy for the sick or disabled, increased sense of responsibility, enhanced self-esteem, greater maturity and coping ability, and increased family closeness. Many of these siblings mature into adults interested in the caring professions, such as medicine, social work, or teaching. Character can grow from confronting a personal crisis, and many parents speak of their healthy children with admiration and pride.

Brothers and sisters of those with cancer go through much adversity, as we parents do. At times, much is overlooked, unintentionally of course, because of the many changes in our lives that we experience at such a difficult time. Well, today, I want to pay a small tribute to Tommy's 15-year-old brother, Matt. From the time Tommy was diagnosed, Matt has been by his side. The first night Matt wouldn't go to bed, just so he could stand by Tommy's bedside and be close to him. When we got back home, Matt took over and made sure Tommy would get his "daily laugh." Every evening, even when Tommy felt too sick to sit up, Matt would be there and always made us smile and laugh. As we all know, the siblings sacrifice much of their own lives during this time. Whether it be their social activities or school work, much of their "normal" lifestyle is changed. They even show their courage through the wide range of emotions, including much sorrow, that they experience. It is said, "Angels shine their light on us that we may see more clearly." So as our angel on earth, thank you Matt for shining your light on your brother Tommy, and may you also be blessed with the light of angels.

Chapter 16

Family and Friends

Shared joy is double joy,
shared sorrow is half sorrow.

— Swedish proverb

THE INTERACTIONS BETWEEN the parents of a child with cancer and their family members, and friends are complex. Potential exists for loving support and generous help, as well as for bitter disappointment and disputes. The diagnosis of a brain or spinal cord tumor creates a ripple effect, first touching the immediate family, then extended family, friends, coworkers, schoolmates, church/synagogue/mosque members, and, sometimes, the entire community.

This chapter begins with how family life needs to be restructured to cope with treatment. It then provides scores of ideas for helpful things extended family members and friends can do to support the family of a child with a brain or spinal cord tumor during this difficult time. To prevent possible misunderstandings, parents of children with cancer also share their thoughts about things that are not helpful.

Restructuring family life

Every family of a child with a brain or spinal cord tumor needs massive assistance. It helps if parents recognize this early and learn not only to accept aid gracefully but also to ask for help when its needed. As discussed later in this chapter, many family members, friends, and neighbors want to help, but they need direction from the family about what is helpful but not intrusive.

Jobs

In families where both parents are employed, decisions must be made about their jobs. It is better, if possible, to use all available sick leave and vacation days prior to deciding whether one parent needs to terminate employment. Parents need to be able to evaluate their financial situation and insurance availability; this requires time and clarity of thought—both of which are in short supply in the weeks following diagnosis.

When Garrett got sick, I used up all of my vacation. At that time, our head of Human Resources called me in and informed me that I now had to take unpaid leave if I wanted to stay out of the office any longer. He then added that in order to continue my benefits, I had to pay "my share" of all benefits costs during this leave. This included insurance, retirement, and other contributions. The weekly outlay was not insignificant. I was dismayed to say the least.

Fortunately, our senior management and common sense prevailed. We came to an informal arrangement where I "made up" lost time by working weekends and extended days when Garrett was home and doing okay. When he was inpatient (most of the first year and the first 3 months of the second), I would stay with him in the hospital on the weekends (Friday night through Sunday evening) and on Tuesday night and all day Wednesday. This would give my wife a break from the hospital and let me spend time with my son.

It worked very well. Pam later calculated that I worked more hours in make-up than I missed for Garrett. The company came out ahead. Every situation is different and every solution will be different in these circumstances. There is only one constant: You will never ever regret the precious time you spent with your child.

In August 1993, the Family and Medical Leave Act (FMLA) became federal law in the United States. FMLA protects the job security of employees of large companies who:

- Take a leave of absence to care for a seriously ill child
- Take medical leave because the employee is unable to work because of his or her own medical condition
- Take leave after the birth or adoption of a child for adoption

The FMLA:

- Applies to employers with 50 or more employees within a 75-mile radius.
- Provides 12 weeks of unpaid leave during any 12-month period to care for a seriously ill spouse, child, or parent, or to care for oneself. In certain instances, the employee may take intermittent leave, such as reducing his or her normal work schedule's hours.
- Requires employers to continue providing benefits, including health insurance, during the leave period.
- Requires employers to return employees to the same or equivalent positions upon return from the leave. Some benefits, such as seniority, need not accrue during periods of unpaid FMLA leave.
- Requires employees to give 30-day notice of the need to take FMLA leave, when the need is foreseeable.

- Is enforced by the Wage and Hour Division, U.S. Department of Labor, or by private lawsuit. You can locate the nearest office of the Wage and Hour Division by calling (866)-4-USWAGE (487-9243) or visiting its website at *www.dol.gov/whd/america2.htm*.

In Canada, a parent may be entitled to benefits under the Employment Insurance Act. Consideration is provided in the act for a parent having to leave work to care for an ill child. Entitlement to benefits is made on a case-by-case basis. Should a parent qualify, benefits are determined by the number of hours the parent has worked prior to making the claim. For further information, parents should contact the nearest Employment and Social Development Canada office, listed in the Government of Canada pages of the telephone directory, or visit its website at *www.hrsdc.gc.ca/eng/home.shtml*.

Marriage

Diagnosis and treatment place enormous pressure on a marriage. Couples may be separated for long periods of time, emotions run high, and coping styles and skills may differ. Initially, family life may be shattered; couples then must work together to rearrange the pieces into a new pattern. Following are parents' suggestions and stories about how they managed.

- Share medical decisions.

    My husband and I shared decision-making by keeping a joint medical journal. The days that my husband stayed at the hospital, he would write down all medicines given, side effects, fever, vital signs, food consumed, sleep patterns, and any questions that needed to be asked at the next rounds. This way, I knew exactly what had been happening. Decisions were made as we traded shifts at our son's bedside.

    • • • • •

    I made most of the medical decisions. My husband did not know what a protocol was, nor did he ever learn the names of the medicines. He came with me to medical conferences, however, and his presence gave me strength.

    • • • • •

    Curt and I discuss every detail of the medical issues. It is so helpful to hash things over together to get a clearer idea of what our main concerns are.

- Take turns staying in the hospital with your child.

    We took turns going in with our son for painful procedures. The doctors loved to see my husband come in because he's a friendly, easygoing person who never asked them any medical questions. We shared hospital duty, also. I would be there during any crisis because I was the person better able to be a strong advocate, but he went when our son was feeling better and needed entertaining company. It worked out well.

⋅ ⋅ ⋅ ⋅ ⋅

My husband fell apart emotionally when our daughter was diagnosed, and he never really recovered. He stayed with her once in the hospital and cried almost the whole time. She never wanted him there again, so I did all of the hospital duty.

⋅ ⋅ ⋅ ⋅ ⋅

Whenever Brian was in the hospital, we both wanted to be there. We were able to be there most of the time because our children have a wonderful aunt and uncle who stayed with them when needed. During Brian's second extended stay in the hospital, we both let go a little, and we each took turns sleeping at the Ronald McDonald House. That way we each got a decent night's sleep (or some sleep) every other night.

⋅ ⋅ ⋅ ⋅ ⋅

My wife took care of most of the medical information gathering because she had a scientific background. But my work schedule was more flexible, so I took my son for almost all of his treatments and hospitalizations. I cherish my memories of those long hours in the car and waiting room.

⋅ ⋅ ⋅ ⋅ ⋅

My husband does about 75 percent of the hospital/clinic/radiation visits. In fact, he does all of them when he is in town. I take care of the rest of the children and float in when I get a chance. I keep in touch with the doctors via email.

- Share responsibility for home care.

  We had a traditional relationship in which I took care of the kids and he worked. I didn't expect him to cook or clean when I was staying at the hospital—it was all he could do to ferry our daughter to her various activities and go to work.

  ⋅ ⋅ ⋅ ⋅ ⋅

  We both worked full time, so we staggered our shifts. He worked 7 to 3 during the day; I worked 3 to 11 at night. He did every single dressing change for the Hickman® catheter—584 changes, we counted them up. Wherever I left off during the day, he took over. He was great, and it really worked out well for us. We shared it all.

  ⋅ ⋅ ⋅ ⋅ ⋅

  My husband really didn't help at all. I couldn't even go out because he wouldn't give the pills. He kept saying that he was afraid he would make a mistake.

- Accept differences in coping styles.

  We both coped differently, but we learned to work around it. I didn't want to deal with "what if" questions, but he was a pessimist and constantly asked the fellow questions about things that might happen. I felt that it was a waste of energy to worry about things that might never happen. I didn't want to hear it and felt that it just added to my burden. It was all I could do to survive every day. We worked it out by going to conferences together, but I would ask my questions and then leave. He stayed behind to ask all of his questions.

• • • • •

My husband didn't have the desire to read as much as I did. However, whenever I read something that I felt he should read, he always took the time to do so and then we discussed it.

• • • • •

My husband and I have always been a team. We complement the strengths and weaknesses of each other and I think that was the reason we managed to hold everything together. When I was down, he would bring me up. When he was down, I would do the same for him. With the exception of the initial trauma when our son was diagnosed, we handled things in that manner throughout treatment.

• Seek counseling.

I went for counseling because I couldn't sleep. At night, I got stuck thinking the same things over and over and worrying. I ended up spending 2 years on antidepressants, which I think really saved my life. They helped me sleep and kept me on an even keel. I'm off them now, my son is off treatment, and everything is looking up.

• • • • •

My husband and I went to counseling to try to work out a way to split up the child rearing and household duties because I was overwhelmed and resenting it. I guess it helped a little bit, but the best thing that came out of it was that I kept seeing the counselor by myself. My son wanted to go to a "feelings doctor," too. I received a lot of very helpful, practical advice on the many behavior problems my son developed. And my son had an objective, safe person to talk things over with.

Most marriages survive, but some don't. It is usually marriages with serious pre-existing problems that are further strained by cancer treatment.

My husband had a lot of problems that really brought my daughter and me down. The cancer really opened my eyes to what was important in life. We stayed together through treatment, but we divorced after the transplant. I just realized that life is too short to spend it in a bad relationship.

• • • • •

My husband went to work rather than go with us to Children's when our son was diagnosed. It went downhill from there. He started using drugs and mistreating us, so we divorced.

Blended families

Many children diagnosed with cancer live in blended families. Parents may be separated or divorced, remarried, or living as single parents. There may be foster parents, biological parents, stepparents, or legal guardians. Communication between involved adults may be open and amiable or strained. It is best for the child when all parents/guardians involved put their differences aside and work together to provide an environment focused on caring and supporting the ill child. Counseling helps, too.

> My son has been treated off and on for 10 years for a brainstem tumor. He is now paralyzed and on a respirator in a care facility. In the beginning, my ex-husband was overseas, so my husband and I made all the appointments, took turns in the hospital, and tucked Brendon in at night. Over the years, my ex-husband has become more and more a part of our family care network. He goes to the care facility every day after work and on weekends. I stay with Brendon the days my husband has off, and my husband stays two evenings a week. My ex-husband will babysit my three other children so my husband and I can go to see Brendon or go on vacation. His mother also helps out enormously with visiting at the care facility and babysitting the three younger children. It's become a community effort. It works out well because we all love our son and we've chosen to work it out rather than bicker.

If the child with cancer has two homes due to a blended family, it often helps to have a journal that goes with the child to each set of parents. It keeps everyone involved up to date. It can contain information about medications given, dose changes, doctor's appointments, blood test results, and current symptoms.

Unfortunately, the diagnosis of cancer in a child can make strained family relations even worse. It is important that all parents/guardians with a legal right to information about all aspects of the illness receive that information and are able to participate in the decision-making process. In some situations a social worker, nurse practitioner, primary care physician, or psychologist will work with all parties to set up family meetings (together as a group or separately, depending on family dynamics) with healthcare providers to make this possible.

The extended family

Extended family—grandparents, aunts, uncles, cousins—can cushion the shock of diagnosis and treatment with loving words and actions. Extended family members sometimes drop their own lives to rush to the side of the newly diagnosed child, and often remain steadfast throughout the months or years of treatment. Regrettably, some family members are not helpful, either out of ignorance about what your family needs or simply because they are frightened by the diagnosis or overwhelmed by events in their own lives.

Some extended families, and even entire communities, rally around the family, but for other families, support never materializes. Several factors affect the strength of support that is offered: well-established community ties, good communication within the extended family, physical proximity to the extended family, and clear exchange of information about the needs of the affected family. If any of these elements are missing, support may dissipate or never appear.

> We had just moved 3,000 miles away from family and friends for my husband to accept a new job. We had no family close by, no friends. Each family member and some close friends used their vacations to fly out and take 2-week shifts at our new house to help out. Thankfully, they got us through the first months, but the rest of treatment was lonely.

Families with strong community ties often receive support throughout treatment.

> Shortly after Jesse's medulloblastoma returned, I was praying with my Bible study group. With four children ages 1 to 9, I just didn't know how we would manage with one parent 100 miles away at the hospital and one parent working. The group decided to collect enough money to allow my sister to quit her job and move in to take care of our other three children while I was at the hospital with Jesse. She stayed for 8 months. It was such a wonderful thing. They didn't even ask us; they just said they would support her financially so she could care for my children and keep the household running.

Grandparents

Grandparents grieve deeply when a grandchild has cancer. They are concerned not only for their grandchild, but also for their own child (the parent). Cancer wreaks havoc with grandparents' expectations, reversing the natural order of life and death. Grandparents frequently say, "Why not me? I'm the one who is old." A brain or spinal cord tumor in a grandchild is a major shock to bear.

Many parents reported that the grandparents responded to the crisis with tremendous emotional, physical, and financial support.

> My mother was a rock. She lived far away, but she put her busy life on hold to come help. She took care of the baby and kept the household running when I was living at the hospital with my very ill child. She was strong, and it gave me strength.

Some parents express tremendous gratitude for the role played by the grandparents in providing much-needed stability to the family rocked by cancer. When the grandparents care for the siblings at home and run the household, the parents can care for the sick child and return to work.

John is Grampa's only grandchild. He's always there to play a board game, tell jokes, or watch his favorite video with him for the 1,000th time. I wish he'd hide his fears a little better, but that may be too much to expect from a truly loving grandfather.

Other families are not as fortunate. Many grandparents are too old, too ill, or simply unable to cope with a crisis of this magnitude. Some simply fall apart.

My mother-in-law became hysterical when my daughter was diagnosed. She called every day, sobbing. Luckily, she lived far away, and this minimized the disruption. We had to ask her not to come, because we just couldn't handle the catastrophe at home and her neediness too. It hurt her feelings, but we just couldn't cope with it.

Other grandparents allow pre-existing problems with their adult child to color their perceptions of what the family needs or what role they should take on during the crisis. For example, sometimes cancer allows grandparents to renew criticism of the way grandchildren are being raised.

While we stayed at the hospital, the grandparents moved into our house to care for our 8-year-old daughter. They decided that this was their chance to "whip her into shape, teach her some manners, and get her room cleaned up." Our daughter was in tears, and we ended up saying, "We appreciate your help, but we will take over."

It is hard to predict how anyone will react to the diagnosis of childhood cancer. Grandparents are no exception. Some respond with the wisdom gleaned from decades of living, others become needy or overbearing, and some withdraw. It is natural in a time of grave crisis to look to your parents for support and help, but it is important to remember that grandparents' ability to respond also depends on events in their own lives. If problems between family members develop, help can be obtained from hospital social workers or through individual counseling.

Helpful things for extended family members to do

Families differ in what is truly helpful for them. The suggestions in this chapter are snapshots of what some families appreciated. True listening and working on maintaining your relationships are paramount. Connections can be made in many different, unique, and personally meaningful ways. Extended family members of the family dealing with cancer should try to support them in ways that respect their wishes, while also honoring their privacy.

Parents of the ill child may want to share the following suggestions with their extended family and friends so they have a better idea of how to help.

- Be sensitive to the emotional state of both the sick child and the parents. Sometimes parents want to talk about the illness; sometimes they just need a hand to hold.

- Encourage all members of the extended family to keep in touch through visits, calls, mail, email, text messages, videos, or pictures. When visits are welcome, make them brief and cheerful. Not only do long visits sometimes distress sick children, but they can also overtax a tired parent.

> Our relatives who lived close to the hospital had teenagers. One was a candy striper at Children's on Saturdays. The aunts, uncles, and cousins came to visit several times a week any time he was in the hospital during his years of treatment. They were all very supportive, very positive, and fun to be around.

- Be understanding if the parents do not want phone calls while in the hospital. Remember that the child can often hear phone conversations when parents talk on the phone in the room.

> The first 3 days in the hospital I spent much of my time crying on the phone when talking to friends and relatives. Then I realized how frightening this must be to my 2-year-old. So I just took the phone off the hook and left it there. Now, each time Jennifer is hospitalized, I call one friend and have her spread the news. Then I take the phone off the hook again and concentrate on my daughter.

- A cheerful hospital room really boosts a child's spirits. Encourage sending balloon bouquets, funny cards, posters, toys, or humorous books. Be aware that some hospitals do not allow rubber balloons, only mylar. Flowers are usually not allowed in children's rooms.

> We plastered the walls with pictures of family and friends, and so many people sent balloons that the ceiling was covered. It was a lovely sight.

- Laughter helps heal the mind and body, so send funny videos or arrive with a good joke if you think it is appropriate.

> My brother Bill and his wonderful girlfriend, Cathleen, created an exciting "trip" for my 4-year-old daughter. She was bald, big-bellied from prednisone, and her counts were too low to leave the house, but her interest in fashion was as sharp as ever. Bill and Cathleen bought 10 outfits, rigged up a dressing room, and with Cathleen as saleswoman, turned Katy's bedroom into a fashion salon. She tried on outfits, discussed all of their merits and shortcomings, and had a fabulous time. It was a real high point for her.

- Puzzles, games, picture books, coloring books, age-appropriate computer games, and crafts are welcome.

> *A friend who was a nurse came to my son's room shortly before Christmas and brought an entire gingerbread house kit, including confectioner's sugar for the icing. We had a very good time putting it together.*

- Offer to give the parent(s) a break from the hospital room. A walk outside, shopping trip, haircut, dinner out, or just a long shower can be very refreshing.

- Donate frequent flyer miles to distant family members who have the time but not the money to help.

> *A close friend (who lived 3,000 miles away) had just lost her job and wished she could be there for us. My parents gave her their frequent flyer miles. She flew in for 3 weeks during a hard part of treatment and helped enormously.*

- Donate blood. Your blood may not be used specifically for the ill child, but it will replenish the general supply, which is depleted by children with cancer.

> *Our family friend John is terrified of needles. John always avoided giving blood. John doesn't like going to the doctor. But John showed up to donate platelets once, early on, and we found that he was a great platelet match for Deli. So he kept returning to that awful two-needle machine that you stay hooked onto for 3 hours at a time, probably a couple dozen times, because we needed him. Then we had Beth, who was one of my professional acquaintances. Beth was always pretty nice to us, but she found out that she too was a good "sticky" platelet donor. Probably at least a dozen times she took hours out of her work day and donated platelets whenever Deli needed some. We concentrated on the few "star" friends and relatives, the one or two people whose attitude, abilities, and circumstances allowed them to be the most helpful.*

Friends

Like family, friends can cushion the shock of diagnosis and ease the difficulties of treatment with their words and actions. Mother Theresa once said, "We can do no great things—only small things with great love." It is a given that the family of a child being treated for a brain or spinal cord tumor is overwhelmed.

Helpful things for friends to do

The list of helpful things to do is endless, but here are some suggestions from parents who have traveled this hard road.

Household

- Provide meals. It is helpful to call in advance to see if anyone in the family has food allergies or if there is something special the child with cancer or the siblings would like to eat.

  We found that the most helpful thing was when people brought us food to eat while in the hospital (where food is scarce for everyone but the patient), and also while recuperating at home. Often feeding ourselves took a back seat to caring for Ayla. This is not conducive to garnering energy to care for someone else!

  • • • • •

  Our closest friends invited us for dinner every Friday night for the year and a half that Ethan was in treatment. She said that she knew we wouldn't feel like it, but we needed to get out and practice being normal until we actually felt more normal. At first it was horrible—I was so anxious and sleep deprived that I could barely function, but as the year progressed, it was the thing I looked forward to most each week. I wasn't sorry to see treatment end, but I really did miss those Fridays night dinners.

- Take care of pets or livestock.
- Mow grass, shovel snow, rake leaves, water plants, and weed gardens.

  We came home from the hospital one evening right before Christmas, and found a freshly cut, fragrant Christmas tree leaning next to our door. I'll never forget that kindness.

- Clean the house or hire a cleaning service.

  My husband's cousin sent her cleaning lady over to our house. It was so neat and such a luxury to come home to find the stove and windows sparkling clean.

- Grocery shop (especially when the family is due home from the hospital).
- Do laundry or drop off and pick up dry cleaning.
- Provide a place to stay near the hospital.

  One of the ladies from the school where I worked came up to the ICU (intensive care unit) waiting room where we were sleeping and pressed her house key into my hand. She lived 5 minutes from the hospital. She said, "My basement is made up, there's a futon, there's a TV; you are coming and staying at my house." I hardly knew her, but we accepted. Every day when we came in from the hospital there was some cute little treat waiting for us like a bowl of cookies, or two packages of hot chocolate and a thermos of hot milk.

A child life specialist shared the following suggestion:

> *For many of the families I work with, allowing acquaintances into the home to clean and cook is just too personal and uncomfortable to allow during such a private time in their lives. It's just too intrusive. However, these families have shared many stories of anonymous giving. For instance, the following were very welcome: restaurant/fast food certificate, baskets of beauty products mysteriously left on the doorstep, journals, phone cards, movie rental cards, gas cards, and Polaroid film and camera left at the doorstep. The anonymity helped prevent the family from feeling indebted.*

Siblings

An entire chapter of this book is devoted to the complex feelings that siblings experience when their brother or sister has cancer. Chapter 15, *Siblings,* provides an in-depth examination of the issues from the perspective of both siblings and parents. Below is a list of suggestions about how family and friends can help the siblings.

• Baby-sit younger siblings whenever parents go to the clinic or emergency room, or need to be with their child for a prolonged hospital stay.

• When parents are home with a sick child, take sibling(s) somewhere fun to get their minds off of the stresses at home. Find out what they would enjoy, such as going to the park, a sports event, miniature golfing, bowling, the zoo, or a movie.

• Invite sibling(s) over for meals.

• If you bring a gift for the sick child, bring something for the sibling(s), too.

> *Friends from home sent boxes of art supplies to us when the whole family spent those first 10 weeks at a Ronald McDonald house far from our home. They sent scissors, paints, paper, and colored pens. It was a great help for Carrie Beth and her two sisters. One friend even sent an Easter package with straw hats for each girl, and flowers, ribbons, and glue to decorate them with.*

• Offer to help sibling(s) with homework.

• Drive sibling(s) to lessons, games, or school.

• Listen to how they are feeling and coping. Siblings' lives have been disrupted; they have limited time with their parents, and they need support and care.

Psychological support

There is much that can be done to help the family maintain an even emotional keel.

• Call frequently, and be open to listening if the parents want to talk about their feelings. Also, talk about non-cancer-related topics, such as sharing neighborhood and school news.

What I wished for most was that friends and family had been able to call more often to see how we were doing; that someone could have handled my confidence on the good days and my tears on the bad days. It somehow took too much emotional energy to make a call myself, but I valued any phone call I received.

- Visit the hospital and bring fun stuff such as bubbles, silly string, water pistols, joke books, funny videos, rub-on tattoos, and board games.

- If one parent has to leave work to stay in the hospital with the sick child, coworkers can send messages by mail, email, or social media.

- If you think the family might be interested, ask the social worker at the hospital to find out whether there are support groups for parents and/or kids in your area.

- Offer to take the children to the support groups or go with the parents. For most families, the parent support group becomes a second family with ties of shared experience as deep and strong as blood relations.

- Drive the parent and child to clinic visits.

- Buy books for the family if they enjoy reading.

- Send email, cards, or letters.

Word got around my parents' hometown, and I received cards from many high school acquaintances who still cared enough to call or write and say we're praying for you, please let us know how things are going. It was so neat to get so many cards out of the blue that said, "I'm thinking about you."

- Baby-sit the sick child so the parents can go out to eat, exercise, take a walk, or just get out of the hospital or house.

Constance and Michael and their son Byron were the only friends who always said, "Whenever you'd like us to watch Jamie, you just let us know," but because his seizures weren't controlled, we hesitated. It was literally 2 years later that we finally took them up on their offer.

- Ask what needs to be done, then do it.

A close friend asked what I needed the day after Michelle was diagnosed. I asked if she could drive our second car the 100 miles to the hospital so my husband could return in it to work. She came with her family to the Ronald McDonald House with two big bags containing snack foods, a large box of stationery, envelopes, stamps, books to read, a book handmade by her 3-year-old daughter containing dozens of cut-out pictures of children's clothing pasted on construction paper (which my daughter adored looking at), and a beautiful, new, handmade, lace-trimmed dress for my daughter. It was full-length and baggy enough to cover all bandages and tubing. She wore it almost every day for a year. It was a wonderful thing for my friend to do.

- Give lots of hugs.

Financial support

Helping families avoid financial difficulties can be the next greatest gift after the life of the child and the strength of the family. It is estimated that even fully insured families spend 25 percent or more of their income on co-payments, travel, motels, meals, and other uncovered items. Uninsured or underinsured families may lose their savings or even their homes. Even families with full health insurance, such as those in Canada, have additional expenses that are not covered. Most families need financial assistance, so following are some suggestions for ways to help.

- Start a support fund.

   A friend of mine called and asked very tentatively if we would mind if she started a support fund. We felt awkward, but we needed help, so we said okay. She did everything herself, and the money she raised was very, very helpful. We did ask her to stop the fund when people started calling us to ask if they could use giving to the fund as an advertisement for their business.

- Share leave with a coworker. Governments and some companies have leave banks that permit people who are ill, or taking care of someone who is ill, to use other coworkers' leave so they won't have their pay docked.

   My husband's coworkers didn't collect money, they did something even more valuable. They donated sick leave hours so he was able to be at the hospital frequently during those first few months without losing a paycheck.

- Job share. Some companies allow job-share arrangements in which a coworker donates time to perform part of the parent's job; this way the parent can spend extra time at the hospital. Job sharing allows the job to get done, keeps peace at the job site, and prevents financial losses for the family. Another possibility is for one or more friends with similar skills (e.g., word processing, filing, sales) to rotate through the job on a volunteer basis to cover for the parent of the ill child.

- Collect money at church or work to give the family informally.

   The day my daughter was diagnosed, my husband's coworkers passed the hat and gave us over $250. I was embarrassed, but it paid for gas, meals, and the motel until there was an opening in the Ronald McDonald House.

• • • • •

Finances were a main concern for us because I wanted to cut back on work to be at home with Meagan. Sometimes my coworkers would pool money and present it with a card saying, "Here's a couple of days work that you won't have to worry about."

• Collect money by organizing a bake sale, dance, or raffle.

Coworkers of my husband held a Halloween party and charged admission, which they donated to us. We were very uncomfortable with the idea at first, but they were looking for an excuse to have a party, and it helped us out.

• Offer to help keep track of medical bills. Keeping track of these bills is time-consuming, frustrating, and exhausting for the parents. If you are a close relative or friend, you could offer to review, organize, and file (or enter into a computer) the voluminous paperwork. Making the calls and writing the letters over contested claims or errors in billing can also be very helpful.

I am the one handling all of the administrative duties for the family. We have learned when Kevin gets his MRI to ask the techs to make a copy for us right then and there. I have to keep copies of everything regarding Kevin's treatment and surgery, including pathology reports, second opinion consults, lab reports, etc. I now have copies of all MRI films, all of the hospital records, every report that was ever written, and all of the radiological reports. I make tons of copies of these in case they're ever needed.

• • • • •

Talking to insurance people really hits a sore spot with me; right from the beginning of the call, there is a menu with many options to choose from, and it can take 10 minutes if you are lucky to get a real live person on the phone. I have, many times, asked for supervisors, demanded and insisted that expediency is necessary. I have learned to take the person's name, their title, and write down time and date on every conversation I have. It is a time-consuming job.

Help from schoolmates

The friendships and social lives of children often revolve around school. Trying to maintain ties with school, teachers, and friends will help your child make a smooth transition back as soon as he is able.

• Encourage visits (if appropriate), cards, emails, text messages, and phone calls from classmates.

Our son had a rough time with fever and seizures during chemo, and he was really missing his routine. His preschool teachers, Kate and Ellie, surprised him one time with a homemade book. They had all the kids pose for an instant picture for the cover, and each one drew a picture for the inside. He loved it.

- Ask the teacher to send the school newspaper and other news along with assignments.

On a Thursday, our second grade son Christopher was diagnosed with a pilocytic astrocytoma of the cerebellum the size of an orange. By Friday morning, Christopher's classroom, Room 35 at Carpenter Avenue Elementary School, was already making Get Well Pizza cards for him. One of his teachers sat down with the kids and talked about what it would be like in the hospital, and an appointed person from the school community called us regularly for updates and passed on prayers and loving regards from families and staff. We had amazingly touching responses from many school parents, teachers, coaches, and even our principal.

The PTA president came to visit and brought a huge card signed by all of Christopher's classmates, teachers, and other Carpenter friends. She had also lined up parents from Room 35 to bring dinners to my husband Jim and I for the entire upcoming week. As the weeks went on, the love and support just escalated. Christopher found his greatest joy throughout the whole hospital ordeal was receiving more incredible Beanie Babies than he could have ever imagined getting.

Our whole family has a view of Carpenter Avenue Elementary School that has changed us forever. They are an extraordinary community of families that I wish every family in need can experience.

- Classmates can sign a brightly colored banner or poster to send to the hospital.

Brent's kindergarten class sent a packet containing a picture drawn for him by each child in the class. They also made him a book. Another time they sent him a letter written on huge poster board. He couldn't wait to get back to school.

- School friends and civic groups can show their support by doing volunteer work at their local hospital or by participating in, or organizing, cancer- awareness events.

Ethan's school read Sadako and the Thousand Paper Cranes, which is a story about a Japanese girl from Hiroshima who contracted leukemia after World War II. The crane is the sign of health, good fortune, and long life in Japan. There is a legend that if you fold a thousand origami cranes, you will be granted one wish. Sadako's wish was that she live a long and healthy life, but she died of cancer 386 cranes short of her goal. Her classmates finished her cranes for her, and paper cranes subsequently became a symbol of peace.

So, the kids at Ethan's school began to fold cranes for him. Each crane has a wish written on the wing (things like "Cancer Be Gone" and "Ethan, I love your spirit"). Some are the size of a robin, and some are smaller than a dime.

They reached their goal of a thousand last week and they are now hanging (on strands, from one to 10 cranes per strand) on the ceiling over Ethan's bed. They are absolutely magical to look at, all rotating and casting shadows; and you can actually read each one's wish on the lower hanging ones. I thought it was a beautiful thing to do.

Religious support

Following are a few suggestions for families who have religious affiliations:

- Arrange for church/synagogue/mosque members and clergy to visit the hospital, if that is what the family wants.

- Arrange prayer services for the sick child.

> *The day our son was diagnosed, we raced next door to ask our wonderful neighbors to take care of our dog. The news of our son's diagnosis quickly spread, and we found out later that five neighborhood families gathered that very night to pray for Brent.*

- Have your child's religious education class send pictures, posters, letters, balloons, or audio or video tapes.

Accepting help (for parents)

As a parent of a child with cancer, one of the kindest things you can do for your friends is to let them help you. Let them channel their time and worry into things that will make your life easier. Think of the many times you have visited a sick friend, made a meal for a new mom, baby-sat someone else's child in an emergency, or just pitched in to do what needed to be done. These actions probably made you feel great and provided a good example for your children. When your child is diagnosed with cancer, both you and your friends will benefit immensely if you let them help you and if you give them guidance about what you need.

One father's thoughts about accepting help:

> *Fathers have a deep-seated need to protect their family. Yet here I was with a child with cancer, and there wasn't a single thing that I could do about it. The loss of control really bothered me. The very hardest thing I had to learn was to let go enough to let people help us.*

One mother's thoughts about accepting help:

> *The most important advice I received as the parent of a child newly diagnosed with cancer came from a hospital nurse whom I turned to when I was overwhelmed with all the advice being offered by family and friends. This wise nurse said, "Don't discount anything. You're going to need all the help you can get." I think it is very*

important for families to remain open and accept the help that is offered. It often comes when least expected and from unlikely sources. I was totally unprepared at diagnosis for how much help I would need, and I'm glad that I remained open to offers of kindness. This is not the time to show the world how strong you are.

What to say (for friends)

Following are some suggestions for friends about what to say and how to offer help. Of course, much depends on the type of relationship that already exists between you and the family you want to help; but a specific offer can always be accepted or graciously declined.

- "Our family would like do your yard work. It will make us feel as if we are helping in a small way."

- "We want to clean your house for you once a week. What day would be convenient? "

- "Would it help if we took care of your dog (or cat, or bird)? We would love to do it. "

- "I walk my dog three times a day. May I walk yours, too? "

- "The church is setting up a system to deliver meals to your house. When is the best time to drop them off? "

- "I will take care of Jimmy whenever you need to take John to the hospital. Call us anytime, day or night, and we will come pick Jimmy up. "

Things that do not help

Sometimes people say things to parents of children with cancer that aren't helpful. If you are a family member or friend of a parent in this situation, please do not say any of the following:

- "God only gives people what they can handle." (Some people cannot handle the stress of childhood cancer.)

- "I know just how you feel." (Unless you have a child with cancer, you simply don't know.)

- "You are so brave," or "so strong," etc. (Parents are not heroes; they are normal people struggling with extraordinary stress.)

- "They are doing such wonderful things to save children with cancer these days." (The prognosis might be good, but what parents and children are going through is not wonderful.)

- "Well, we're all going to die one day." (True, but parents do not need to be reminded of this fact.)

- "It's God's will" or "Everything happens for a reason." (These are just not helpful things to hear.)

- "At least you have other kids," or "Thank goodness you are still young enough to have other children." (A child cannot be replaced.)

> *A woman whom I worked with, but did not know well, came up to me one day and out of the blue said, "When Erica gets to heaven to be with Jesus, He will love her." All I could think to say was, "Well, I'm sorry, but Jesus can't have her right now."*

Parents also suggest the following things:

- Rather than say, "Let us know if there is anything we can do," make a specific suggestion.

> *Many well-wishing friends always said, "Let me know what I can do." I wish they had just "done," instead of asking for direction. It took too much energy to decide, call them, make arrangements, etc. I wish someone would have said, "When is your clinic day? I'll bring dinner," or "I'll baby-sit Sunday afternoon so you two can go out to lunch."*

- Do not make personal comments about sick children in front of them. For instance, "When will his hair grow back in?" "He's lost so much weight." or "She's so pale."

> *When in the mall or other public place, strangers had no qualms about staring at Ayla (age 3) who had an eye patch, tubes that sometimes snuck out from under her shirt, and no hair. We combated this by telling her that she was so absolutely stunningly beautiful that people just could not help but stare at her. We really played this up and tied it in to her belief in Snow White, Cinderella, etc. Many times we let her and her sister Jasmine wear their princess costumes out in public. Then they really got a kick out of people staring. I also did not hesitate to tell people that she had cancer when they asked what was wrong with her. I never minimized what she was going through. We talk about cancer freely and how doctors are there to fix you up if you get this.*

- Do not do things that require the parents to support you (for example, repeatedly calling them up and crying about their child's illness).

- Do not ask "what if" questions: "What if he can't go to school?" "What if your insurance won't cover it?" Or, "What if she dies?" The present is really all the parents can deal with.

- Refrain from saying, "I don't know how you do it," or "You're so strong."

> *Whenever someone says: "You're so strong" or "I don't know how you do it," answer: "I don't do it alone," or "With lots of help" or (if it's true) "I'm pretty close to losing*

it completely." There's a thin line between being honest about your situation and being oppressive, for want of a better word. In my more cynical moments, I am convinced the world wants us (i.e., the cancer kids/families) to valiantly triumph over hardship with the Movie-of-the-Week-attitude. Well if that gets them to wash my floors, it's a small price!

I think some of the most supported families I've seen on treatment had a knack at keeping people informed about the current situation. I updated the outgoing message on our answering machine every couple of days and people could call our home for current news (a hospice nurse/neighbor gave me that idea). Other friends from the hospital used newsletters, phone chains, announcements in church, etc. Again, my cynical side recognizes that you're opening up your most personal moments to the public (anyone who called my house and heard the message the day after my son's stroke probably felt like an intruder) but it's a way to help people feel invested in your family.

Losing friends

It is an unfortunate reality that most parents of children with cancer lose some of their friends. For a variety of reasons, some friends just can't cope and either suddenly disappear or gradually fade away.

My daughter Lauren was diagnosed with a very rare and aggressive cancer. We finished treatment in April of this year, and since that time I have been feeling an overwhelming series of emotions, most of which lie at the bottom of the happiness scale. This past weekend, I finally met with my best friend, who had her first baby in March. Needless to say, I have not been overly involved with her life of late. My own was often more than I could hack. This friend did prove to be a true friend throughout the cancer trip as she visited us often at the hospital. She confessed to me that she missed me so much, and that she sometimes mistook my silence for indifference. I didn't take offense, as I might have, but rather, this seemed to be the "invite" that I needed to re-enter the world that I had left when Lauren was diagnosed. The fact that I had value as a friend, and not just as a caregiver, was a wake-up call. Throughout the past year, I had isolated myself from everyone from my old life, and was starting to think that maybe I would never make it back. Maybe now I can pull back the cobwebs and struggle back.

· · · · ·

We had friends and family we thought would be the greatest sources of support in the world. Yet, they pulled away from us and provided nothing in the way of help, emotional or otherwise. We also had friends that we never expected to understand step up in surprising ways. My wife's friend, Leslie, a busy single woman who we would never expect to do such a thing, actually negotiated time off with a new employer so she could fly from her home in Tampa and help out after Garrett's transplant. She stayed with us for over a week, then came back a few months later to do it again.

A couple of my SCUBA diving buddies who we liked, but didn't know well, have since become our best friends. They would visit us in the hospital, bringing both our kids gifts, and giving us a much-needed break. They were the only folks who regularly came by when Garrett was home after the transplant and who always followed our strict rules without complaint.

Of course, the best support we had was from other parents of kids with serious illnesses or problems.

Telling your friends about cancer is difficult, but it's not as hard as keeping it a secret would be. Fighting this cancer has been a family effort and, frequently, an effort involving our larger circle of friends. The more people we've been able to call on for support, the better. We've had to keep in mind that we've had an opportunity to adjust. But, the news is brand new to our friends, and it can be a shock. People often don't know what to do or say when they've been told that someone they care about has cancer.

After we've given them some time, and when they ask what they can do, we tell them something constructive: mow the lawn, take back the recyclables, go to the store, bring over a pizza on Friday night, whatever would help.

Before my son was diagnosed, I had no idea what this experience was like, and I try to remember that my friends don't really know either, unless I tell them. They can't know the sleepless nights, the anxiety over tests, the fear when your child says he doesn't feel well, or the terror that we might lose our precious child. Some of us have found great support and others none. I hope your family and friends come to your side.

I want to say that I hope that cancer does not become your life. For us, it used to be an "elephant in the living room," and now it's maybe a "zebra in the kitchen." There are times when it demands everything you can give, no doubt, but there will be moments when there is time for the rest of your life.

Chapter 17

Communication and Behavior

When I approach a child, he inspires in me two sentiments: tenderness for what he is, and respect for what he may become.

— Louis Pasteur

UNDER THE BEST OF CIRCUMSTANCES, child rearing is a daunting task. When parenting is complicated by an overwhelming crisis such as cancer, communication within the family may suffer, and both children and parents may have difficulty adjusting to the new stressors in their lives.

Prior to a cancer diagnosis, children usually know the family rules and the consequences for breaking them. After diagnosis, normal family life is disrupted, and all sorts of confusing and distressing feelings and behaviors may appear. When people are under great stress, they often behave in ways they would not under normal circumstances. In response, parenting styles may need to change to the frequently shifting needs and behaviors of the ill child and affected siblings.

This chapter covers feelings that many children have about their disease and some emotional and behavioral changes that may arise in both children and parents. Suggestions for maintaining effective communication and appropriate behavior within the family are also offered. The stories included describe what many parents experienced and how they coped with their and their ill child's powerful, and sometimes overwhelming, emotions. For stories about the emotions of siblings, please see Chapter 15, *Siblings*.

Communication

Chapter 1, *Diagnosis*, lists many of the feelings parents may experience after their child's diagnosis of a brain or spinal cord tumor. It is helpful to remember that children, both the ill child and siblings, are also overwhelmed by strong feelings, and they generally have fewer coping skills than do adults. At different times and to varying degrees, children and teens may feel fearful, angry, resentful, powerless, violated, lonely, weird, inferior, incompetent, or betrayed. Children have to learn strategies to deal with these strong feelings to prevent "acting out" behaviors (aggression, risk taking) or "acting in" behaviors (depression, withdrawal).

Good communication is the first step toward helping your family identify how behavior and family functioning are being impacted and how family members can work with each other, and with professionals, to restore order and a nurturing climate. Clear and loving communication with your children or teens is the foundation for trust. Children need to know from the very beginning that you will answer questions truthfully and take the time to talk about feelings.

Honesty

Above all else, children need to be able to trust their parents. They can face almost anything, as long as they know their parents will be at their side. Trust requires honesty. For your ill child and her siblings to feel secure, they must always know that they can depend on you to tell them the truth, be it good news or bad. This trust you build with your children reduces feelings of isolation and disconnection within the family.

> We were always very honest. We felt that if she couldn't trust us to tell her the truth, how scary that would be. I've seen a few incidents in the clinic of people with totally different styles who don't tell their kids the truth. I ran into the bathroom at the clinic crying after overhearing a mother who had deceived her child into coming to the clinic. Then he found out he needed a back poke and completely lost it. It makes me cringe. Children just have to be prepared. If they can't trust their parents, who can they trust?

Listening

Just trying to get through each day consumes most of a parent's time, attention, and energy. Consequently, one of the greatest gifts parents can give their children is time— when they really focus on what children are saying and pay attention to the feelings that generate the words.

> When my daughter was 7 years old (3 years after her treatment ended), I realized how important it was to keep listening. She was complaining about a hangnail and I told her that I would cut it for her. She started to yell that I would hurt her. I asked her, "When have I ever hurt you?" and she said, "In the hospital." I sat down with her in my arms, rocked her, and explained what had happened in the hospital during her treatment, why we had to bring her, and how we felt about it. I told her how I felt when she was hurt by procedures. I asked her to tell me about her memories and feelings about being in the hospital. We cleared the air that day, and I expect we will need to talk about it many more times in the future. Then she held out her hand so I could cut off her hangnail.

Talking

If you are not in the habit of sharing your feelings with your children, it is hard to start doing so in a crisis. But now, more than ever, it's important to try. Parents can create an opening for discussion by simply stating how they are feeling, for example, "I have lots of different feelings at the same time. Sometimes I really get mad at the tumor because it is making your life so tough, but I am also happy that the medicine is working." Telling your healthy children what you're feeling can strengthen your connection and reassure them of your love: "I really miss you when I have to take your sister to the hospital. I'll call you every night just so I can hear your voice," or "I wish the family didn't have to be separated so much, and I feel sad that you have to go through this." Such statements reassure children of your continued love for them and distress about being separated from them; they also create an opportunity for children to share with you how they feel about what is happening to the family.

> My daughter, diagnosed at 1 year old and now entering fifth grade, has three older siblings, so we have been through many developmental stages as far as communication goes. I try to answer their questions honestly, but I only tell them what I think they can understand without overwhelming them with information. I remember one of my boys, soon after my daughter's diagnosis, asked me if she was going to die, and I said "no" emphatically. I regretted it immediately, and realized that I would have to deal with my fears about the possibility of her dying, then go back and tell him the truth. So, later, I told him that I hadn't given an accurate answer because I was scared and that we didn't know if she was going to die. We hoped not, but we would have to wait and see. I have found that as their understanding deepens, they come back with more questions, needing more detailed answers. So, my motto is, be honest, but don't scare them. If you say everything is okay, but you are crying, they know something is wrong, and that they can't trust you for the truth.

It is also helpful to tell your sick child how the illness is affecting her siblings, for example, "It is very hard for Jim to stay at home with a babysitter when I bring you to the hospital. Let's try to think of something nice to do for him."

Common behavioral changes in children

Discipline can be challenging, even when family life is going well. But when a child has cancer, parents are stressed, siblings may be angry or worried, and the ill child is scared and upset. Parents may find themselves reaching their emotional breaking points, and children may begin behaving in negative ways, making the situation unmanageable. The first step to reestablishing order is to decide whether the ill child is going to be treated as if she only has a few months to live, or as if she will survive and needs to learn strategies for how to self-regulate difficult emotions. Step two is to examine your own behavior to see if you are modeling the conduct that you expect from your children. If your child becomes angry or destructive, step three is to develop a consistent, healthy response to the behaviors to help her develop social and emotional competence.

Barbara Sourkes, a respected child psychologist, wrote in her book *Armfuls of Time: The Psychological Experience of the Child with a Life-Threatening Illness:*

> While loss of control extends over emotional issues, and ultimately over life itself, its emergence is most vivid in the child's day-to-day experience of the illness, in the barrage of intrusive, uncomfortable, or painful procedures that he or she must endure. The child strives desperately to regain a measure of control, often expressed through resistant, noncompliant behavior or aggressive outbursts. Too often, the source of the anger—the loss of control—goes unrecognized by parents and caregivers. However, once its meaning is acknowledged, an explicit distinction may be drawn for the child between what he or she can or cannot dictate. In order to maximize the child's sense of control, the environment can be structured to allow for as much choice as is feasible. Even options that appear small or inconsequential serve as an antidote to loss, and their impact is often reflected in dramatic improvements in behavior.

In the following sections, parents share how they handled their children's range of emotions and behaviors.

Anger

Parents sometimes respond to the diagnosis of childhood brain and spinal cord tumors with anger, and so do children. Not only is the child angry at the disease, but also at the parents for bringing her in to be hurt, at having to take medicine that makes her feel terrible, at losing her hair, at losing her friends, and on and on. Children with brain or spinal cord tumors and their siblings have good reasons to be angry.

> I think that much anger can be avoided by giving choices and letting kids have some control. Parents need to clearly explain that there are some things that simply have to be done (spinal taps) but that the child or teen is in control of positions, people present, music, even timing. For example, if your teen gets bad headaches after spinals, help him negotiate the date and time when the spinal will be done so that sports or social life will not be impacted.

· · · · ·

> We have a case of the halo or the horns. Our son is either very defiant or an absolute angel. He argues about every single thing. I really think that it is because he has had so little control in his life. I have very clear rules, am very firm, and put my foot down. But I also try to choose my battles wisely so we can have good times, too. My husband reminds me when I get aggravated that if he weren't this type of tough kid, he wouldn't have made it through so many setbacks. Then I am just glad to still have him with us.

If you talk to Ezra (age 13), he'd tell you he's angry that everything is so hard now. Because of the medulloblastoma and because of treatment, his life is hard every day. Even eating and drinking are work for him.

Tantrums

Healthy children have tantrums when they are overwhelmed by strong feelings, and so do children with brain or spinal cord tumors. In some cases, tantrums can be predicted by parents paying close attention to what triggers the outburst (for example, a missed nap or anxiety about an upcoming procedure). This knowledge can help parents prevent tantrums by avoiding situations that create emotional overload for their child; but sometimes there is no warning of the impending tantrum. Knowledge can also help parents understand that many tantrums and behavioral changes are due to medication side effects (for example, steroids) and are out of the child's control.

> *We never knew what would set off 3-year-old Rachel, and to tell the truth, she didn't know what the problem was herself. She was very verbal and aware in many ways, but she had no idea what was bothering her and causing the anger. I would just hold her with her blanket, hug her, and rock until she calmed down. Later she would say, "I was out of control," but she still didn't know why.*

Of course, if the child is destructive, he needs help learning safer ways to vent his anger. For a child who is frequently destructive, professional counseling is necessary. *The Misunderstood Child* by Larry Silver has a chapter that explains in detail how parents can initiate a behavior modification program at home.

> *My 5-year-old's behavior always intensified at clinic during treatment. He was hyperactive and defiant, to put it nicely. On his very last chemo day, he was hooked up to an infusion pump with a low battery, so his movement was limited to the bed. By the end of the session, he was so mad at being unable to move around, he was screaming at the top of his lungs, and throwing toys. First I tried to calm him, but then I got angry: I told him that he could just forget about the balloon we had in the car, it was gone. Of course, that just made it worse. We were both out of control, and they'll remember us there for quite some time, I'm sure.*

> • • • • •

> *My daughter had frequent, violent rages that sometimes caused damage (toys thrown at the walls, books ripped up). She was small, but strong. I talked to her when she was calm about how the tantrums would be handled. Tantrums with no damage would be ignored; afterwards we would cuddle and talk about what prompted the anger and other ways for her to handle the anger. If she began to break things or hurt people, I would wrap her in a blanket and rock her until she relaxed. I would*

tell her, "I need to hold you because you are out of control. This is so hard. I know. I love you." All of the tantrums ended after she went off treatment, but dealing with her destructive anger was one of the hardest things I have ever experienced.

· · · · ·

When my son needed to get out a good old temper tantrum just to unload, I'd let him. Then he'd fall into my reassuring arms and soak up some good ole momma lovin' and just whimper till he slept...my hand stroking his hair, and I'm whispering things like, "I know, honey, I know. It's just so wrong. I'm here, baby. I love you. I know. I know. Just sleep for now. I'll be here when you wake. I'm not moving. I'm not going anywhere. I love you. There now."

Withdrawal

Some children deal with their feelings by withdrawing rather than blowing up in anger. Like denial, withdrawal can temporarily be helpful as a way to come to grips with strong feelings. However, too much withdrawal is not good for children, and it can be a sign of depression. Parents or counselors need to find gentle ways to allow withdrawn children to express how they feel.

The day for our family band gig started out badly. Ez (age 13) was downhearted, green, looked very small, felt nauseated, and hadn't eaten much breakfast. He just sorta sat and stared for an hour as Hannah and I bustled around practicing, writing up the set list and deciding on introductions, and putting gear in the car. I kept asking him did he want to play trumpet a bit with us and he said no. We got to the site, it was a glorious day, the band before us was wonderful, everybody was smiling, but Ez sat hunched on a bench. I was in despair. I also was, practically, fearing he might throw up on stage. So we got up there and this is what happened: he played badly, but he was a good presence. He introduced some of the songs and was so funny the audience howled. He was relaxed and smiling even as at one point he dropped the bomb, saying through the microphone: "I just want you to know I used to play trumpet better than this before I had cancer." He rallied for the last couple songs, and nailed the ending of the last piece wonderfully. The most amazing thing, though, was that he was instantly in a wonderful smiley proud mood as we got off stage and had a huge appetite after.

· · · · ·

My daughter became very depressed and withdrawn as treatment continued. She started to talk only about a fantasy world that she created in her imagination. She seemed to be less and less in the real world. She didn't ever talk to her therapist about her feelings, but they did lots of art work together. At the beginning, she only drew pictures of herself with her body filling the whole page. After EMLA® (local anesthetic) became available, and she was less terrified of being hurt, she began to draw her body more normal sized. As she got better, she began to draw the family again. When she drew a beautiful sun shining on the family, I cried. She just couldn't talk about it, but she worked so much out through her art.

The emotional impact of cancer is very pronounced during the teenage years, a time when appearance is particularly important. When adolescents look different from their peers, they may feel sad, angry, embarrassed, bewildered, helpless, and scared. Thus, depression is common during and after treatment. Children and teens may go through a period of withdrawal and/or grieving; it is crucial that children and teens receive support and counseling during these times.

I had cancer when I was 15. I tried so hard as a freshman in college to put it all behind me and get on with my life. It just didn't work. Next to treatment, that was the worst year of my life. It showed me that if I didn't deal with it consciously, I was going to deal with it subconsciously. I had nightmares every night. I'd wake up feeling that I had needles in my arms. I decided to start taking better care of myself in a different kind of way. I do something fun every day. I try to see the positive side of situations. I read more and write a lot. I unplug from the cancer community whenever I feel overwhelmed. I try to explore my feelings with my counselor rather than shove them in the back corner. It's like garbage; if you don't take it out, it starts to stink. Once I started dealing with these feelings, things really improved.

Comfort objects

Many parents worry when, after diagnosis, children regress to using a special comfort object. Many young children ask to return to using a bottle, or cling to a favorite toy or blanket. It is reasonable to allow your child to use whatever he can to find comfort against the difficult realities of treatment. The behaviors usually stop either when the child starts feeling better or when treatment ends.

My daughter was a hair twirler. Whenever she was nervous, she would twirl a bit of her hair around her finger. As her hair fell out, she kept grabbing at her head to find a wisp to curl. I told her that she could twirl mine until hers grew back. She spent a lot of time next to me or in my lap with her hand in my hair. It was annoying for me sometimes, but it had a great calming effect on her. When hers grew back, I would gently remind her that she had her own hair to twirl. She also went back to a bottle, although we did limit the bottle use to home or hospital. Both behaviors, hair twirling and drinking from a bottle, disappeared within 6 months of the end of treatment, when she was 6 years old.

When Ayla (32 months) finally came home from the hospital after treatment for medulloblastoma, I decided to sleep with her. We were crammed into a small bed but I got to spend more time with her (you never know what the future may hold) and she knew that if she needed love all she had to do was open her eyes and see me there. Love has healing qualities. I think that the physical closeness somehow trans-fers the love. As we sleep and our bodies let down their defenses, the love can flow back and forth much easier. So despite what our American culture believes, I think that if your child wants you to sleep right beside her, you should.

Talking about death

Part of effective parenting is allowing children to talk about topics that may cause feel-ings of discomfort in parents and children. No parent wants to talk, or even think, about the possibility of a child's death. In some cultures, the subject of death is taboo. But a diagnosis of cancer forces both parents and children to acknowledge that death is a very real possibility. Even children as young as age 3 may think about death and what it means. They need to be able to talk about their feelings, fears, or questions without their parents shutting down the conversation.

Eighteen months into treatment, 5-year-old Katy said, "Mommy, sometimes I think about my spirit leaving my body. I think my spirit is here (gesturing to the back of her head) and my body is here (pointing to her belly button). I just wanted you to know that I think about it sometimes."

My son is a teenager and has to face some difficult issues with death. Just as my son finished treatment for medulloblastoma, another boy a year ahead of my son in our school was diagnosed with a glioblastoma multiforme brain tumor and died within 9 months. It was very hard for my son and one of his teachers even said to him after the death, "I guess this puts things into perspective for you." Like he needed to be reminded. Also, three of his roommates from cancer camp have died in the past year and they were all brain tumor kids. It is like they are being put face-to-face with their own mortality. These kids are extremely intuitive, they know the score. All you can do is be there for them, to listen, to support, to hold and love them.

Trusting your child

Sometimes children will tell you what they need to do to persevere through this trial. Their coping choices may not be what the parents would choose—the decisions may even make the parents nervous. But, it is the child or teen's way to make peace with the day-to-day reality of diagnosis and treatment.

Early one summer morning, 12-year-old Preston and I left the hospital after a week-long stay for chemotherapy. He had been heavily sedated and was groggy and shaky on his feet. My husband and daughter were getting ready to go on a boat trip, and I felt Preston was too sick to go. We sadly saw them off, then returned to the car. Preston said, "Mom, I really need to go fishing. I know you don't understand, but I really need to do this."

It made me very uncomfortable, but we went home to get his equipment. We then drove up to the mountains to a very deserted spot on the river, and Preston said that he needed to be out of my sight. So I watched him put on his waders, walk into the swift river, and disappear around a bend upstream. I went out into the river and sat on a rock. I waited for 2 hours before Preston came back. He said, "That's what I needed; I feel much better now."

There is a fine line between providing adequate protection for our children or teens and becoming overly controlling because of worry about the disease. You might ask yourself, "If she didn't have cancer, would I let her do this?"

Coping

Many children develop emotional competence from facing and coping with the difficulties of cancer. Others, because of both temperament and the environments in which they have lived, are blessed with good coping abilities. They understand what is required, and they do it.

I'll be finishing my last round of radiation today. I have an oligodendroglioma tumor on my right temporal lobe. I've been having some crazy feeling aura seizures. I do feel like I'm losing it at times. I definitely feel it's okay to worry. Believe me, I have my times for sure! I like to get together with as many friends as I can and go to the beach and check out the waves and smell the air. Definitely have to be listening to music. Talk to as many people as I can surround myself with and of course be alone to hit up the computer and sleep. The telephone seems to be a good friend too. I feel that I have too many lives to touch before I'm all said and done.

Many parents express great admiration for their child's strength and grace in the face of adversity.

Stephan has not had any behavior problems while being treated for his initial diagnosis (age 5) or his relapse (age 7). He has never complained about going to the hospital and views the medical staff as his friends. He has never argued or fought about painful treatments. Unlike many of the parents in the support group, we've never had to deal with any emotional issues. We are fortunate that he has that confident personality. He just says, "We've got to do it, so let's just get it done."

Common behavioral changes in parents

It's impossible to talk about children's behavior without discussing parental behavior. Your child's development does not occur in a vacuum; it occurs within the context of your family, and you set the tone for your home's atmosphere. At different times during their child's treatment, parents may be under enormous physical, emotional, financial, and existential stress. The crisis can cause parents to behave in ways of which they are not always proud—ways in which they would not behave under normal circumstances. Some of the common problem behaviors mentioned by parents follow.

Dishonesty

As stated earlier, children feel safe when their parents are honest with them. If parents start to keep secrets from a child to protect her from distressing news, she may feel isolated and fearful. She might think, "If mom and dad won't tell me, it must be really bad," or, "Mom won't talk about it. I guess there's nobody I can talk with about how scared I am."

Denial is a type of unconscious dishonesty. This occurs when parents say things to children such as, "Everything will be just fine," or, "It won't hurt a bit." This type of pretending just increases the distance between child and parent, leaving the child with no support. However horrible the truth, it seldom is as terrifying to a child as a half-truth upon which his imagination builds.

> I try so hard to be honest with my 5-year-old son, but blood draws, which he thinks of as "shots," are just so hard for him. Every doctor's visit, that's his first question, "I'm going to get a shot?" and I just want to say no. My husband's the one who started saying, "It'll be fine," but the anxiety that came up later at the appointment was so much worse that I put an end to that pretty quickly. Now I say, "Yes, but just once," because if I say, "I don't know," it just makes him worry.

Depression

Parents of children with cancer often feel sad or depressed. If you are consistently experiencing any of the following symptoms, it is often helpful to get professional help:

- Changes in sleeping patterns (sleeping too much, waking up frequently during the night, early morning awakening),

- Appetite disturbances (eating too little or too much)

- Loss of sex drive

- Fatigue

- Panic attacks

- Inability to experience pleasure
- Feelings of sadness and despair
- Poor concentration
- Social withdrawal
- Feelings of worthlessness
- Suicidal thoughts
- Drug or alcohol abuse

Depression is extremely common and very treatable, and it should be dealt with early.

> *Find a counselor you click with. Stick with that person until you truly feel some peace about your experiences and strength for dealing with the ongoing stress of treatment or whatever else might come up. I regret that I toughed it out and didn't recognize the depression I was experiencing for such a long time. I think finding sources of support in a variety of ways at the earliest moment possible can greatly mitigate long-term difficulties in coping.*

• • • • •

> *It was 2 years after my son finished treatment that my depression became severe enough that I recognized it. I actually had a lot of suicidal thoughts and my husband urged me to see a doctor. He started me on Zoloft® and it has helped me tremendously.*

Losing your temper excessively

All parents lose their temper sometimes. They lose their tempers with spouses, healthy children, pets, and even strangers. But it is especially painful for parents, the sick child, and siblings when the target of the anger is a very sick child or a brother or sister.

Abuse of children and spouses increases at times when either or both spouses feel incompetent and powerless. If you find yourself unable to manage your temper, seek professional counseling immediately.

> *I had my share of temper tantrums. The worst was when he was having his radiation. I tried to make him eat because it would be so many hours before he could have any more food. He always threw up all over himself and me, several times, every morning. It seemed like we changed clothing at least three times before we even got out of the house each day. I remember one day just screaming at him, "Can't you even learn how to throw up? Can't you just bend over to barf?" I really flunked mother of the year that day. I can't believe that I was screaming at this sick little kid, who I love so much.*

. . . . .

I had always taught my children that feeling anger was okay, but we had to make good choices about what to do with it. Hitting other people or breaking things was a bad choice; hitting pillows, running around outside, or punching pillows were good choices. But, as with everything else, they learned the most from watching how I handled my anger, and during the hard months of treatment my temper was short. When I found myself thinking of hitting them, I'd say, in a very loud voice, "I'm afraid I'm going to hurt somebody so I'm going in my room for a time-out." If my husband was home, I'd take a warm shower to calm down; if he wasn't, I'd just sit on the bed and take as many deep breaths as it took to calm down.

Unequal application of household rules

You will guarantee family problems if the ill child enjoys favored status while the siblings must do extra chores. Granted, it is hard to know the right time to insist that your ill child resume making his bed or setting the table, but it must be done. Siblings need to know from the beginning that any child in the family, if sick, will be excused from chores, but that this child will have do them again as soon as she is physically able.

I spoiled my sick daughter and tried to enforce the rules for my son. That didn't work, so I gave up on him and spoiled them both. He was really acting out at school. What he needed was structure and more attention, but what he got was more and more things. They both ended up thinking the whole world revolved around them, and it was my fault.

A child life specialist commented:

It's hard for parents to learn that saying "No" is okay, especially when there is only one child. One mom told me the other day that it's easier for her because there are two kids, and if it was just the child undergoing treatment, he'd get away with a lot more, but the sister has to do 'X, Y, and Z' and so her brother does, too. But it's hard to learn to say, "No, you don't get everything you want when we go to the grocery store," or "No, you don't get a new toy every single time you leave clinic."

Overindulgence of the ill child

Overindulgence is a very common behavior of parents of children with cancer.

I bought my daughter everything I saw that was pretty and lovely. I kept thinking that if she died she would die happy because she'd be surrounded by all these beautiful things. Even when I couldn't really afford it, I kept buying. I realize now that I was doing it to make me feel better, not her. She needed cuddling and loving, not clothes and dolls.

Four days into Selah's diagnosis, we were doing anything to keep her happy. Our sweet little 4 year old had turned into a demon child in that short time. Luckily, my very dear friend took me outside into the hallway, pushed me against the wall, and demanded to know exactly what I was doing. I just looked at her and said, "I have no idea." I just didn't want my daughter to die and that was my only focus. She then told me I was giving my daughter no boundaries, no behavior expectations, and she had no respect for anyone who walked into the room. She was so right, and I couldn't see it for fear that Selah would die. Through my tears and our hugs, she assured me that the way we were going, if she didn't die from cancer, we were going to want to kill her because of the monster we were creating. I am still so grateful that she wasn't afraid to tell me what I needed to hear.

One aspect of overindulgence that is quite common is parents' reluctance to teach life skills to sick children. After years of dealing with a physically weak and sometimes emotionally demanding child, parents may forget to expect age-appropriate behaviors.

I realized that I had formed a habit of treating my child as if she were still young and sick. I was still treating her like a 3 year old, and she was 7. One day, when I was pouring her juice, I thought, "Why am I doing this? She's 7. She needs to learn to make her own sandwiches and pour her own drinks. She needs to be encouraged to grow up." Boy, it has been hard. But I've stuck to my guns, and made other extended family members do it, too. I want her to grow up to be an independent adult, not a demanding, overgrown kid.

Overprotection of a sick child

For a child to feel normal, he needs to be treated as if he is normal. Ask the doctor what changes in physical activity are necessary for safety, and do not impose any additional restrictions on your child. Let your child be involved in sports or neighborhood play. And even though it is hard, stop yourself from constantly reminding your child to be careful.

Life seemed to be finally returning to "normal": surgery to remove tumor regrowth went great, all visible tumor removed. Only slight peripheral vision deficit, off all the meds, physically growing like crazy. Life was great!

Then, Michael (now 16) goes off snowboarding with some adult friends a couple of hours away from home. Sent that insurance card along, just in case. Hardly an hour or two goes by and the phone rings. Michael has "wiped out" and is on the way to the hospital in an ambulance! (My stomach does one of those nosedives again, the kind I thought we could leave behind, at least for a while). He doesn't remember why he wiped out and of course the first aid attendants flipped out when they removed his helmet and saw that nice big scar. After an hour ride to the hospital and several hours sitting in waiting rooms (hasn't this poor boy done his lifetime's worth of doctor visits yet?), a CT scan reveals no problems—ruled out a concussion and sent back to the slopes—too late to do any more snowboarding. But I am devastated. Here come the sleepless nights again. I will start worrying why he wiped out—was it a focal seizure? It's almost PMS (pre-MRI syndrome) time anyways; scan to be done at the end of the month. Perhaps we ditched the Dilanti® too soon. Michael hates to be on it, so he pushes the doctor to get him off as soon as possible.

Can't life ever be normal for this family again? And Michael! The one time he gets a chance to leave the doctors and the tests and the waiting rooms and the crazy, nervous mom behind and now his special day is ruined.

$$\cdot \ \cdot \ \cdot \ \cdot \ \cdot$$

My 6-year-old son finished his radiation and is still on chemo for his medulloblastoma. I feel like I have to lighten up in order for life to go on. So I just let the nanny take all four kids on a 4-hour drive to spend 8 hours at Six Flags®. It just about drove us nuts with worry, but they all came home safe and sound. They felt like they had a normal sibling outing.

$$\cdot \ \cdot \ \cdot \ \cdot \ \cdot$$

Alissa (age 8) has metal rods to support her spine following multiple operations for spinal astrocytoma. She uses a wheelchair right now. We don't protect Alissa like she's going to break. On Fourth of July, she sat in the middle of the stands with all her friends for the fireworks, and then she cruised the field later like everybody else. The mayor of our city gave her an award for being the first and only person in a wheelchair to perform the pledge of allegiance at the city council meeting (she went with her Brownie troop), and she will be participating in a fashion show with her Brownie troop to raise funds for our neurological institute.

Not spending enough time with the sibling(s)

While acknowledging that there are only so many hours in a day, parents interviewed for this book felt the most guilt about the effect that diagnosis and treatment had on the siblings. They wished they had asked family and friends to stay with the sick child more often, allowing them to spend more of their precious time with the siblings. Many expressed pain that they didn't know how severely affected the siblings had been.

I try to find some time in each holiday, weekend, or whenever it is just for Christopher and me. No matter how ill Michael is, someone else can cope with it for an hour or two, and nothing is allowed to interfere with that. We still go out, even if it is only Christopher and me at McDonald's®.

Bottom line is that all mothers have to accept that along with the baby is delivered a large package of guilt, and whatever we do for one we will wish we had done for the other.

But I don't think you can put one child on hold for the duration of the other's illness, because the year that Christopher has lost while Michael has been ill won't ever come again. He'll only be 11 once, just as surely as Michael will only be 14 once (or possibly forever), and we owe it to our healthy kids to allow them to be just that.

Using substances to cope

Some parents find themselves turning to alcohol or drugs to help them cope. Some parents use illegal drugs, and some overuse prescription medications or over-the-counter sleeping pills. If you find yourself drinking so much that your behavior is affected, or using drugs to get through the day or night, seek professional help.

Coping

Many parents find unexpected reserves of strength and are able to ask for help from friends and family when they need it. They realize that different needs arise when there is a great stress to the family, and they alter their expectations and parenting accordingly. These families usually had strong and effective communication prior to the illness and pull together as a unit to deal with it.

The majority of families, however, have periods of calm alternating with times when nerves are frayed and tempers are short. In the end, most families survive intact and are often strengthened by the years of dealing with cancer.

After 12 years living with Jen's glioma, I have made my own peace with the fact that I may not be able to prevent or choose what Jen has to deal with. I can, however, make a difference in how we go through it so she finds peace and comfort.

We have been truly blessed by most of the care Jen has received. We have felt the compassion of those who have been willing to recognize the feelings of this process as a part of the medicine and were willing to communicate and acknowledge that to Jen and to us. For her that makes a tremendous difference in how she responds.

Improving communication

Parents suggest the following ways to keep the family more emotionally balanced.

- Make sure the family rules are clearly understood by all of the children. Stressed children feel safe in homes with regular, predictable routines.

   After yet another rage by my daughter with cancer, we held a family meeting to clarify the rules and consequences for breaking them. We asked the kids (both preschoolers) to dictate a list of what they thought the rules were. The following was the result, and we posted copies of the list all over the house (which created much merriment among our friends):

   1. *No peeing on rug.*

   2. *No jumping on bed.*

   3. *No hitting or pinching.*

   4. *No name calling.*

   5. *No breaking things.*

   6. *No writing on walls.*

   If they broke a rule, we would gently lead them to the list and remind them of the house rules. It really helped.

- Have all caretakers consistently enforce the family rules.

   We kept the same household rules. I was determined that we needed to start with the expectation that Rachel was going to survive. I never wanted her to be treated like a "poor little sick kid," because I was afraid she would become one. We had to be careful about babysitters, because we didn't want anyone to feel sorry for her or treat her differently. I do feel that we avoided many long-term behavior problems by adopting this attitude early.

- Give all the kids some power by offering choices and letting them completely control some aspects of their lives, as appropriate.

   For a few months we ignored Shawn's two brothers as we struggled to get a handle on the situation. We just shuttled them around with no consideration for their feelings. When we realized how unfair we were being, we made a list of places to stay, and let them choose each time we had to go off to the hospital. We worked it out together, and things went much smoother.

·　·　·　·　·

*My bald, angry, 4-year-old daughter asked me for some scissors one day. I asked
what she was going to do, and she said "Cut off all the Barbies® hair." I told her
those were her dolls and she could cut off their hair if she chose. I asked her to consider leaving one or two with hair, because when she had long hair again, she might
want dolls that looked like her then, too. But I said it was up to her. She cut off the
hair (down to the plastic skull!) of all but one of the dolls. It really seemed to make
her feel better. A few months later, she dismembered them. Fifteen years later, we
occasionally find Barbie® legs and arms lying around the house, and we all laugh.*

- Take control of the incoming gifts. Too many gifts make the ill child worry excessively
  ("If I'm getting all of these great presents, things must be really bad") and the siblings
  feel jealous. Be specific if you prefer that people not bring or send gifts, or if you prefer
  gifts for each child, not just the sick one.

- Recognize that some problems are caused solely by treatment. It helps to remember
  that children with cancer are not naturally defiant or destructive. They are feeling sick,
  powerless, and altered by surgery, radiation, and/or drugs, and parents need to try to
  help by sympathizing, yet setting limits. Remember, with time, their real personalities
  will return.

  *In the beginning, my 2-year-old daughter was incredibly angry. She would have
  massive temper tantrums, and I would just hold her and tell her that I wouldn't let
  her hurt anybody. I would continue to hold her until she changed from angry to sad.
  When she was on certain chemotherapy drugs, she would either be hugging me or
  pinching, biting, or sucking my neck. It drove me crazy. Now she's not having as
  many fits, but she still pushes her sisters off swings or the trampoline. She has a
  general lack of control. Sometimes, when I can't stand it anymore, I swat her on the
  bottom, and then I feel really bad.*

- If your child likes to draw, paint, knit, collage, or do other artwork or crafts, encourage it. Art is both soothing and therapeutic, and it gives children a positive outlet for
  feelings and creativity.

  *Recently, when Cami was going through another "This-is-the-last-time-I'm-going-
  to-the-doctor" outburst, we spent the waiting time writing a list of all the horrible
  things we want to do to cancer (step on it; put needles in its eye; not let it have cake).
  I also draw cells—good and bad. We give lollipops to the good cells and scribble out
  the bad ones. It sounds simplistic, but it really helps.*

- Allow your child to be totally in charge of her art. Do not make suggestions or criti-
  cisms (e.g., "stay inside the lines" or "skies need to be blue not orange"). Rather,
  encourage her and praise her efforts. Display the artwork in your home. Listen

carefully if your child offers an explanation about the art, but do not pry if he says it is private. Above all, do not interpret it yourself or disagree with your child about what the art represents. Being supportive will allow your child to explore ways to soothe himself and clarify strong feelings.

> *Jody was continually making projects. We kept him supplied with a fishing box full of materials, and he glued and taped and constructed all sorts of sculptures. He did beautiful drawings full of color, and every person he drew always had hands shaped like hearts. If we asked him what he was making, he always answered, "I'll show you when I'm done."*

- If your child does artwork or likes to write, recognize that powerful emotions may surface for both child and parents.

> *At my daughter's preschool, once a week each child would tell the teacher a story, which the teacher wrote down for the child to take home. Most of my daughter's pre-diagnosis stories were like this: "There was a rhinoceros. He lived in the jungle. Then he went in the pool. Then he decided to take a walk. And then he ate some strawberries. Then he visited his friend." But during treatment, she would dictate frightening stories (and this from a kid who wasn't allowed to watch TV and had never seen any violence). Two examples are: "Once there were some bees and they stung someone and this someone was allergic to them and then they got hurt by some monkeybars and the monkeybars had needles on them and the lightning came and hit the bees," and, "Once upon a time there were six stars and they twinkled at night and then the sun started to come up. And then they had a serious problem. They shot their heads and they had blood dripping down."*

- Come up with acceptable ways for your child to physically release her anger. Some options are: ride a bike, run around the house, swing, play basketball or soccer, pound nails into wood, mold clay, punch pillows, yell, take a shower or bath, or draw angry pictures. In addition, teach your child to use words to express his anger, for example, "It makes me so angry when you do that," or "I am so mad I feel like hitting you." Releasing anger physically and expressing anger verbally in appropriate ways are both valuable life skills to master.

> *Our kids go along okay for a while, dealing with stuff. Then suddenly (because they're tired, have reached a new point developmentally, or are not feeling well in a way they can't describe), they lose it. It seems that every kid needs something different at these times, but what works best for Cami is for us to help her find words for her frustration. We talk about how unfair cancer is, how terrible treatment is, how no one else really knows what she's going through. Sometimes she just bursts out crying with relief that someone understands!*

Shawn was very, very angry many times. We had clear rules that it was okay to be angry, but he couldn't hit people. We bought a punching bag, which he really pounded sometimes. Play-Doh® helped, too. We had a machine to make Play-Doh® shapes, which took a lot of effort. He would hit it, pound it, push it, roll it. Then he would press it through the machine and keep turning that handle. It seemed to really help him with his aggression.

• Treat your ill child as normally as possible.

When Justin was in the hospital, I could never stand to see him in those little hospital gowns. I asked if we could dress him in his own outfits, and they said yes. So even when he was in the ICU [intensive care unit] with all the tubes coming out of his body, we dressed him every day in something cute. It just felt better to see him in his clothes. Several months later my mother said she really admired us for doing that, because we were sending the message to Justin that everything was going to be okay. That even though he couldn't breathe on his own, he was still going to get up every day and get dressed. Now I think it probably did communicate to him that things were going to be normal again.

• Get professional help whenever you are concerned or run out of ideas about how to handle emotional problems. Mental health care professionals (see Chapter 19, *Sources of Support*) have spent years learning how to help resolve these kinds of problems, so let them help your family.

My daughter and I both went to wonderful therapists throughout most of her treatment. My daughter was a very sensitive, easily overwhelmed child, who withdrew more and more into a world of fantasy as cancer treatment progressed. Her therapist was skilled at drawing out her feelings through artwork and play. My therapist helped me with very specific suggestions on parenting. For instance, when I told the therapist that my daughter thought that treatment would never end (a reasonable assumption for a preschooler), she suggested that I put two jars on my daughter's desk. One was labeled "ALL DONE," and the other was labeled "TO DO." We put a rock for every procedure and treatment already completed in the ALL DONE jar, and one rock for every one yet to do in the TO DO jar. (Only recommended if the child is more than halfway through treatment.) Then, each time we came home, my daughter would move a rock into the ALL DONE jar. It gave her a concrete way to visualize the approach of the end of treatment. She could see the dwindling number of pebbles left. On the last day of treatment, when she moved the last pebble over and the TO DO jar was empty, I cried, but she danced.

- Most emotional problems resulting from cancer treatment can be resolved through professional counseling. However, some children and parents also need medications to get them through particularly rough times.

    My daughter was doing really well throughout treatment until a combination of events occurred that was more than she could handle. Her grandmother died from cancer during the summer, one of her friends with cancer died on December 27, then another friend relapsed for the second time. She was fine during the day, but at night she constantly woke up stressed and upset. She had dreams about trapdoors, witches brewing potions to give to little children, and saw people coming into her room to take her away. She would wake up smelling smoke. She was awake 3 or 4 hours in the middle of the night, every night. Her doctor put her on sleeping pills and anti-anxiety medications, and the social worker came out to the house twice a month.

- Teach children relaxation or visualization skills to help them cope better with strong feelings. (See Appendix C, *Books and Websites*, for additional information about developing such skills.)

- Have reasonable expectations. If you are expecting a sick 4 year old to act like a healthy 6 year old, or a teenager to act like an adult, you are setting your child up to fail.

    It seemed like we spent most of the years of treatment waiting to see a doctor who was running hours behind schedule. Since my child had trouble sitting still and was always hungry, I came well prepared. I always carried a large bag containing an assortment of things to eat and drink, toys to play with, coloring books and markers, books to read aloud, and Play-Doh®. He stayed occupied and we avoided many problems. I saw too many parents in the waiting room expecting their bored children to sit still and be quiet for long periods of time.

- As often as possible, try to end the day on a positive note. If your child is being disruptive, or if you are having negative feelings about your child, here is an exercise you can use to end the day in a pleasant way. At bedtime, parent and child each tell one another something they did that day that made them proud of themselves, something they like about themselves, something they like about each other, and something they are looking forward to the next day. Then a hug and a sincere "I love you" bring the day to a calm and loving close.

Checklist for parenting stressed children

A group of parents compiled the following suggestions for ways to parent stressed children.

- Model the type of behavior you desire. If you talk respectfully and take time-outs when angry, you are teaching your children to do so. If you scream or hit, that is how your children will handle their anger.

- Seek professional help (for you and/or your children) for any behaviors that trouble you.

- Teach your children to talk about their feelings.

- Listen to your children with understanding and empathy.

- Be honest and admit your mistakes.

- Help your children examine why they are behaving the way they are.

- Distinguish between having feelings (always okay) and acting on strong feelings in destructive or hurtful ways (not okay).

- Have clear rules and consequences for acting on destructive feelings.

- Teach children to recognize when they are losing control.

- Discuss acceptable outlets for anger.

- Give frequent reassurances of your love.

- Provide plenty of hugs and physical affection.

- Notice and compliment your child's good behaviors.

- Recognize that the disturbing behaviors result from stress, pain, and drugs.

- Remember that with lots of structure, love, time, and sometimes professional help, the problems will become more manageable.

> *Every possible grouping of our family has been in therapy at one point or another. We have all done individual therapy, family therapy, and my husband and I did couples therapy. I feel that each of these sessions was a gift to our family. It helped us vent, cry, plan, and forge stronger bonds. We are all happy together many years after our daughter's cure, and every single penny we spent was worth it.*

Our children look to us to learn how to handle adversity. They learn how to cope from us. Although it is extremely difficult to live through your child's diagnosis and treatment, it must be done. So we each need to reach deep into our hearts and minds to help our children endure and grow.

Children Learn What They Live

If a child lives with criticism, he learns to condemn.
If a child lives with hostility, he learns to fight.
If a child lives with ridicule, he learns to be shy.
If a child lives with shame, he learns to feel guilty.
If a child lives with tolerance, he learns to be patient.
If a child lives with encouragement, he learns confidence.
If a child lives with praise, he learns to appreciate.
If a child lives with fairness, he learns justice.
If a child lives with security, he learns to have faith.
If a child lives with approval, he learns to like himself.
If a child lives with acceptance and friendship,
He learns to find love in the world.

— Dorothy Law Nolte

Chapter 18

School

*Most of us had two feelings at the same time: wanting
to go back to school and being scared of going back.*

— Eleven children with cancer
There Is a Rainbow Behind Every Dark Cloud

CHILDREN WITH BRAIN AND SPINAL CORD TUMORS often experience disruptions in their education because of repeated hospitalizations or side effects from the disease or treatment. As their health improves, and when their treatment schedule allows, returning to school can be either a relief or a challenge.

For many children, school is a refuge from the world of hospitals and procedures—a place for fun, friendship, and learning. School is the defining structure of children's daily lives and going back to school can signal hope for the future and a return to normalcy. Some children, however, especially teens, may dread returning to school because of temporary or permanent changes to their appearance or concerns that prolonged absences may have changed their social standing with friends.

In addition, physical disabilities caused by the tumors or cancer treatment may prevent children from participating in games, gym class, athletics, or other activities. These physical impairments sometimes require time out from the regular classroom for physical, occupational, and speech therapies. School can also become a major source of frustration for children who learn differently as a result of the tumor and/or treatment. Many children who survive brain or spinal cord tumors require specialized education and rehabilitation services.

Although educating children who have or had brain or spinal cord tumors can be a complex process, many issues can be successfully managed through careful planning and good communication. This chapter covers educational issues your child may encounter during and after treatment, a short section about avoiding communicable illnesses at school, and stories full of advice and experiences from many families of children with brain or spinal cord tumors.

Keeping the school informed

After a school-aged child is diagnosed with a brain or spinal cord tumor, she is usually rushed to a children's hospital (sometimes far from home) and is no longer able to attend school. To prevent your child from being dropped from school rolls due to non-attendance, you need to notify the school in writing about your child's medical situation. This notification allows planning to begin for your child to receive home-based schooling once he is able to resume his studies. Following is a sample letter, reprinted with permission from Sharon Grandinette, Exceptional Education Services.

> Date
>
> Dear [Name of Principal],
>
> Our son, John Doe [date of birth], a student at [name of school], was diagnosed with a brain tumor in [month] and had surgery to remove the tumor. He is still hospitalized. He is unable to attend school at this time, and may undergo treatment with chemotherapy or radiation.
>
> We are requesting that a Student Study Team meeting be scheduled with the school nurse in attendance. The purpose of the meeting is to discuss John's current medical status and how it may impact his school attendance and functioning. John may require school interventions or special education services, and we would like to discuss those options at the meeting. Depending on John's medical status, we may be able to attend the meeting in person, but if not, we request that it take place by phone.
>
> Please send us the appropriate release forms so that we may authorize an exchange of information between the school and the medical/rehabilitation professionals treating John.
>
> Sincerely,
>
> [Parent/guardian name(s)]

Because treatments for brain and spinal cord tumors (e.g., surgery, chemotherapy, radiation, and stem cell transplantation) cause changes in children's behavior and ability to function in school, both during and after treatment, the study team meeting can lay the foundation for any needed accommodations or interventions.

At the meeting, you may wish to distribute booklets about how to help children with brain and spinal cord tumors in the classroom, as well as age-appropriate information that can be shared with the classmates. You can formulate a communicable disease notification strategy, if necessary, and do your best to establish a rapport with the entire school staff. Take this opportunity to express appreciation for the school's help and your hopes for a close collaboration in the future to create a supportive climate for your child.

At the meeting, the school will designate a person (e.g., child's teacher, guidance counselor, special education expert) to communicate with a designated person at the hospital (e.g., school liaison, child life specialist, social worker). To read about how St. Jude Children's Research Hospital manages this process, visit *www.stjude.org* and enter the search term "School program."

> I still feel unbelievable gratitude when I think of the school principal and my daughter's kindergarten teacher that first year. The principal's eyes filled with tears when I told her what was happening, and she said, "You tell us what you need and I'll move the earth to get it for you." She hand-picked a wonderful teacher for her, made sure that an illness notification plan was in place, and kept in touch with me for feedback. She recently retired, and I sent her a glowing letter, which I copied to the school superintendent and school board. Words can't express how wonderful they were.

The designated liaisons will work to keep information flowing between the hospital and school and will help pave the way for a successful school reentry for your child. The liaison from the hospital should encourage questions and address any concerns the school staff have about having a seriously ill child in the school. Privacy laws prohibit liaisons from communicating unless parents sign a release form authorizing the school and hospital to share information. These forms are available at schools and hospitals.

In the months and years that follow, maintaining an open and amicable relationship with the school will ensure that your child, who may be emotionally or physically fragile, continues to be welcomed and nurtured at school.

Keeping the teacher and classmates involved

While your child is hospitalized, it helps to stay connected with his teacher and classmates. Parents can help by calling the teacher periodically and bringing notes or taped messages from the sick child to her classmates. Following are some suggestions for keeping the teacher and classmates involved with your child's life:

- Give the teacher a copy of the booklet *Living and Learning with Cancer* (listed in Appendix C, *Books and Websites*).

- Have the hospital's pediatric oncology nurse, social worker, or child life specialist give a presentation to your child's class about what is happening to their classmate and how he will look and feel when he returns. This talk should include a question and answer session to clear up misconceptions and alleviate fears. All children, especially teenagers, should be involved in deciding what information should be discussed with classmates and whether or not the child/teen wants to be present.

- Encourage your child's classmates to keep in touch. The class can make a card or banner or send a group photo. Individual students can call on the phone or send notes, emails, text messages, or pictures.

- If your child is old enough, allow her to establish a page on a social network site so she can communicate with her friends, express her feelings and thoughts, post photos, and remain connected.

- If possible, use Skype® or a similar webcam software program to allow your child to interact "face-to-face" with classmates on the Internet, a smartphone, or another electronic device.

Keeping up with schoolwork

As treatment progresses, your child will probably return to school either part time or full time, but extended absences due to infections or complications from treatment might occur. A child who is out of school longer than 2 weeks for any medical reason is entitled by law to instruction at home or in the hospital. It is a good idea to request off-site instruction as soon as you find out your child may be out of school for longer than 2 weeks. The school will require a letter from the doctor stating the reason and expected length of time this service will be needed.

> We used Skype® and had a weekly time set up so that Patrik could see his classmates, and they could see him. If an oral presentation was due, he heard a few of theirs, and presented his. If nothing shareable was due, they just traded jokes or did a show and tell of something that had happened that week. Both Patrik and his classmates enjoyed collecting jokes all year. If he was not feeling well or was hospitalized, it was cancelled for that week. It sure helped make him still feel a part of his class, and the teacher said it really helped his classmates to see he was still okay, and still himself. He wasn't allowed to attend school at all for frontline treatment (almost 10 months).

> Patrik started the first day of 5th grade this year. He was able to walk in the building, feel welcome, and step right back into his friendships. No problems at all with that. I really thank his teacher last year for keeping him a part of his class despite not being in school.

In some children's hospitals in large cities, teachers are located onsite. If your child is at home, the home school district provides the teacher. The teacher is responsible for gathering materials from the school and judging how much schoolwork your child can do.

Helping siblings

The diagnosis of cancer affects all members of the family. Siblings can be overlooked when the parents need to spend most of their time caring for the ill child. Many siblings feel frustrated, angry, frightened, neglected, or guilty, and they may try to keep their feelings bottled up to prevent placing additional burdens on their parents. Often, the place where these complicated feelings emerge is at school. Siblings may cry easily, fall behind in classwork, do poorly on tests, cut classes, challenge teachers, withdraw from friends or school activities, or disrupt the classroom.

To help prevent these problems from developing, you can send a letter to each sibling's school principal that requests teachers, counselors, and nurses be informed of the cancer diagnosis in the family and that asks for their help with and support for the siblings.

> *At the time when Matt was in treatment and his older brother Joey was 5, we knew Joey needed some support, too. He would hide behind the couch with his blanket and suck his thumb when home health nurses, equipment company personnel, or respiratory therapists came to our home. We were fortunate that a reputable counselor was near our home and, under our challenging and chaotic circumstances, we could take him for a few sessions without adding further commotion to our life. The support gave Joey the benefit of knowing he had a helper, too, and that he felt cared for as much as his brother did.*

If possible, try to include the siblings' teachers in some of the school discussions concerning the ill child. Teachers of siblings need to be aware that the stresses facing the family may cause the siblings' feelings to bubble to the surface during class. Parents must advocate just as strongly for their healthy children's emotional and educational needs as they do for their sick child's needs. Chapter 15, *Siblings*, deals exclusively with siblings and contains suggestions about how to help them cope.

Returning to school

Parents may not even think about school during the early efforts to save their child's life, but a quick return to school helps children regain a sense of normalcy and provides a lifeline of hope for the future.

> *Kids are fantastic with Alissa (age 8) who has had multiple surgeries for spinal astrocytoma. They can also be brutally honest. The best therapy for Alissa is being around her friends. School offered us home teaching when Alissa was diagnosed, but we said no. Alissa looks forward to school; it helps her. The people and the teachers rally around her. Alissa would be able to have a major back operation on a Friday,*

and she would be back to school by Tuesday. The most important thing is to get them back into real life as soon as possible.

Preparation is the key to a successful return to school. You and hospital staff (e.g., hospital school liaison, social worker, child life specialist) may want to prepare a package for the school staff that contains the following information:

- A doctor's statement that addresses your child's health status; ability to safely return to the school environment; physical restrictions, including any limits to physical education or recess; and probable attendance disruptions.

- Whether your child will attend full or half days.

- A description of any changes in her physical appearance, such as weight gain or hair loss, and suggestions about how to help the other children handle it appropriately.

- A request that the school administration is willing to bend the rules about head coverings so your bald child can wear a wig, hat, or scarf to school.

- The possible effects of medications on academic performance and any medications or other health services that will need to be given at school (see section later in this chapter called "Individual health care plan").

- A list of signs and symptoms requiring parent notification (e.g., fever, nausea, vomiting, pain, swelling, bruising, or nosebleeds) and, if parents are divorced or separated, what notification procedures should be followed.

- Concerns about exposure to communicable diseases, if necessary.

- Any special accommodations, such as extra snacks, rest periods, extra time to get from class to class, use of the nearest restroom (even if it is the staff restroom), and the need to leave for the restroom without permission. This list should also include any requests for academic accommodations such as extended time for tests and reduced workload. These services are discussed in greater detail later in this chapter.

The following are parent suggestions about how to prevent problems through preparation and communication:

- Keep the school informed and involved from the beginning to foster a spirit that "we're all in this together."

- Explain to classmates what is happening and reassure them that cancer is not contagious.

> *Elizabeth was in preschool at the time of her diagnosis. The manager did a wonderful job of integrating her back into the fold. All of the other children at the school were taught what was happening to Elizabeth and what would be happening (such*

as hair loss). They learned that they had to be gentle with her when playing. The manager was a former home health nurse, so I was very confident that she would be able to take care of my daughter in the event of an emergency. She was already familiar with central lines and side effects from chemotherapy. She was a gem!

- Arrange for places that your child can rest if she is too tired to participate in class.

  Robby was diagnosed in January of his kindergarten year. He returned to kindergarten the same day he got out of the hospital. His teacher was wonderful. She moved the desks around in the classroom so that if Robby got tired, she would go get his cot and put it in the center of the classroom so he could lay down and still listen. If a child had a cold, she would move him/her to the other side of the classroom. The kids washed their hands at least four times a day. The teacher's aide would sit in the rocking chair holding Robby if he was sad.

- Bring a pediatric oncology nurse or school liaison into the class to talk about brain and spinal cord tumors and answer questions. If treatment is lengthy, this should be done at the beginning of each new school year to prepare the new classmates. Because the sick child may be given special privileges that could cause other students to feel upset or jealous, the nurse or school liaison should also explain the reasons for different rules or privileges.

  My 16-year-old son was allowed to leave each textbook in his various classrooms. This prevented him from having to carry a heavy backpack all day. They also let him out of class a few minutes early, because he was slower moving from room to room.

- For elementary school children, enlist the aid of the school liaison or school counselor to help select the teacher for the upcoming year. You have no legal right to choose a particular teacher, but you are entitled to write to the administration to discuss your child's particular needs and request that these needs be considered when making assignments for the upcoming year.

  Because my son has had such a hard third-grade year, I have really researched the fourth-grade teachers. I sat in class and observed three teachers. I sent a letter to the principal, outlining the issues, and requested a specific teacher. The principal called me and said, "You can't just request who you want. What would happen if all the parents did that? You'll have to give me three choices just like everybody else." I said, "My son has a seizure disorder, behavior problems, and learning disabilities. Can you think of a child who has a greater need for special consideration?" My husband and I then requested a meeting with him, and at the meeting he finally agreed to honor our teacher request.

- Prepare the teacher(s) and your child for the upcoming year.

  I asked for a spring conference with the teacher selected for the next fall and explained what my child was going through, what his learning style was, and what type of classroom situation seemed to work best. Then, I brought my son in to meet the teacher several times, and let him explore the classroom where he would be the next year. This helped my son and the future teacher get to know to one another.

- Have a mental health therapist talk with your child about his emotions and his life both inside and outside of school.

  My daughter went to a psychotherapist for the years of treatment. It provided a safe haven for frank discussions of what was happening, and also provided a place to practice social skills, which were a big problem for her at school.

- Realize that teachers and other school staff can be frightened, overwhelmed, and discouraged by having a child in their classroom with a life-threatening illness. Accurate information and words of appreciation can provide much-needed support.

  It can be so helpful for the school staff to have periodic meetings to address concerns, fears, progress, or to learn about upcoming procedures. I don't think enough parents know they can request meetings (Individualized Education Program [IEP] or otherwise) as they feel the need, and so can school staff. When Matt started school (elementary), I requested monthly inclusion meetings for the first semester and then every other month during the second semester with his IEP team. We wrote this in his IEP so it actually happened. I learned to do this from a parent much wiser than me!

Avoiding communicable diseases

The dangers of communicable diseases to immunosuppressed children are discussed in Chapter 12, *Common Side Effects of Chemotherapy*. The following information applies to children whose blood counts are very low, which only occurs with some types of treatment.

Parents of children with low blood counts need to work closely with the school to develop a chicken pox, whooping cough, measles, and flu outbreak plan if the school does not already have a communicable disease notification plan in place. The school should notify you immediately if your child has been exposed to chicken pox so she can receive the varicella zoster immune globulin (VZIG) injection within 72 hours of exposure.

Several methods can be used to ensure prompt reporting of outbreaks. Some parents notify all the classmates' parents by letter to ask them for prompt reports of illness. If you have a good rapport with the teacher, you can ask the teacher to immediately report to you any cases of communicable disease.

> My daughter's preschool was very concerned and organized about the chicken pox reporting. They noted on each child's folder whether he or she had already had chicken pox. They told each parent individually about the dangers to Katy, and then frequently reminded everyone in the monthly newsletters. The parents were absolutely great, and we always had time to keep her out of school until there were no new cases. With the help of these parents, teachers, our neighbors, and friends, Katy dodged exposure for almost 3 years. She caught chicken pox 7 months after treatment ended and had a perfectly normal case.

· · · · ·

> My son was diagnosed at age 14. He was starting ninth grade, the last year of junior high. He missed about a third of that year. He was able to keep up, thanks to some terrific teachers and a very cooperative administration, not to mention being a really motivated kid. He hated missing school and would go even when he didn't feel very good, just to say he'd been to school that day, even if only for two periods. Our oncologists gave him the okay to be in school, saying that infection in kids his age was usually from bacteria they were already carrying around, so other kids were not a big threat, provided they weren't sick.

Other parents enlist the help of the office staff who answer the phone calls from parents of absent children.

> We asked the two ladies in the office to write down the illness of any child in Mrs. Williams' class. That way the teacher could check daily and call me if any of the kids in her class were ill.

Section 504 of the Rehabilitation Act of 1973

Some children, whether on or off treatment, may be eligible for services under Section 504 of the Rehabilitation Act. This civil rights law applies when a child has a physical or mental impairment that substantially limits one or more major life activity. The Section 504 team at the school determines whether a child is eligible based on the findings and recommendations of the treatment team about how the illness and treatment affects functions required for school participation. For example, a child in treatment might need a Section 504 Accommodation Plan that provides:

- Exemption from regular attendance/tardy policies
- A school-based health plan
- Reduced homework when ill or hospitalized
- Occupational, physical, or speech therapy

The list above describes accommodations made during treatment. However, Section 504 is also frequently used when a child who is off treatment has disabilities that do not meet the requirements of the Individuals with Disabilities Education Act (IDEA) (described below) but who do have impairments that limit one or more major life activity. For example, a child with processing problems might need a Section 504 Plan to obtain necessary accommodations, such as elimination of timed tests, more time to finish written assignments, and less homework. A written 504 Plan should specifically lay out all of the accommodations and educational services that will be provided to your child.

Individuals with Disabilities Education Act

The cornerstone of all federal special education legislation in the United States is the Individuals with Disabilities Education Act (IDEA). This law, first passed in 1990, has been amended several times. It covers children and their families from birth to age 3, preschoolers, and school-aged children through age 21. The major provisions of this legislation are the following:

- All children, regardless of disability, are entitled to a free and appropriate public education and necessary related services in the least restrictive environment.

- Children will receive fair testing to determine whether they need special education services.

- Parents can challenge the decisions of the school system, and disputes will be resolved by an impartial third party.

- Parents of a child with disabilities participate in the planning and decision-making for their child's special education.

You should check the school district website or contact the school superintendent, director of special education, or special education advisory committee in your school district to obtain a copy of the school system's procedures for special education. Depending on the district, this document may range from two to several hundred pages.

> Our son has multiple late effects from his chemotherapy, radiation, and stem cell transplant. He has an FM unit to help him hear his teacher. The school system was great about providing physical therapy, occupational therapy, and speech therapy. But they wanted to put him in a special needs school, but I wanted him to have support in the classroom. They said they had no staff, so I put an ad in the newspaper at a university graduate school near his school. We found a second-year grad student in special ed to help him in the classroom. The school district refused to hire her, so we appealed and had a hearing. We won. The aide is wonderful and helps Michael stay on task, understand instructions, and keep organized. I'm an effective, but exhausted, advocate.

Several online sources provide reliable information about learning disabilities and parents' rights under special education law. Two that many parents find especially useful are Wrightslaw at *www.wrightslaw.com* and the National Center for Learning Disabilities at *www.ncld.org*.

Referral for services

State-of-the-art treatment for childhood brain and spinal cord tumors has resulted in greater numbers of long-term survivors, but not without cost. Surgery, radiation, chemotherapy, and stem cell transplants can cause changes in learning abilities, motor skills, vision, hearing, and social skills. Parents and educators need to remain vigilant for these issues that affect learning so intervention can occur quickly. Signs of learning disabilities include problems with:

- Handwriting

- Spelling

- Reading or reading comprehension

- Understanding math concepts, remembering math facts, comprehending math symbols, sequencing, and working with columns and graphs

- Auditory or visual language processing, which includes trouble with vocabulary, blending sounds, and syntax

- Attention deficits

- Short-term memory and information retrieval

- Planning and organizational skills

- Social maturity and social skills

The first step to get your child educational support is called "referral for services." Every child who had a brain or spinal cord tumor should be referred for services. To make a referral for services, a parent or the child's teacher writes to the school principal specifically requesting special education testing and stating that the child is "health impaired" due to treatment for cancer. Do not ask for a referral verbally; you must request testing and services in writing. Obtain written notification of the date the school received the letter, because school staff are legally required to hold a meeting within 30 days of receipt of your request.

> My son had problems as soon as he entered kindergarten while on treatment. He couldn't hold a pencil, and he developed difficulties with math and reading. By second grade, I was asking the school for extra help, and they tested him. They did an IEP and gave him special attention in small remedial groups. The school system also provided weekly physical therapy, which really helped him.

The next steps in the special education process are evaluation, eligibility, IEP development, annual review, and 3-year assessments. You will need to become an advocate for your child as your family goes through the necessary steps to determine what placement, modifications, and services will be used to help your child learn.

> We have had an excellent experience with the school district throughout preschool and now in kindergarten. We went to them with the first neuropsychological results, which were dismal. They retested him and suggested a special developmental preschool and occupational therapy. Both helped him enormously. He had an evaluation for special education services done and now has a full-time aide in kindergarten. He is getting the help he needs.

Evaluation

Once the referral is made, an evaluation is needed to find out whether the school district agrees that the child needs additional help, and if so, what types of help would be most beneficial. Usually, a team composed of the teacher, school nurse, district psychologist, speech and language therapist, resource specialist, and Section 504 coordinator attend the first meeting. The evaluation usually includes educational, medical, social, and psychological areas.

Children with a history of surgery, radiation, or chemotherapy to the brain require thorough neuropsychological testing, which is best administered by pediatric neuropsychologists experienced in testing children with cancer. The results should be shared with the school system, which must consider the findings but may also conduct its own assessment. If parents disagree with the findings from the school's evaluation, they have the legal right to request an independent educational evaluation by a neuropsychologist, which is paid for by the school district.

> Zach has a brain injury because of his treatment. While he is not impulsive, he is not his "age," either. But we expect that he should still be able to do his own best. We had an advocate who knew where the best place for school for him would be. She helps all brain-injured kids (not only ones with tumors). We also had a neuropsychological evaluation done on Zach and it was very, very detailed. It told his strengths, weaknesses, and the best ways for him to learn.

Children with brain or spinal cord tumors are often evaluated for the need for specific therapies or services in identified areas (called "related services"). Examples of related services are physical therapy, occupation therapy, adaptive physical education, and assistive technology.

> Initially, the school was reluctant to test Gina because they thought she was too young (6 years old). But she had been getting occupational therapy at the hospital

for 2 years, and I wanted the school to take over. I brought in articles and spoke to the teacher, principal, nurse, and counselor. Gina had a dynamite teacher who really listened, and she helped get permission to have Gina tested. Her tests showed her to be very strong in some areas, and very weak in others. Together, we put together an IEP, which we have updated every spring. Originally, she received weekly occupational therapy and daily help from the special education teacher. She's now in fourth grade and is doing so well that she no longer needs occupational therapy; she only gets extra help during study hall.

School districts have 60 days from the time the parents agree to the evaluation to complete the evaluation and present the findings. A meeting (including the parents and often the child or teen) is held to discuss the evaluation results and make a determination about whether a child is eligible for services.

Eligibility for special education

The IDEA law requires that your child meet two requirements to be eligible for special education services: 1) The child must have one (or more) of the 14 disabilities listed in the law; and, 2) as a result of the disability, the child needs special education services to benefit from the general education program. The 14 eligibility categories for special education under the federal law are:

- Autism
- Deaf/blindness
- Deafness
- Developmental delay
- Emotional disturbance
- Hearing impairment
- Intellectual disability
- Multiple disabilities
- Orthopedic impairment
- Other health impairment (OHI)
- Specific learning disability
- Speech or language impairment
- Traumatic brain injury (TBI)
- Visual impairment, including blindness

Most children with effects from treatment for brain or spinal cord tumors qualify for services under the category of OHI and often a secondary eligibility (e.g., hearing impairment, speech or language impairment, orthopedic impairment, TBI).

Individual education program (IEP)

After eligibility is determined, an IEP is developed. An IEP details the special education program and any other related services that will be provided to meet the individual needs of your child. The IEP describes what your child will be taught, how and when the school will teach it, and any educational accommodations that will be made for your child.

Students with disabilities need to learn the same things as other students: reading, writing, mathematics, history, and other subjects that help them prepare for vocational training or college. The difference is that with an IEP in place, many specialized services, such as small classes, speech therapy, physical therapy, counseling, and instruction by special education teachers, are used.

The IEP has five parts:

1. **A description of the child.** This section includes your child's present level of social, behavioral, and physical functioning, academic performance, learning style, and medical history.

2. **Goals and objectives.** This section lists skills and behaviors that your child is expected to master in a specific time period. These goals should not be vague like "John will learn to write a report," but rather, "John will prepare and present an oral book report with two general education students by May 1." Each goal should answer the following questions: Who? What? How? Where? When? How often? When will the service start and end?

> There came a time when my husband and I had to decide if we would continue to pursue an academic path for our son or focus more on life skills. This was difficult for us. We did not want to "give up" on our child, but it was clear that because the tumor and treatment had impacted him so severely, he had reached the highest level of classroom learning he could attain. At age 15 he had the math and reading skills of a third grader. As we began to think of his adult life, we saw that his energy was better spent preparing for jobs and independent living than learning how to multiply fractions or write a 3-page book report.

3. **Related services.** Many specialized services that will be provided at no cost to the family can be mandated by the IEP, including:

   - Speech therapy
   - Physical therapy and adaptive physical education

- Occupational therapy
- Social skills training
- Mental health services
- Assistive technology assessment
- Behavioral plans and functional behavior assessment
- Transportation to and from school and therapy sessions

For each of these services, the IEP should list the frequency, duration, start date, end date, and whether the services will be group or individual, for example, "Jane will receive individual speech therapy sessions twice a week, for 60 minutes a session, from September through December, when her needs will be reevaluated."

As discussed in Chapter 10, *Surgery,* rehabilitation services help many children make a full or near full recovery. Children who have a long-term need for rehab can access some of these services from the school system. To advocate for these services, parents should obtain letters of medical necessity from individual therapists, the physiatrist, and the primary treating doctor and present them as supporting documentation during the IEP meeting.

Formal rehabilitation in the outpatient or school setting is frequently enhanced by recreational activities. Community and school athletic teams are excellent therapy for children who can participate in them. Participation in the arts, such as music, art, drama, and dance, are also helpful.

4. **Placement.** The term *placement* refers to the least restrictive setting in which the IEP goals and objectives can be met. For example, one student may be in the regular classroom all day with an aide present, and another might leave the classroom for part of each day to receive specialized instruction in a resource room. The IEP should state the percentage of time the child will be in the general education program and the frequency and duration of any special services.

5. **Evaluating the IEP.** A meeting with all members of your child's IEP team is held periodically to review your child's progress toward attaining the short- and long-term goals and objectives of the IEP. To ensure the IEP is working for your child, an annual IEP meeting is required, and parents can request more meetings, if needed, to address any concerns.

If at any time communication deteriorates and you feel your child's IEP is inadequate or not being followed, here are several facts you need to know:

- Changes to the IEP cannot be made without parental consent.

- If parents disagree about the content of the IEP, they can withdraw consent and request (in writing) a meeting to draft a new IEP; or they can consent only to the portions of the IEP with which they agree.

- Parents can request to have the disagreement settled by an independent mediator and hearing officer.

- The IEP is a legal document and schools are required to comply with what is written in the IEP.

> We've set up goals and objectives in Victoria's IEP so that she succeeds at her level. She is graded against these requirements. We have two or three meetings each year to determine the appropriate level of her capabilities. We've negotiated for all her classwork to be done during school hours with one-to-one help in the resource room. Victoria, who has seizures and cognitive issues due to a hypothalamic hamartoma, is on her school's Honor Roll for grades! Her name was published in our town newspaper along with others who excelled and she received a nice certificate. This is how an IEP is supposed to work, grades being determined upon achievable goals outlined in an IEP, and hard work. She knows of course that grading for her is different than for other kids, and attempted to downplay her accomplishment, but secretly I think that she was quite proud and it has motivated her to work even harder.

IDEA does not describe specific types of educational placement, modifications, and related services. Because options are open, your child's IEP should reflect those programs and services uniquely appropriate for his needs. Advocates, disability organizations, and your child's medical team, teachers, and therapists can assist you in determining which options best suit your child, although ultimately you know your child best.

> This year (third grade) has been a nightmare. My son has an IEP that focuses on problems with short-term memory, concentration, writing, and reading comprehension. The teacher, even though she is special ed qualified, has been rigid and used lots of timed tests. She told me in one conference that she thought my son's behavior problems were because he was "spoiled." The IEP required that she send a note home with my son if he has a seizure, and she has never done it. She even questions him when he tells her that he had a seizure at recess. I learned that the IEP is only as valuable as the teacher who is applying it.

Hundreds of accommodations are available through an IEP. A few examples are:

- Preferential seating
- Study groups with discussion for learning/memory
- Taping of classes for reinforcement
- Reduction in reading load

- Books on tape

- A copy of notes from a peer to increase listening in class and reduce the need for writing

- A copy of teacher's planning notes prior to instruction

- Reduction in writing load

- Use of computer for written assignments

- Keyboard training (kindergartners are not too young to learn)

- Use of planning organizers

- Calculator use permitted after mastery of concepts demonstrated

- Extended time for tests

- Oral tests rather than written tests

- Extra time to travel between classes

- Locker placement consideration

- Key locks instead of combination locks

- An assignment check-off system

- Breakdown of large assignments into steps

> *Nettie recently was tested for auditory processing disorder. She did very well with the testing, but the ability to score it only goes down to 7 years and developmentally she is lower than that in some areas. Therefore, certain aspects of the test were unable to be administered. However, based upon what testing was done, Nettie does demonstrate a great deal of difficulty processing things presented auditorily. It was suggested that we try using a device called an "Easy Listener." She would wear a little box with headphones. The teacher would wear a microphone which links right to the box Nettie is wearing. That would mean that no matter what the noise level in the room, or where the teacher is, the teacher's voice will always sound only 6 inches away from Nettie's ears. We are also going to try using a computer program called Earobics® to try and retrain parts of her brain to "listen" better. Auditory processing disorder is sort of like having dyslexia of the ears. The ears hear fine, but the brain doesn't receive the message properly. So we'll see if any of these things help her.*

To learn about other accommodations used by survivors and children on treatment, visit the American Childhood Cancer Organization website (*www.acco.org/Information/Resources/Books.aspx*) to order a free copy of the book *Educating the Child with Cancer, 2nd edition.*

Transition services

Transition planning, starting no later than age 14, is required for students with IEPs, because special education students have the right to be prepared for graduation, higher education, and/or employment in ways that fit their needs. U.S. high schools may have a Department of Rehabilitative Services (DRS) vocational counselor on staff who helps students with disabilities plan for life after high school, or as part of the student's transition services, the school can connect the student with the DRS. The DRS can provide:

- Career guidance and counseling

- Diagnostic evaluations

- Supported employment and training

> *Part of Ben's transition plan was, at age 16, to travel to the local vocational school 4 days each week to learn basic skills in hotel and retail occupations. He was paid a small amount for each hour of onsite work at participating companies. He received high school credit and by the time he left the school he had two certificates that described his skills and experiences.*

For more information about transition planning, visit *www.wrightslaw.com/info/trans. index.htm.*

> *As my son grew older, we could see he was ready to interact with a world that was bigger than his high school. With my assistance during his application, interview, and training, a local grocery store hired him as courtesy clerk. Easter Seals® arranged for a job coach who watched Ben on the job to make sure he was safe in the parking lot and who came to our home to teach him how to bag groceries (from the options in my kitchen pantry!) He has worked about 20 hours per week for 7 years now. He is proud of his job and his managers always say he is their hardest worker. There have been bumps along the way, though. Sometimes employees and customers do not understand that Ben is hearing impaired or is a very concrete thinker. He is inflexible and his social skills are not great. On a few occasions I have had to facilitate conversations between him and his coworkers. Despite these issues, this job had been a great thing for him.*

IDEA Part C—Early intervention services

Part C of the IDEA mandates early intervention services for disabled infants and toddlers (from birth to the child's third birthday), and, in some cases, children at risk for developmental delays. These services are administered either by the school system or the state health department, and the services are usually provided in the family home. You can find out which agency to contact by asking the hospital social worker or by calling the special education director for your school district.

The law requires services not only for the eligible infant or toddler, but for the eligible family, as well. Therefore, an Individualized Family Service Plan (IFSP) is developed. This plan includes:

- A description of the child's physical, cognitive, language, speech, psychosocial, and other developmental levels
- Goals and objectives for the family and child
- The description, frequency, and delivery of services needed, such as speech, vision, occupational, and physical therapy; health and medical services; and family training and counseling
- A caseworker who locates and coordinates all necessary services
- Steps to support transition to other programs and services

At age 3, children are transitioned to the school district for assessment of the need for special education services. If eligible, the school district provides early childhood special education services. For more information, visit *http://nichcy.org/schoolage/preschoolers*.

Differences between IDEA and Section 504

	IDEA	Section 504
Type of law	A federal education law.	A civil rights law.
Who is covered	Children ages 3–21 whose disability affects their ability to benefit from general education. Part C covers infants and toddlers.	Any student with a disability in an educational setting.
Types of disabilities	Child must have one or more of the 14 disabilities listed in the law.	Any physical or mental disability (including cancer) that substantially limits one or more major life activity.
Person in charge	Special education director.	Section 504 coordinator.
Evaluation of eligibility	Several assessment tools are used to determine whether the child has a disability. Written consent from a parent or guardian is needed before evaluation begins. A reevaluation every 3 years is required.	Evaluation is conducted in the area of concern. Written consent of a parent or guardian is not necessary before evaluation is done, but notice must be provided. Yearly reevaluation or review is required.
Tools used to implement law	Individualized Education Program (IEP) and a Behavior Intervention Plan (BIP) for any child with a disability who also has a behavioral issue.	Section 504 Plan.
Change in placement	IEP meeting is required before any change in placement or services is made.	Meeting is not required for a change of placement or services.

	IDEA	Section 504
Due process	School district must provide resolution sessions and due process hearings for parents/guardians who disagree with evaluation, implementation, or placement.	School district must provide a grievance procedure for parents/guardians who disagree with evaluation, implementation, or placement; due process hearing is not required.

Individual Health Care Plan (IHCP)

If your child has any medical needs that must be managed at school (e.g., management of seizures, headaches, shunts, or medication), your child's doctor should write a letter to the principal with written orders for care. The school nurse will develop an IHCP to ensure that your child's medical needs are appropriately managed at school. The IHCP is incorporated into either an IEP or Section 504 Plan, and it includes a brief medical history, medications and side effects, student health goals, clear descriptions of health services that will be provided by the school, and contact numbers for emergencies. Parents and school personnel must sign the plan before it is implemented, and it should be updated every year.

Your legal rights (Canada)

Each Canadian province and territory has its own ministry or department of education and establishes its own laws, policies, procedures, and budgets pertaining to educational requirements and services. The Council of Ministers of Education operates on a voluntary basis to advocate for educational services, establish common goals, and improve the quality of education across the country. One of the shared goals of this group in recent years has been to improve the delivery of special education services to children across Canada.

Most provinces and territories have an evaluation process similar to the one used in the United States. Canada also employs a similar IEP process, although the specific rules vary by province. For a list of province-specific special education legislation, contacts, and resources, visit *www.cps.ca/en/issues-questions/map/provincial-special-education-legislation-and-contacts*.

The terminally ill child and school

In the sad event that a child's health continues to deteriorate and all possible treatments have been exhausted, it is time for the students and staff to discuss ways to be supportive during the child's final days. Students need timely information about their ill classmate so they can deal with his declining health and prepare for his death. The possibility of death from a brain or spinal cord tumor should have been sensitively raised in the initial class presentation before the child's return to school, but additional information is needed as the child's health declines. The following are suggestions about how to prepare classmates and school personnel for the death of a student:

- The school staff needs to be reassured that death will not suddenly occur at school; rather, the child will either die at home or in the hospital.

- Staff needs to be aware that going to school is vital to a sick child's well-being. School staff members should welcome and support the child's need to attend school for as long as possible.

- Staff can design flexible programs for the ill student.

   Jody was lucky because he went to a private school, and there were only 16 children in his class. Whenever he could come to school, they made him welcome. Because children worked at their own pace, he never had the feeling that he was getting behind in his classwork. He really felt like he belonged there. Sometimes he could only manage to stay an hour, but he loved to go. Toward the end when he was in a wheelchair, the kids would fight over whose turn it was to push him. The teacher was wonderful, and the kids really helped him and supported him until the end.

- It is helpful to provide reading materials about death and dying for the ill child's classmates, siblings' classmates, teachers, and school staff.

- Extraordinary efforts should be made to keep in touch when the child can no longer attend school. Cards, banners, tapes, texts, emails, telephone calls, and webcam or conference calls (e.g., on the principal's speaker phone) from the entire class or individual classmates are good ways to share thoughts and best wishes.

- Classmates can visit the hospital or child's home, if appropriate. If the child is too sick to entertain visitors, the class can come wave at the front window and drop off cards or gifts.

- The class can send books, video games, or a basket of small gifts and cards to the hospital or home.

- The class can decorate the family's front door, mailbox, and yard when the child will be returning home from the hospital.

All of the above activities encourage empathy and concern in classmates, as well as help them adjust to the decline and imminent death of their friend. The activities also help the sick child know she has not been forgotten by her teachers, friends, and classmates, even if she cannot attend school.

When the child dies, a memorial service at school gives students a chance to grieve. School counselors or psychologists should be available to talk to the classmates to allow them to express their feelings. Parents usually very much appreciate receiving stories or poems about their child from classmates. Scholastic® has a webpage with many excellent suggestions for classmates to remember their friend at *www.scholastic.com/browse/ article.jsp?id=3754883.*

As I sit here, almost 18 years since Matt's diagnosis, helping him learn the home row on the computer keyboard, I can't help but feel gratitude and pain, all at the same time.

Matt took 3 years of computer classes in high school and can scoot his way around a Word® document and the Internet like no one's business, and he is presently taking a keyboarding class at the community college. I thought it would be a walk in the park. I didn't realize getting his fingers to relax and curl so they could stay positioned on the home row would be so difficult, but he's making amazing progress. I forgot the real meaning of practice.

He has always wanted to go to college, but he is quite limited academically. I am so grateful that there are some courses he can take, as difficult as they are for him. I often reflect on the many teachers and assistants who have worked with him over the school years. Their patience, their energy, their creativity, their passion, their time, their love, and above all, their wisdom to know that everything they invested in my son is so well worth it.

Chapter 19

Sources of Support

The effort to "put up a front" is draining, isolating, and counterproductive. Support groups can be a powerful way of letting down these fronts a bit at a time among people who understand and feel the same conflicting pressure— to act as though everything is all right when it is not.

— David Spiegel, MD
Living Beyond Limits

THE DIAGNOSIS OF CANCER CAN BE a frightening and isolating experience. Every parent of a child with cancer has a story to tell of lost or strained relationships. Yet we are social creatures, reliant on a web of support from family, friends, neighbors, and religious communities. We need the presence of people who not only care for us, but who sincerely try to understand what we are feeling. Many parents of children with cancer experience deep loneliness after the first rush of visits, cards, and phone calls ends—when the rest of the world goes back to normal life.

Members of families struck by childhood cancer—parents, the child with cancer, and siblings—often turn to support groups and various other forms of psychological and emotional help. Families join support groups to dispel isolation, share suggestions for dealing with the illness and its side effects, and talk to others who are living through the same crisis. Individual and family counseling can help address shifting responsibilities within the family, explore methods to improve communication, and help find ways to channel strong feelings constructively.

This chapter offers resources that can help families regain a sense of control over their lives and find wonderful new friends who understand what they are going through.

Hospital social workers

Although the need for skilled pediatric social workers is widely recognized, shrinking hospital budgets often prevent adequate staffing. If your child is treated at a children's hospital staffed with social workers, child life specialists, and psychologists, consider yourself lucky. Sadly, millions of dollars are spent on technology, while programs that help people cope emotionally are often the first to be discarded. If your pediatric center offers no emotional support, get help through some of the other methods described in this chapter.

Pediatric oncology social workers usually have a master's degree in social work, with additional training in oncology and pediatrics. They serve as guides through unfamiliar territory by mediating between staff and families, helping with emotional or financial problems, locating resources, and easing the young patient back into school. Many social workers form close, long-lasting bonds with families and continue to answer questions and provide support long after treatment ends.

> Over the course of my son's treatment, I became very close to the hospital's social worker. I came to see her as not only a person who was very good at her job and providing me with wonderful support, but also as a friend. She was very much in tune with my personality, and seemed to sense when I was having a rough day, even if I had been doing my best to hide it. So many times she would stop by my son's room and invite me to join her for coffee in the cafeteria, her treat. And we would sit and talk about anything and everything. She seemed to have a natural talent for making me laugh when I really needed to most. And she never expressed discomfort when I needed to cry or curse the unfairness of the situation we were in. She was a very good listener.

· · · · ·

> We went to a children's hospital that was renowned in the pediatric cancer field. The medical treatment was excellent, but psychosocial support was nonexistent. The day after diagnosis, we were interviewed for 20 minutes by a psychiatric resident, and that was it. I never met a social worker, and the physicians were so busy they never asked anything other than medical questions. If I started crying, they usually left the room. I didn't know any parents of a child with my daughter's diagnosis; I didn't know there was a local support group; I didn't know there was a summer camp for the kids. I felt totally isolated.

In addition to social workers, some hospitals have child life specialists, psychiatric nurses, psychiatrists, psychiatric residents, and psychologists on staff who can help you deal with problems while your child is inpatient. Ask your child's nurse, treating physician, or the hospital social worker to help you access these resources.

Support groups for parents

Support groups offer a special perspective for parents of children with cancer and fill the void left by the withdrawal or misunderstanding of family and friends. Parents in similar circumstances can share practical information learned through personal experience, provide emotional support, give hope for the future, and truly listen and empathize.

> The countless heartfelt consultations, gestures, and visits from the nurses, doctors, hospital staff, and program developers were amazing. They gave me strength and they guided me through this. I was not in control. I was lost in a world I did not know and had no experience with. But they gave me hope, they told me I could do it, and they kept me informed and made me part of their process. The parent support group was instrumental in that movement from helpless to hopeful. I was not alone and I realized that no matter how bad we had it, we were lucky that our children were alive and fighting. I had to pull myself and our lives back together. We built a life and routines around this unfortunate situation and we began to adapt.

Coping with a life-threatening illness requires a unique perspective—the ability to focus on the grave situation at hand while balancing other aspects of daily life. In support groups, many families find this frame of reference and are better able to find emotional balance. Just meeting people who have lived through the same situation is profoundly reassuring.

> The group was a real lifeline for us, especially when Justin was so sick. We looked forward to the meetings and were there for every one. It was a real escape; it was a place to go where people were rooting for us. People from the group would always swing by the ICU to see us whenever they were bringing their own kids in for treatment. They always stopped by to visit and chat. We amassed a tremendous library of children's books that the group members would drop off. The support was wonderful.

. . . . .

> I felt like I was always putting up a front for my family and friends. I acted like I was strong and in control. This act was draining and counterproductive. With the other parents, though, I really felt free to laugh as well as cry. I felt like I could tell them how bad things were without causing them any pain. I just couldn't do that with my family. If I told them what was really going on, they just looked stricken, because they didn't know what to do. But the other parents did.

. . . . .

> Our Tuesday gatherings were an anchor for us. It was a time to meet with parents who truly understood what living with cancer meant. These parents had been in the

trenches. They knew the midnight terrors, the frustrations of dealing with the medical establishment; after all, it was an alien world to most of us. They knew about chemo, hair loss, friend loss, and they knew the bittersweet side of cherishing a child more than one thought one could cherish anyone. We gathered to cry, to laugh, to whine, to comfort one another, to share shelter from a frightening world. It was a haven.

Cancer can be a very isolating experience. For the parents of a child with a brain or spinal cord tumor, the issues that other parents in their social circles are dealing with seem light years away. But the moms and dads in the kitchen at a Ronald McDonald House or the ped-onc lounge can offer practical advice about things such as burnt skin from radiation and how long it will be before it really resolves. They understand each other's feelings and emotions, because they are sharing the same experience. It is a bond that cuts across all social, economic, cultural, and racial differences.

My 2-year-old daughter was diagnosed 1 week after I gave birth to a new baby girl. I remember early in her treatment, I was sitting with Gina on my lap, and my husband sat next to me, holding the new baby. The doctor breezed in and said in a cheerful voice, "How are you feeling?" I burst into sobs and could not stop. He said "Just a minute" and dashed out. A few minutes later a woman came in with her 8-year-old daughter who had finished treatment and looked great. She put her arms around me and talked to me. She told me that everyone feels horrible in the beginning; and it might be hard to believe, but treatment would soon become a way of life for us. She was a great comfort, and of course, she was right.

· · · · ·

Families from all over the world stay at the Children's Inn during treatment or follow-up. The kitchen areas, the large open-air playroom, and the computer room are frequently places to meet parents or their kids and siblings, and the Inn's supporters are always hosting game nights or family-style dinners. Everyone at the Inn, the managers and volunteers, shuttle drivers and house staff, makes a real effort. Our son feels completely at home staying there.

Many wonderful national and regional organizations exist to help families of children with brain and spinal cord tumors. Several of them are listed in Appendix B, *Resource Organizations*. In addition to these organizations, there are dozens of different types of support groups, ranging from those with hundreds of members and formal bylaws to three moms who meet for coffee once a week. Some groups deal only with the emotional aspects of the disease, while others may focus on education, advocacy, social opportunities, or crisis intervention. Some groups are facilitated by trained mental health practitioners, while others are self-help groups led by parents. And, naturally, as older members drop out and new families join, the needs and interests of the group may shift.

Parents are horrified by acute postoperative recovery and afraid for their child's life; disoriented by the "foreign land" of the hospital: new language, seemingly arbitrary rules, strange sounds and smells, rotating teams of doctors and nurses; confused by medical and treatment decisions that need to be made quickly; disheartened by their feeling of incompetence; isolated and alone; angry at God, at themselves and even at the sick child, for which they immediately feel guilty. A family whose child is newly diagnosed with a brain tumor is hit with these emotions almost immediately. Most parents don't realize these reactions are normal, and their sense of desperation is enhanced by the conviction that they aren't "doing a good job handling things."

Meeting other families who are going through the same thing, or who have already been through it successfully, can greatly relieve the stress of a family new to the world of pediatric brain tumors. The emotional benefits are obvious, and much needed information can be shared. Families who belong to a support group have the means to reorient themselves to the new world they find themselves in. More experienced families can help them learn the language, rules and customs, and offer an example of a functioning family unit that has successfully navigated diagnosis and recovery. Firsthand, from-the-trenches strategies for dealing with this disease can be invaluable, and what a relief to know that you are not alone!

It is important to remember, however, that support group members are not infallible. One person may say something thoughtless or hurtful. Someone else may provide incorrect information. It is best to accept the support in the spirit in which it is given, but to always take any concerns or questions you have to your child's doctor or nurse practitioner.

Online support

Parents from small, isolated communities may have a difficult time finding a support group in their area that fits their needs, as may single parents, parents who aren't able to attend support group meetings, or parents who prefer some anonymity. For these parents and families, finding emotional support is possible via the Internet. Many online discussion groups exist for families dealing with childhood cancer. Such groups can provide parents with the understanding that only another parent of a child with cancer can give. Topics might include coping skills that have been effective for other families or helpful medical information you can use in your fight against childhood cancer.

The support I have gained through online discussion groups is priceless. I have received a great deal of comfort from my participation in these groups. They have enabled me to connect with families from all over the world, many of whom are fighting the exact same disease. I have often come to my computer in the middle of the night, when everyone else in the house was asleep. I can express my fears at

3:00 a.m. and know someone will always be there to reassure me with the knowledge that they have felt these things, too. That's one of the most beautiful things about these groups. Someone is always there, even in the middle of the night.

· · · · ·

How ironic that we subscribed to this list in a moment of panic, with a black cloud lined with despair lingering above. But now we can say we have lassoed cyberspace, and here, among new friends, we have found and we have shared love, hope, support, informative information, mutual stories, mutual questions, thoughtful and sincere answers, honesty, disagreement, pain, inspiration, fundraising, friendship, humor, and enjoyment, as well as understanding. This list reflects the roller coaster of life. Activity on this list enables individuals to place that initial black cloud in their back pocket, hold sunshine in their hand, and watch hope dance above.

To find brain tumor discussion groups (or electronic mailing list services), parents can start by consulting the following websites: *www.acor.org*, *www.braintrust.org*, and *www.yahoogroups.com* (see Appendix C, *Books and Websites*). Electronic chat rooms often are not monitored, but some lists are carefully monitored by moderators. One of the largest lists, composed of almost 2,200 members and dedicated to brain tumor caregivers, health specialists, and patients, is the Braintmr list, which is sponsored by T.H.E. Brain Trust and available at *www.braintrust.org*.

Support groups for children with cancer

Many pediatric hospitals have ongoing support groups for children with cancer. Often these groups are run by experienced pediatric social workers who know how to balance having fun with sharing feelings. For many children, these groups are the only place where they feel completely accepted, and where most of the other kids are bald and have to take lots of medicine. The group is a place where children or adolescents can say how they really feel, without worrying that they are causing their parents more pain. Many children form wonderful and lasting friendships in peer groups.

All four of my kids have been going to the support groups for over 7 years now. We have one group for the kids with cancer, which is run by a social worker. The siblings group is run by a woman who specializes in early childhood development. Both groups do a lot of art therapy, relaxation therapy, playing, and talking. They meet twice a month, and I will continue to take my children until they ask to stop. I think it has really helped all of them. We also have two teen nights out a year. All of the teenagers with cancer get together for an activity such as watching a hockey game or basketball game, or going bowling, to the movies, or out for pizza. They also see each other at our local camp for children surviving cancer (Camp Watcha-Wanna-Do) each year.

Support groups for siblings

Many hospitals have responded to the growing awareness of siblings' natural concerns and worries by creating hospital visiting days for them. This allows both parent time with the siblings and the opportunity for the siblings to explore and become familiar with the hospital environment. Sibling days allow interaction with other kids who have a sibling with cancer and with staff, and a time to have questions answered and concerns addressed. Some hospitals have expanded these 1-day programs into ongoing support groups to improve communication, education, and support for siblings.

> *Our local brain tumor support group has just started a monthly meeting for siblings. They have pizza, there's a counselor involved, and parents attend their own meeting in another room.*

> • • • • •

> *Annie went to Camp Goodtimes long after her brother stopped going and attended camp as many years as they would allow. She intends to be on the staff at camp next summer.*

Parent-to-parent programs

Some pediatric hospitals, in conjunction with parent support groups, have developed parent-to-parent visitation programs. The purpose of these visits is for veteran parents to provide one-on-one support to parents of newly diagnosed children. The services provided by the veteran parent can be informational, emotional, or logistical. The visiting parent can:

- Empathize with the parents
- Help notify family and friends
- Ease feelings of isolation
- Provide hospital tours
- Write down parents' questions for the medical team
- Offer advice about sources of financial aid
- Explain unfamiliar medical terms
- Be available by phone for any problems that arise
- Supply lots of smiles and hugs, and (above all) hope

Families of newly diagnosed children can ask whether the hospital has a parent-to-parent program. If not, ask to speak to the parent leader of the local support group.

Often, this person will ask a parent to visit you at the hospital. Many parents are more than willing to visit, as they know only too well what those first weeks in the hospital are like. They are often accompanied by their child who has completed therapy and is rosy-cheeked and full of energy—a living beacon of hope.

> *I am the parent consultant for our region. Among the services I provide are: meet with all newly diagnosed families; give a packet of information to each child or teen with cancer; continue to visit the families whenever they return to the hospital; educate families about the various local resources; provide moral support; stay with children during painful procedures if the parents can't; organize and present all of the school programs; liaison with schools for school reentry; organize and send out monthly reminders for parent support group meetings, child support group meetings, and sibling group meetings; send out birthday cards to kids on treatment; serve as activities director at the summer camp; and generally try to help out each family in any way possible. My job is a part-time, paid position funded through the local independent agency, Cancer Services of Allen County, Inc.*

Hospital resource rooms

Hospital resource rooms are now becoming more widely available, and they are designed to help patients and their families find information—electronic or print—about specific conditions.

> *I think I first learned from a medical librarian about www.nih.gov and Medline, where you can find current research on chemotherapy and other treatments. If your local hospital is a teaching facility, they often have all the major medical journals, so we were able to get full-text versions of papers that we needed. Until we had our own home access to the Internet, most of our research was done through our local hospital's medical library.*

· · · · ·

> *Patient resource rooms are wonderful places. They usually have basic information on your child's illness, listings of agencies and cancer organizations, online access, and a person available to answer questions and help get you started if you're unfamiliar with doing Internet searches. It should be one of the first places families are directed to.*

Brain tumor conferences

Most of the major brain tumor organizations offer annual or biannual multi-day conferences for patients and families, and it may be worthwhile to attend one. These conferences often bring to one location a number of experts in brain tumor research, neurosurgery, and neuro-oncology, as well as present panel discussions by specialists, caregivers, and long-term survivors. They offer an opportunity to gather information, network with other families, and find hope.

Many pediatric cancer facilities and organizations also sponsor workshops, teleconferences, and web-based presentations about topics such as long-term effects of treatment, school issues, and updates about brain tumor treatments.

I would like to share my thoughts on the very first brain tumor conference that my family attended. The connection began with the people: I reached out to others for feedback, asked for information and embraced the intellect, experience, wisdom, and courage of friends. I left the conference knowing that it is okay to continue to dream, and although we showed our hurt, and cried, we learned we need to search, and try. We smiled too: for every tear, every pain and suffering, we united and became electrified.

Clergy and religious community

Religion is a source of strength for many people. Some parents and children find that their faith is strengthened by the cancer ordeal, while some begin to question their beliefs. Others, who have not relied on religion in the past, may now turn to it for solace.

Most hospitals have staff chaplains who are available for counseling, religious services, prayer, and other types of spiritual guidance. The chaplain often visits families soon after diagnosis and is available on an on-call basis. As with all types of emotional support, approaches that work well with one family may not be helpful for others.

The day after my daughter was diagnosed, a chaplain started coming to the room every day. She was very nice, but I felt like she wanted me to talk about the cancer, and I just couldn't. I clearly remember feeling as if my body parts were being held together by the weakest of threads. I felt if I started talking, or even said the word cancer, that those threads holding me together would break and I would fly apart into a million pieces. So we chatted about inconsequential things until one day I thanked her for coming, but said I felt strong enough to start talking to my family and friends.

When Shawn was first diagnosed, Father Ron came in, and we all just really bonded with him. Shawn was in the hospital most of the first year, so we had a chance to become very close. Often Shawn would ask for Father Ron before he had to have a painful procedure. Father Ron would talk to him, give him a little stuffed animal and a big hug, and then Shawn would feel better.

When Shawn was very ill, I began to worry about the fact that he had never been baptized, and I asked Father Ron to baptize him in the chapel. We ended up going to his own little church nearby, and we had a private service with just godparents and family, because Shawn's counts were so low. It was a wonderful, special service; I'll never forget it.

Parents who were members of a church, synagogue, or mosque prior to their child's diagnosis may derive great comfort from the clergy and members of their religious community. Members of the congregation usually rally around the family, providing meals, babysitting, prayers, and support. Regular visits from clergy provide spiritual sustenance throughout the initial crisis and subsequent years of treatment.

We belong to a religious study group that has met weekly for 8 years. In our group, during that time, there have been three cancer diagnoses and one of multiple sclerosis. We have all become an incredibly supportive family, and we share the burdens. I cannot begin to list the many wonderful things these people have done for us. They consistently put their lives on hold to help. They fill the freezer, clean the house, support us financially, parent our children. They do the laundry covered with vomit. They quietly appear, help, then disappear. I can call any one of them at 3:00 a.m. in the depths of despair and find comfort.

Individual and family counseling

Cancer is a major crisis for even the strongest of families. Many find it helpful to seek out sensitive, objective mental health professionals to explore the difficult feelings—fear, anger, depression, anxiety, resentment, guilt—that cancer arouses.

Family dynamics undergo profound changes when a child is diagnosed with a brain or spinal cord tumor. Seeking professional counseling for ways to adjust and manage is a sign of strength. When a child has cancer, problems may be too complex and family members may be too exhausted to manage on their own. Seeking professional help sends children a message that the parents care about what is happening to them and want to help face it together.

One of the first questions that arises is, "Who should we talk to?" There are numerous individuals in the cancer community who can make referrals and valuable recommendations, including:

- Other parents who have sought counseling

- Pediatricians

- Oncologists

- Nurse practitioners

- Clinic social workers

- School psychologists or counselors

- Health department social workers

You can ask the people listed above for a short list of mental health professionals who have experience working with the issues your family's is struggling with, for example, traumatized children, marital problems, stress reduction, or family conflicts. Generally, the names of the most well-respected clinicians in the community will appear on several of the lists.

> The whole treatment experience put an enormous strain on our marriage. My wife has always been easy to excite, whereas I've always been very "laid back." There were moments when I was afraid that it would completely fall apart. Counseling really helped. We managed to survive, and I think in many ways, it has even brought us closer together.

In making your decision, it helps to understand the various types of mental health professionals and their different levels of education and liscensure. The following disciplines train individuals to offer psychological services:

- **Psychology (EdD, MA, PhD, PsyD).** Marriage and family psychotherapists have either a master's degree or a doctorate; clinical and research psychologists have a doctorate.

- **Social work (MSW, DSW, PhD).** Clinical social workers have either a master's degree or a doctorate in a program with a clinical emphasis.

- **Pastoral care (MA, MDiv, DMin, PhD, DDiv).** These are laymen or clergy who receive specialized training in counseling.

- **Medicine (MD, RN, ARNP, PA).** Psychiatrists are medical doctors who completed a residency in psychiatry. Physician assistants and advanced practice nurses have the equivalent of master's level training in medicine with additional training in mental health. These three specialists are the only mental health professionals who can prescribe medications. In addition, some nurses obtain postgraduate training in psychotherapy.

- **Counseling (MA).** In most states, individuals must have a master's degree and a year of internship before they can work as counselors.

You may hear all of the above professionals referred to as "counselors" or "therapists." The following designations refer to licensure by state professional boards, not academic degrees:

- LCSW (Licensed Clinical Social Worker)

- LSW (Licensed Social Worker)

- LMFCC (Licensed Marriage, Family, Child Counselor)

- LPC (Licensed Professional Counselor)

- LMFT (Licensed Marriage and Family Therapist)

These initials usually follow others that indicate an academic degree (e.g., PhD); if they don't, inquire about the therapist's academic training. Most states require licensure or certification in order for professionals to practice independently; unlicensed professionals are allowed to practice only under the supervision of a licensed professional (typically as an "intern" or "assistant" in a clinic or licensed professional's private practice).

When you are seeking a mental health professional, ask the professional how long she has been in practice. A licensed marriage and family therapist who has been seeing patients for 10 years may be a better clinician for your needs than a licensed psychologist or psychiatrist in his first year of practice.

Another method for finding a suitable counselor is to contact the American Association for Marriage and Family Therapy in Alexandria, VA, at (703) 838-9808, or online at *www.aamft.org*. This is a national professional organization of licensed/certified marriage and family therapists. It represents more than 50,000 therapists in the United States and Canada, and its membership also includes licensed clinical social workers, pastoral counselors, psychologists, and psychiatrists.

A psychiatrist who is the mother of a child with cancer offers a few thoughts:

> *Counseling helps, preferably from someone who regularly deals with parents of seriously ill children. This therapy is almost always short—although there may be some pre-cancer problems complicating the cancer issues that need to be hammered out.*

> *Antidepressants definitely have a role in the "so your child has cancer" coping strategy. They cannot make the diagnosis go away. They can improve concentration, energy, sleep, appetite, ability to get pleasure in life, and hope for the future—all*

of which you, your child with cancer, your spouse, and your other kids need you to have! They are not a magic bullet. They take 2 to 8 weeks to work, and you may need to change once before you get the right medication, but it can make all the difference.

Also, nurture yourself. Take bubble baths. Buy flowers. Let people pamper you. Say yes when people offer to help. Redefine normal so things can be good again. Make time for yourself. Spend time with your spouse (even an hour to walk and talk and hold hands). Find time for your non-cancer kids, reveling in their accomplishments. Celebrate what is good about your life.

Pick out things that you feel are important to keep up with and do them. (For me it was laundry.) Ignore things that don't matter for the time being. (For me it was tidy rooms and cooking.) Make peace with your decisions and follow them.

To find a therapist, a good first step is to call two or three therapists who appear on several of your lists of recommendations. Following are some suggested questions to ask during your telephone interviews:

- What are your fees? Do you bill the insurance company directly? Do you accept my insurance?

- Are you accepting new clients?

- Do you charge for an initial consultation?

- What training and experience do you have working with ill or traumatized children?

- How many years have you been working with families?

- What is your approach to resolving the problems families develop from trauma? Do you use a brief or long-term approach?

- What evaluation and assessment procedures will be used to define the problem?

- How and when will treatment goals be set?

The next step is to make an appointment with one or two of the therapists you think might best address your needs. Be honest about the fact that you are interviewing several therapists prior to making a decision. The purpose of the introductory meeting is to see whether you feel comfortable with the therapist. After all, credentials do not guarantee that a given therapist is a good fit for you. Compatibility, trust, and a feeling of genuine caring are essential. It is worth the effort to continue your search until you find a good match.

I called several therapists out of desperation about my daughter's withdrawal and violent tantrums. I made appointments with two. The first I just didn't feel comfortable with at all, but the second felt like an old friend after 1 hour. I have been to see her dozens of times over the years, and she has always helped me. I wasn't interested in theory; I wanted practical suggestions about how to deal with the behavior problems. My 8-year-old daughter asked why I was going to see the therapist, and I said that Hilda was a doctor, but instead of taking care of my body, she helped care for my feelings.

· · · · ·

We went to family counseling because I was concerned that my son seemed to be increasingly withdrawn and depressed. It was a disaster. The kids clammed up, I talked too much, and my husband was offended by some of the remarks the counselor made. She was not a good choice for our family. It's a hard decision to change counselors when you know you need help, but it's better to make a move than to stay in an uncomfortable situation.

· · · · ·

We went into family therapy because every member of my family experienced misdirected anger. When they were angry, they aimed it at me—the nice person who took care of them and loved them no matter what. But I was dissolving. I needed to learn to say "ouch," and they needed to learn other ways to handle their angry feelings.

Children need to be prepared for counseling, just as they do for any unknown event. Following are several parents' suggestions about how to prepare your child:

- Explain who the therapist is and what you hope to accomplish. If you are bringing your child in for therapy, explain why you think talking to an objective person might benefit him.

- Older children should be involved in the process of choosing a counselor. Younger children's likes and dislikes should be respected. If your young child does not get along well with one counselor, change counselors.

- Make the experience positive (e.g., describe the therapist as "the talking doctor").

- Reassure young children that the visit is for talking, drawing, or playing games, not for anything that is painful.

   In the beginning of treatment, my son had terrible problems with going to sleep and then having nightmares, primarily about snakes. We took him to a counselor, who worked with him for several weeks and completely resolved the problem. The counselor had him befriend the snake, talk to it, and explain that it was keeping him awake. He would tell the snake, "I want you to stop bothering me because I need to go to sleep." The snake never returned.

- Ask the therapist to explain the rules of confidentiality to both you and your child. Do not quiz your child after a visit to the therapist.

David had a very difficult time dealing with his brother's cancer. Realizing that we were unable to provide him with the help he needed, we sought professional help for him. I think the reason he feels so comfortable with his therapist is that he is aware of the rules of confidentiality. After his sessions, I'll always ask him how it went. Sometimes he'll just grin and say it was fine, and other times he might share a little of his conversation with me. I never push or question him about it. If it is something he needs to discuss, I wait until he decides to broach the subject.

- Make sure your child does not think she is being punished; assure her that therapists help both adults and children understand and deal with feelings.

- Go yourself for individual or family counseling or to support group meetings. You not only will be taking care of yourself, but you will be a good role model for your children.

Some other types of therapy used to help children with cancer or their siblings are music therapy (*www.musictherapy.org*), art therapy (*www.arttherapy.org*), and dance therapy (*www.adta.org*).

In *Armfuls of Time*, psychologist Barbara Sourkes quotes Jonathan, a boy with cancer, who told her, "Thank you for giving me aliveness." She discusses the importance of psychotherapy for children with a life-threatening illness:

Even when life itself cannot be guaranteed, psychotherapy can at least "give aliveness" to the child for however long that life may last. Through the extraordinary challenges posed by life-threatening illness, a precocious inner wisdom of life and its fragility emerges. Yet even in the struggle for survival, the spirit of childhood shines through.

Camps

Summer camps for children with cancer, and often their siblings, are becoming increasingly popular. These camps provide an opportunity for children with cancer and their siblings to have fun, meet friends, and talk with others in the same situation. Counselors are usually cancer survivors and siblings of children with cancer, or sometimes oncology nurses and residents. At these camps, children can have their concerns addressed in a safe, supportive environment that is supervised by experts. These camps provide a carefree time away from the sadness and stress at home or from the all-too-frequent hospital visits.

Of all the ways to get support, I think the camp really helps the most. You are all there together for enough time to break down the barriers. Although camp does not focus on cancer, many times we really got down to talking about how we really felt. I have been a counselor at the camp for eight summers now. Most of the campers know that I relapsed three times and I'm doing great many years later. They see the many other long-term survivors who are counselors, and it gives them what they need the most—hope. The best support is meeting survivors, because nobody else truly understands.

· · · · ·

When we went to pick up 7 ½-year-old Kristin from camp, she told us how wonderful it had been and exclaimed, "I want to come back every year until I am old enough to be a counselor." That said it all to me.

· · · · ·

Caitlin went to camp, and this was a dream come true for her. As we pulled into the parking lot, she exhaled a deep breath and said, "I made it. I am finally normal!"

Some camps are set up to accommodate not only the child who has undergone treatment, but also their siblings and parents. Many other camps offer separate weeklong camping experiences just for siblings.

There was not a chance my husband would have gone last summer, and all my exhortations about how much fun he could have with our children were in vain. He can't stand the thought of going to a place for fun where "cancer" is the binding element, so I went alone last year and had the best 6 days since diagnosis! In fact, it was the only time I was really happy since Danny's brain and spinal tumors were discovered in April. The staff went out of their way to ensure that parents had as much fun as kids, there was constant companionship for the kids, even at meals, and they created such a warm environment for everyone. It is a truly wonderful experience, and it was so hard to leave and come back to normal life and clinics, chemo, decisions. I have been looking forward to this coming summer since I left camp in August.

· · · · ·

Thank God for the programs offered in partnership with our hospital such as summer camp, the sibling support programs, and karate. They helped me help 5-year-old Kyle maintain his sanity and mine. One of my biggest worries as a single mom was how I would give one of my children what they deserved without cheating the other. How would I give Kyle a great summer, without excluding Mia (2-year-old being treated for medulloblastoma)? How would I care for Mia without cheating Kyle? Without the staff, the programs, and my mom and sister, I probably would have had a nervous breakdown.

Appendix B, *Resource Organizations*, contains a short list of camps with contact information. To view a comprehensive list, visit *www.acor.org/ped-onc/cfissues/camps.html*.

It's like your psyche has been hit by a truck. Some days the pain is worse than others. Some days your threshold is stronger than others, but allow yourself the help that is available to get back to stable. Take it from me; it is next to impossible to pull from a dry well. So unlike children, we can't temper tantrum ourselves out of our feelings, we can't rant and scream and stomp our feet at the unfairness of it all. We can't just sit in momma's arms and have a hug and feel better. We have to handle it with an attitude and the responsibility that is expected of being adult. And we have to be a nurse, teacher, mom, emotional measuring stick for our kids, care for the marriage, pay the bills, and, oh yeah, don't forget about ourselves—all at the same time. It's just far too much. Say "Yes" to yourself, and your needs—get help when you need it. Other things that I found helpful were:

- *Saying "no," "no, thank you," and "I'll take that into consideration when I make my decision."*
- *Saying "yes," "yes, please, that would be a great help," and "sure, if you could drop off a lasagna or pick up some milk on your way over that would be great."*
- *Writing in a journal.*
- *Taking a retreat weekend.*
- *Playing cards with the girls.*
- *Counseling (on occasion with priest, psychologist, social worker).*
- *Having movie night with my sisters (usually a comedy—you are allowed to laugh).*
- *Treating myself to an inside-and-out car wash.*
- *Allowing myself to "cry in my cornflakes," then getting up, splashing some cold water on my face and getting on with the day.*
- *Enjoying a glass of wine, a candle, and Andrea Boccelli.*
- *Gardening.*
- *Having coffee with a friend.*
- *Helping someone else who was in worse shape than I was.*
- *Talking with other cancer kid moms about cancer kid family stuff.*
- *Talking with other non-cancer kid moms about non-cancer family stuff (the kids bickering, too much housework, the latest magazine, and what the women in it are wearing).*
- *Declaring the next 5 minutes was "get the crazies out" time, and tickling, dancing silly, and playing "make me laugh" (you know you're losing it when you do this, and no one else is home).*

- *Being an online (www.acor.org) listserv member.*
- *Going out with my husband. (Even if I had to drag him, we always enjoyed the evening in spite of ourselves.)*

And anything else I deemed necessary to help me get through it.

Chapter 20

Nutrition

Let your food be your medicine
and your medicine be your food.

— Hippocrates

NOW, MORE THAN EVER, it is important for your sick child to eat balanced, healthful, and energy-packed meals. Yet, the reality is that the eating habits of children with brain or spinal cord tumors go haywire. Although, your child's body needs added energy to metabolize medications and repair the damage to healthy cells caused by chemotherapy and radiation, those same treatments can wreak havoc on your child's appetite and taste sensations. This chapter discusses eating problems, explains good nutrition, suggests ways to pack extra calories into small servings, and offers tips about how to make food more appealing to children undergoing treatment.

How treatment affects eating

Eating is tremendously affected by most types of chemotherapy. Listed below are several common side effects of treatment that often prevent good eating. Other side effects that affect eating—nausea, vomiting, diarrhea, constipation, and mouth and throat sores—are covered in detail in Chapter 12, *Common Side Effects of Chemotherapy*. In addition, cranial radiation can change the way food tastes, making previously loved foods bland and undesirable.

Loss of appetite

Loss of appetite is one of the most common problems associated with cancer treatment. Children suffering from nausea and vomiting, diarrhea or constipation, altered sense of smell and taste, mouth sores, and other unpleasant side effects understandably do not feel hungry. Loss of appetite is most pronounced during the intensive periods of treatment. If your child loses more than 10 to 15 percent of her body weight, she may need to be fed intravenously or by nasogastric tube. Sometimes this can be avoided if parents learn how to increase calories in small amounts of food.

My son looked like a skeleton several months into his protocol. I used to dress him in "camouflage" clothes—several layers thick. This kept him warm and prevented stares.

In addition to simple loss of appetite, your child may experience a side effect of chemotherapy called early filling. This means the child has a sense of being full after only a few bites of food. If your child is suffering from early filling and only eats when hungry, she may begin losing weight and become malnourished. This chapter provides dozens of creative ways to encourage your child to eat more.

Increased appetite and weight gain

When children are given high doses of steroids such as prednisone or dexamethasone, they develop voracious appetites. They are hungry all the time, develop food obsessions, and frequently wake parents up during the night begging for another meal.

Jamie's treatment for low-grade astrocytoma called for weekly dexamethasone given intravenously to combat nausea, so we didn't have ravenous hunger like some kids have, but we did have nighttime munch sessions. We'd all get up and pull everything out: drinks, snacks, leftover pizza or pasta or chicken, grocery-cut fruit, precut carrots, almonds or peanuts, crackers and cheese, whatever was quick.

Most parents become very concerned if their child consumes huge quantities of food and gains weight. A moon face with chubby cheeks and a rotund belly are classic features of a child on high-dose steroids. Much of the extra weight is fluid, which steroids cause the body to retain. There are two important points for parents to remember about treatment with steroids. First, when the steroids stop, the extra fluid is excreted and weight drops. Second, the child's appetite may go from voracious to poor after the steroids stop, so it is unwise to limit food when your child is taking steroids. Instead, try to make the most of this brief time of good appetite to encourage consumption of a variety of nutritious foods. A well-balanced diet now will help your child withstand the rigors of the treatments ahead.

My daughter didn't sleep when she was on steroids for weeks, and she gained a lot of weight. She'd sit in bed and demand, all day and all night long, "toast with butter spread on it like icing on a cake." So, I gave it to her. When she was off the steroids, she'd rapidly lose the weight and she'd look skeletal. Both extremes were really hard on all of us emotionally.

If you are concerned about the weight gain, consult your child's oncologist. If the fluid retention is extreme, the doctor may have you restrict your child's salt intake; in some cases, children are given drugs called diuretics to rid the body of excess fluid.

Lactose intolerance

Lactose intolerance is when the body can't absorb the sugar (lactose) contained in milk and other dairy products. Both antibiotics and chemotherapy can cause lactose intolerance in some children. The part of children's intestines that breaks down lactose stops functioning properly, resulting in gas, abdominal pain, bloating, cramping, and diarrhea. If your child develops lactose intolerance, it is important to talk to a nutritionist to learn about low-lactose diets and alternate sources of protein. The following are suggestions for parents of lactose-intolerant children:

- Add special enzyme tablets or drops to dairy products to make them more digestible for children with lactose intolerance. Some of these products are over-the-counter additives, but others require a prescription. Discuss these additives with the oncologist before giving them to your child.

- Children who cannot tolerate the lactose in cow's milk often can manage acidophilus milk, soy milk, rice milk, almond milk, or lactose-free milk. These are easier to digest and come in a variety of flavors.

- Always be sure dairy products are pasteurized, not raw.

- Remember that milk is a common ingredient in other foods, such as bread, candy, processed meats, and salad dressings. Read ingredient lists carefully.

- If your child can't tolerate any dairy products, add calcium to his diet by serving canned salmon, sardines, spinach and other green leafy vegetables, or calcium-fortified fruit juices. Consult your child's oncologist and nutritionist about calcium supplements. Many children like the taste of a chewy calcium supplement called Viactiv®, which is available at most drug stores.

> Calcium supplements interfered with my son's seizure medications, as do antacid supplements (which are usually made from calcium carbonate). We also recently found out Dilantin® may be affected by some chemo drugs. We allow a window of about 2 hours between giving our son his seizure medications and any other meds, including calcium.

Altered taste and smell

One common reason children on treatment do not eat is because, for them, food has no taste or tastes bad. If food tastes bland to your child, try serving spicy cuisines, such as Italian, Mexican, or Greek foods.

Chemotherapy often causes foods, particularly red meats, to taste bitter and metallic. If that happens, avoid using metal pots, pans, and utensils, which can magnify the metallic taste. Serve your child's food with plastic knives, forks, and spoons. You can also replace red meat with tofu, pork, chicken, turkey, eggs, and dairy products.

For some children, taste returns to normal after treatment ends. And for a few children, it takes years before some foods taste pleasant again.

What kids should eat

A good diet includes sufficient calories to ensure a normal rate of growth; fuels the body's efforts to repair and replace healthy cells; and provides the energy the body needs to break down the various chemotherapy drugs given and excrete their by-products. Over the time that chemotherapy is being administered, maintaining weight is the priority over a balanced diet. Research shows that well-nourished children can tolerate more treatment with fewer side effects, recover faster from treatment, and maintain weight better.

When the body becomes malnourished, body fat and muscle decrease. This leads to weakness, lack of energy, weight loss, a decreased ability to digest food, and a diminished ability to fight infection and recover from injury. These health issues often require a reduction in the dose of chemotherapy drugs.

To keep your child's body well-nourished, foods from all six basic food groups are needed. The groups are (1) meat and other proteins; (2) dairy products; (3) bread and cereal; (4) fruits; (5) vegetables; and (6) fats and sweets. Children on chemotherapy also benefit from a higher than average intake of fats, which add needed calories.

Examples of foods contained in each group are listed below, with a small child's serving size in parentheses beside each food. Consult a nutritionist to determine the serving size that is appropriate for your child.

Meat and other proteins (two or three servings per day)

Meat (1 ounce)	Eggs (1)
Fish (1 ounce)	Peanut butter (2 tbsp.)
Poultry (1 ounce)	Dried beans, cooked ($1/2$ cup)
Cheese (1 ounce)	Dried peas, cooked ($1/2$ cup)

These foods provide protein, which helps build and maintain body tissues, supply energy, and form enzymes, hormones, and antibodies. Some typical 1-ounce servings of meat and meat substitutes are: a meatball 1 inch in diameter, a 1-inch cube of meat, one slice of bologna, a 1-inch cube of cheese, or one slice of processed cheese.

Dairy products (two or three servings per day)

Milk ($^1/_2$ cup)	Tofu ($^1/_2$ cup)
Cheese (1 ounce)	Custard ($^1/_2$ cup)
Ice cream ($^1/_2$ cup)	Yogurt ($^1/_2$ cup)

Dairy products provide calcium, vitamin D, and protein. Steroids can weaken bones, so calcium and vitamin D (both necessary for bone growth and strength) are very important.

Breads and cereals (six to 11 servings per day)

Bread ($^1/_2$ slice)	Dry cereal ($^1/_2$ cup)
Oatmeal ($^1/_2$ cup)	Granola ($^1/_2$ cup)
Cream of wheat ($^1/_2$ cup)	Cooked pasta ($^1/_2$ cup)
Graham crackers (1 square)	Saltines (3 squares)
Rice ($^1/_2$ cup)	Potatoes (1 baked)

Breads and cereals supply vitamins, minerals, fiber, and carbohydrates. Try to use only products made with whole wheat flour and limited sugar to get more nutrients per serving. One sandwich made with two slices of bread provides four servings of this food group.

Fruits (two to four servings per day)

Fresh fruit (1 medium piece)	Dried fruits ($^1/_4$ cup)
Canned fruit ($^1/_4$ cup)	Fruit juice ($^1/_2$ cup)

Fruits provide vitamins, minerals, and fiber. Fruits can be camouflaged by puréeing them with ice cream or sherbet in the blender to make a tasty milkshake or smoothie, or by adding them to cookie and muffin recipes.

Vegetables (three to five servings per day)

Raw vegetables ($^1/_4$ cup)	Cooked vegetables ($^1/_4$ cup)

Vegetables, like fruit, are excellent sources of vitamins, minerals, and fiber. If your child does not want vegetables, they can be grated or puréed and added to soups or spaghetti sauce. If you own a juicer, add a vegetable to fruits being juiced. There are also many brownie, cake, bread, and muffin recipes that use vegetables that cannot be tasted, such as zucchini bread, brownies with spinach, carrot cake, and veggie muffins.

Fats and sweets (several servings per day)

Butter or oil	Nuts
Mayonnaise	Whipped cream
Peanut butter	Avocado
Meat fat (in gravy)	Olives
Ice cream	Chocolate

Although the food pyramid calls for fats to be used sparingly, higher consumption of fats is needed for children being treated for cancer. Experiment to find the fats your child enjoys eating and serve them frequently.

Making eating fun and nutritious

In some homes, mealtimes turn into battlegrounds, with worried parents resorting to threats or bribery to get their child to eat. Parents rarely win these battles—eventually they give in, exhausted and frustrated, and serve the sick child whatever she will eat (often to the dismay of the siblings who still have to eat their vegetables). The next several sections are full of methods used successfully by many parents to make mealtimes both fun and nutritious.

How to make eating more appealing

Many children are finicky eaters at the best of times. Cancer and its treatment can make eating especially difficult. Here are some general suggestions for making eating more appealing for your child:

- Give your child small portions throughout the day rather than three large meals. Feed your child whenever she is hungry.

- Remember that your child knows best which foods he can tolerate.

- Explain clearly to your child that eating a balanced diet will help her fight the cancer.

- Make mealtimes pleasant and leisurely.

- Rearrange eating schedules to serve the main meal at the time of day when your child feels best. If he wakes up feeling well most days, make a high-protein, high-calorie breakfast.

- Don't punish your child for not eating.

- Set a good example by eating a large variety of nutritious foods.

- Have nutritious snacks available at all times. Carry them in the car, to all appointments, and in backpacks for school.

- Serve fluids between meals, rather than with meals, to keep your child from feeling full after only a few bites of food.

- Limit the amount of less nutritious foods in the house. Potato chips, corn chips, soda, and sweets with large amounts of sugar may fill your child up with empty calories.

- If your child is interested, include her in making a grocery list, shopping for favorite foods, and food preparation.

Make mealtime fun

Here are some suggestions for making mealtime more fun:

- Try to take the emphasis off the need to eat food "because it's good for you." Focus instead on enjoying each other's company while sharing a meal. Encourage good conversation, tell stories and jokes, and perhaps light some candles.

- Make one night a week "restaurant night." Use a nice tablecloth and candles, allow the children to order from a menu, and pretend the family is out for a night on the town.

- Because any change in setting can encourage eating, consider having a picnic on the floor occasionally. Order pizza or other takeout, spread a tablecloth on the floor, and have an in-home picnic. One parent even sent lunch out to the treehouse.

> My son enjoyed eating in different places around the house and seemed to eat more when he was having fun. I sometimes fed the kids on their own picnic table outdoors in good weather, and at the same picnic table in the garage during the winter. They were thrilled to wear their coats and hats to eat. Occasionally I would let them eat off TV trays while watching a favorite program or tape.

- Some families have theme meals, such as Mexican, Hawaiian, or Chinese. They use decorations, wear costumes, and cook foods with exotic spices.

- Some children seem to eat better if food is attractively arranged on the plate or is decorated in humorous ways. Preschoolers enjoy putting a smiley face on a casserole using strips of cheese, nuts, or raisins. Sandwiches can be cut into funny shapes using knives or cookie cutters.

> My daughter liked to have food decorated. For example, we would make pancakes look like a clown face by using blueberries for eyes, a strawberry for a nose, orange slices for ears, etc. She also enjoyed eating brightly colored food, so we would add a drop of food coloring to applesauce, yogurt, or whatever appealed to her.

How to serve more protein

Because many children cannot tolerate eating meat while on chemotherapy, below are suggestions for increasing protein consumption:

- Add 1 cup of dried milk powder to a quart of whole milk, then blend and chill. Use this extra-strength milk for drinking and cooking.

- Use extra-strength milk (above), whole milk, evaporated milk, or cream instead of water to make hot cereal, cocoa, soup, gravy, custards, or puddings.

- Add powdered milk to casseroles, meat loaf, cream soups, custards, and puddings.

- Add chopped meat to scrambled eggs, soups, and vegetables.

- Add chopped, hard-boiled eggs to soups, salads, sauces, and casseroles.

- Add grated cheese to pizza, vegetables, salads, sauces, omelets, mashed potatoes, meat loaf, and casseroles.

- Serve bagels, English muffins, hamburgers, or hot dogs with a slice of cheese melted on top.

- Spread peanut butter on toast, crackers, and sandwiches. Dip fruit or raw vegetables into peanut butter for a quick snack.

- Spread peanut butter or cream cheese onto celery sticks or carrots.

- Serve nuts for snacks, and mix nuts into salads and soups.

- Serve yogurt and granola bars for extra protein. Top pie, Jell-O®, pudding, or fruit with ice cream or whipped cream.

- Use dried beans and peas to make soups, dips, and casseroles.

- Use tofu (bean curd) in stir-fried vegetable dishes.

- Add wheat germ to hamburgers, meat loaf, breads, muffins, pancakes, waffles, and vegetables, and use it as a topping for casseroles.

Ways to boost calories

Parents need to change their perceptions about what constitutes healthy food when they are struggling to feed a child who is on chemotherapy. Many parents have ingrained habits about serving only low-fat meals and snacks. While your child is on chemotherapy, it is necessary to reverse that focus. Your mission is to find ways to add as many calories as possible to your child's food. Here are some suggestions:

- Add butter or margarine to hot cereal, eggs, pasta, rice, cooked vegetables, mashed potatoes, and soups.

- Use melted butter as a dip for raw vegetables and cooked seafood such as shrimp, crab, and lobster.

- Use sour cream to top meats, baked potatoes, and soups.
- Use mayonnaise instead of salad dressing on salads, sandwiches, and hard-boiled eggs.
- Add mayonnaise or sour cream when making hamburgers or meat loaf.
- Use cream instead of milk over cereal, pudding, Jell-O®, and fruit.
- Make milkshakes, puddings, and custards with cream instead of milk.
- Serve your child whole milk (not 2 percent or skim milk).
- Sauté vegetables in butter.
- Serve bread hot so it will absorb more butter.
- Spread bagels, muffins, or crackers with cream cheese and jelly or honey.
- Make hot chocolate with cream and add marshmallows.
- Add granola to cookie, bread, and muffin batters. Sprinkle granola on ice cream, pudding, and yogurt.
- Serve meat and vegetables with sauces made with cream and pan drippings.
- Combine cooked vegetables with dried fruit.
- Add dried fruits to recipes for cookies, breads, and muffins.

Nutritious snacks

Try to always bring a bag of nutritious snacks whenever you leave home with your child. This allows you to feed her whenever she is hungry and avoid stopping for non-nutritious junk food. Examples of healthful snacks include:

- Apples or applesauce
- Baby foods
- Breakfast bars
- Burritos made from beans or meat
- Buttered popcorn
- Celery sticks filled with cheese or peanut butter
- Cookies made with wheat germ, oatmeal, granola, fruits, or nuts
- Cereal
- Cheese
- Chocolate milk
- Cottage cheese

- Crackers with cheese, peanut butter, or tuna salad
- Custards made with extra eggs and cream
- Dips made with cheese, avocado, butter, beans, or sour cream
- Dried fruit such as apples, raisins, apricots, or prunes
- Fresh fruit
- Granola mixed with dried fruit and nuts
- Hard-boiled and deviled eggs
- Ice cream made with real cream
- Juice made from 100 percent fruit
- Milkshakes made with whole milk or cream
- Fruit smoothies made with frozen fruit, sherbet, or ice cream
- Muffins
- Nuts
- Peanut butter on crackers or whole wheat bread
- Pizza
- Puddings
- Protein bars
- Sandwiches with real mayonnaise or butter
- Vegetables such as carrot sticks or broccoli florets
- Yogurt, regular or frozen

Vitamin supplements

The nutritional needs of kids with cancer are higher than other children's, yet kids on treatment often eat less food. Most children and teens with cancer are unable or unwilling to eat the variety of foods necessary for good health. In addition, damage to the digestive system from chemotherapy alters the body's ability to absorb the nutrients contained in the food your child does manage to eat. As a result, vitamin supplements are usually necessary.

Vitamin supplementation should only be done after consultation with your child's oncologist and nutritionist. Oversupplementation of some vitamins, folic acid for example, can make your child's chemotherapy less effective. But providing other vitamins can make the difference between a pale and listless child and one with bright eyes and a more positive attitude. Vitamin supplements should be individually tailored for your child in consultation with the oncologist and nutritionist.

Halfway through treatment, my daughter just looked awful. Her new hair began to thin out and break easily and her skin felt papery. I had been giving her a multivitamin and mineral tablet every day because her appetite was so poor, but it didn't seem to be enough. I talked to her doctor, then began to give her more of the antioxidant vitamins: betacarotene, E, and C. I bought the C in powder form, which effervesced when mixed with juice. She really liked her "bubble drinks." The betacarotene and E she swallowed along with the rest of her pills. Within a few weeks her hair stopped falling out, her skin stopped peeling, and she felt better.

• • • • •

I gave my teenage daughter supplements of vitamins and some minerals. I also increased her vitamin intake by using the juicer every day. She always drank a big glass of fruit or vegetable juice, and I really think it helped her do as well as she has.

What kids really eat

This chapter has listed ideas for increasing calories and making food more appealing. It also described the wild cravings kids get while taking chemotherapy, usually for foods that are spicy, fatty, salty, or all three. What follows are accounts of what several kids really ate while on chemotherapy. You'll notice how varied the list is, so experiment to see what your child finds palatable. Remember that children's tastes and aversions may change throughout treatment.

Judd craved chicken chow mein and fried rice takeout from a Chinese restaurant. He also loved Spaghetti-Os® and hot dogs.

• • • • •

I let Preston eat whatever tasted good to him, which was usually lots of potatoes and eggs. He liked spicy food (especially Mexican) while on prednisone.

• • • • •

Katy typically only ate one food for days or weeks at a stretch. One time, she ate pesto sauce (made from olive oil, garlic, Parmesan cheese, and basil leaves) on pasta for every meal for weeks. She also went through a spicy barbecue sauce phase, in which she wouldn't eat any food unless it was completely immersed in sauce. She ate no fruits, vegetables (except potatoes), or meat for the entire period of treatment. She ate mostly cereal and beans when she was feeling well, and mostly puréed baby food when she was really sick.

· · · · ·

In the beginning, when Meagan lost so much weight, we snuck Polycose® (a powdered nutritional supplement) into everything. She finally got stuck on cans of mixed nuts. They are high calorie and were instrumental in putting back on the weight. She also craved capers and would eat them by the tablespoonful.

· · · · ·

All Brent asks for are "peanut butter and jelly sandwiches, cut in fours, no crusts, with Fritos®." The only fruit he has eaten for 3 years is an occasional banana, and he eats no vegetables. He always ate everything before his diagnosis at age 6.

· · · · ·

The doctor told me to keep Kim on a low-salt, low-folic-acid diet. She wouldn't eat anything, so he eventually said he didn't care what she ate, as long as she ate. She liked Spaghetti-Os®, Chick-fil-A® nuggets, Chick-fil-A® soup, and McDonald's® sausage and pancakes.

· · · · ·

All Carl ate was dry cereal, dry waffles, oatmeal, and bacon. He ate no other meat or vegetables throughout treatment, but did drink milk. I thought that he would never be healthy, but he's 15 now (diagnosed when 2), eats little junk food, never gets sick, and looks great.

· · · · ·

While Shawn was on prednisone, I felt like I could never get out of the kitchen because he ate nonstop. The rest of the time he ate almost nothing. He survived on bagels, dry cereal, french fries, popcorn, and burritos.

· · · · ·

John (14 months old) craved creamed corn and pork and beans. I would just sit him on a potty chair at the table and let him eat, and it would go in one end and out the other. When on prednisone, he would sit at the table almost all day. He also drank a gallon of apple juice a day. He rarely eats meat to this day (2 years off treatment).

· · · · ·

On prednisone, Rachel ate only hot dogs, bologna, scrambled eggs with cheese, and potato chips. She would eat until she literally threw up. Now, 2 years off treatment, she is gradually expanding her repertoire. She only drinks milk (no water, juice, or soda), eats no sweets, and prefers all salty foods. I really have no idea whether it is learned behavior or a result of the cancer treatment.

Nutritionists and dietitians

It can be very helpful to consult with the hospital nutritionist to obtain more information and ideas about how to add more protein, calories, and vitamins/minerals to your child's diet. You can also consult with a private nutritionist who has experience with both children's nutritional needs and those of cancer patients. The American Dietetic Association (ADA) is the country's largest group representing registered nutrition professionals. It awards the Registered Dietitian credential to those who pass an exam after completing academic coursework and a supervised internship. You can consult the ADA's website at *www.eatright.org* for a list of dietitians near you.

> *I had two quite different experiences with hospital nutritionists. At the children's hospital, I couldn't get the doctors concerned about my daughter's dramatic weight loss. She was so weak she couldn't stand, and her muscles seemed to be wasting away. I finally asked them to please send in a nutritionist. A very young woman came in and talked to me about the major food groups. I felt my cheeks begin to flush, and my eyes glistened as I said, "I know what she is supposed to eat; I need to know how I can make her want to eat." I must have sounded a bit crazy, because she just handed me a booklet and backed out the door.*

> *The next week when my daughter began her radiation, the radiation nurse took one look at her and called the nutritionist right down. This nutritionist was very warm and caring. She helped me understand that I needed to think fat, protein, and calories, and she gave me lots of practical suggestions on how to boost calories. I think that she probably saved my daughter from tube feedings.*

Parent advice

Several parents whose children have completed therapy offer the following suggestions about how to handle the inevitable eating problems of children on therapy.

> *Doctors sometimes reassure parents by saying, "His appetite will return to normal." Don't be surprised if this does not happen until long after the most intensive parts of treatment are completed.*

· · · · ·

> *Let the child control what type of food and how much he wants. In the beginning, any food is good food.*

• • • • •

Buy a juicer and use it every day. This was the only way we got any fruits or vegetables into our daughter. Make apple juice and sneak in a carrot. Sometimes we would make the juice, then blend it in the blender with ice cubes to make an iced drink, which we would serve with a straw.

• • • • •

I solved my daughter's salt cravings by buying sea salt and letting her dip french fries in it once a week. For some reason, that satisfied her and stopped her from begging for regular table salt at every meal.

• • • • •

One magic word: butter, butter, butter. We would make Maddie peanut butter and jelly sandwiches with a layer of butter on each side of the bread first. Milkshakes are great and Häagen Dazs® ice cream has the highest fat content. We also went to an "eat when she's hungry" mode. It was definitely more relaxing.

• • • • •

When your child is on prednisone, don't try to restrict his food intake. It can be hard to watch these rotund little ones just shovel the food in, but once they get off the prednisone, they stop eating and quickly lose the weight. Then you have the opposite problem: how to get them to eat anything!

• • • • •

If you only keep good food in the house, and don't buy junk food, your child will eat more nutritious food.

• • • • •

Take good care of yourself by eating well. We are all under tremendous stress and need good nutrition. I gave my daughter healthy foods and glasses of juiced fresh fruits and vegetables while I was living on lattés (a coffee drink). I now have breast cancer and wish that I had eaten well during my daughter's treatment.

• • • • •

There is reason for hope. My daughter ate almost nothing while on treatment. After treatment ended, she ate more food, but still no variety. She didn't turn the corner until a year off treatment, but now she is gradually trying new foods, including fruits and vegetables again. I'm glad I never made an issue of it.

Commercial nutritional supplements

Many children cannot tolerate solid food or can only eat small amounts each day. Liquid supplements can help provide the necessary calories. The following is a sampling of the variety of supplements that can be purchased at pharmacies or grocery stores. If you are unable to locate a particular brand, your pharmacist may be able to order it for you:

- **Sustacal®.** Lactose-free liquid. Flavors are chocolate, vanilla, eggnog, and strawberry. It also comes in a high-protein or extra-fiber formula. (Mead Johnson)

- **Sustacal Pudding®.** Sustacal® in pudding form. Flavors are chocolate, vanilla, and butterscotch. (Mead Johnson)

- **Sustacal HC®.** Concentrated liquid. Flavors are vanilla, chocolate, strawberry, and eggnog. (Mead Johnson)

- **Ensure®.** Lactose-free liquid. Flavors are chocolate, vanilla, black walnut, coffee, butter pecan, banana, and strawberry. Other formulas have high protein or extra fiber. (Ross Laboratories)

- **Ensure Plus®.** Concentrated liquid. (Ross Laboratories)

- **Isocal®.** Lactose-free, vanilla-flavored liquid. (Mead Johnson)

- **Enrich®.** Lactose-free liquid with fiber. (Ross Laboratories)

- **Instant Breakfast®.** Powder that is added to milk. Variety of flavors. (Carnation)

- **Citrotein®.** Orange-flavored powder that is added to water or juice. (Doyle Pharmaceutical)

- **Polycose®.** Liquid or powder. Powder is added to milk, juice, gravy, or soups. Adds carbohydrates for extra calories. One tablespoon adds 30 calories. (Ross Laboratries)

- **Myoplex® Nutrition Shake.** A liquid that is added to water and a little ice and mixed in a blender. Flavors include orange, piña colada, banana cream pie, chocolate, strawberry, and vanilla. (EAS, Inc.)

- **Boost Kids Essential®.** High in calcium and formulated for kids ages 1 to 10. Flavors are chocolate, strawberry, and vanilla. (Nestle)

- **Nutren Junior®.** Vanilla-flavored liquid formulated for children ages 1 to 10 who need nutritional support. It comes with or without added fiber. It is 50 percent whey and 50 percent casein. (Nestle)

- **Kindercal®.** Lactose-free liquid in vanilla and chocolate flavors. Formulated for children. (Mead Johnson)

We tried all the high-calorie drinks: Pediasure® in three flavors, Boost®, and Scandi-shake®. The one that Emily would drink is called Nutrashake® (tastes like melted ice cream and can also be eaten frozen). Of course Pediasure® and Boost® are available over the counter. We had to get Scandi-shake® (a powder that you mix with milk) at the hospital. I had to do some research to obtain the Nutrashake®. It comes frozen, and Kroger grocery stores carry it. Since there were no Kroger stores near us, I finally found an outfit called American Medical Supply that would ship it.

· · · · · ·

The home health agency I worked for did a study on the nutritional content of Ensure®, Sustacal®, and Carnation Instant Breakfast®. All were basically the same, with Carnation® being much more palatable. The other two have a bit of a medicinal smell and taste to them. You can add calories by throwing it in a blender with ice cream, bananas, or strawberries. My other two non-cancer kids loved this stuff. Mandy would "sip" a tiny bit but would rather eat the spicy food: bologna, Polish sausage, or tomatoes drowning in Catalina dressing. Reese's® peanut butter cups were breakfast for a long time (7 grams of protein!).

Feeding by tube and IV

Sometimes, it becomes necessary to feed children intravenously or through a gastric (G-tube) or nasogastric (NG) tube. Although intravenous (IV) feeding and feeding by tube may require additional hospitalization, it helps if parents understand the benefits clearly. If a child with cancer becomes malnourished, events are set in motion that can have grim consequences. As appetite and weight decrease, the child's ability to tolerate and recover from treatment diminishes. The child becomes progressively weaker and his resistance to infection decreases. Infections and weakness may require interruptions in treatment. To prevent this scenario, most protocols require tube or IV feeding after 10 percent of body weight is lost. The two types of supplemental feeding are described below.

Total parenteral nutrition (TPN)

TPN, also known as hyperalimentation, is a form of IV feeding used to prevent or treat malnutrition in children who cannot eat enough to meet basic nutritional needs. Below are some of the many reasons why your child may require TPN:

• Severe mouth and throat sores that prevent swallowing

• Severe nausea and vomiting

• Severe diarrhea

• Inability to chew or swallow normally

• Loss of more than 10 percent of body weight

TPN ensures that your child receives all the protein, carbohydrates, fats, vitamins, and minerals she needs. TPN is administered through the central venous catheter, but children receiving TPN can also eat solids and drink fluids.

> My daughter needed TPN for 2 weeks after her stem cell transplant. They told us ahead of time that it would be necessary, and they were right. She got terrible sores throughout her GI tract and couldn't drink or eat. They just hooked the bag up to her Broviac®. After a couple of weeks, she started gingerly sipping small amounts of water and apple juice. For some reason, I just didn't worry about her eating. I assumed that when she could eat, she would. She was a robust eater before her illness, so I thought that would help. Before we left for home, she asked for a hospital pizza (yuck!) and ate a few bites. Her eating at home quickly went back to normal, although it took some time to regain the weight she lost.

In most cases, TPN is started in the hospital. Each day the concentrations of glucose, protein, and fat will be increased in a step-wise fashion, and doctors will assess your child's tolerance for the mixture. Generally, TPN is given 8 to 12 hours per day, depending on your child's unique situation. The infusion may be delivered over the hours that work best for your family. If your child attends school, overnight infusions will probably work best. If your child is at home during the day, infusions during these hours will give the entire family a better night's sleep.

Be sure to request a small portable infusion pump and backpack from your home care company so your child can go about his daily activities as usual. Your child's oncologist may need to write a letter to your insurance company to verify your child's malnutrition so this therapy will be covered.

Enteral nutrition

The doctor may recommend enteral feeding if your child requires supplemental nutrition and her bowel and intestines are still functioning well. Enteral feedings are preferred over IV, whenever possible. Enteral nutrition is feeding via a tube placed through the nose and into the stomach or small intestine (NG tube) or via a tube surgically placed directly into the stomach through the abdominal wall (G-tube). Nutritionally complete liquid formulas are fed through the tube. Your child's oncologist and nutritionist will determine the appropriate formula for your child. Infrequent side effects of enteral nutrition are irritated throat, nausea, diarrhea, or constipation.

> Rachel (age 14) used a backpack to carry a G-tube pump and her bag of Ensure® with her when she went out. When chemo was over, she worked for about a month with a psychiatrist who used hypnotherapy to get her to start eating normally again. After about 3 months, she was eating everything she used to. The tube was removed, and the hole closed on its own.

Alan (age 8) is currently finished with chemo and radiation therapy for medulloblastoma, but has weight issues. Alan has never been big on milkshakes since he started treatment. When he was in radiation his teeth were very sensitive to hot and cold. He does get Pediasure® through a G-tube, but we found a juice called Nestle NuBasic®, which is a 5 oz. can of calories and nutrition. The small size is great because it isn't overwhelming for Al to drink, and he has put on almost 4 pounds after 2 weeks. (He is drinking three cans a day in addition to the Pediasure® at night, but not eating much "real" food yet.)

Enteral feedings are usually started in the hospital. If your child's malnutrition is profound, he may initially require continuous feeding at a slow rate. These feedings will be increased as tolerated, with the eventual goal being four to six feedings per day. Blood tests can help the oncologist determine whether your child is malnourished in spite of the obvious weight gain that results from steroid therapy.

I feel good nutrition is very important to good health, but the reality of the situation with our child was that he hated anything nutritious when he was on chemotherapy. I could doctor it up, add the best toppings, make it look terrific, season it just right, and it would still be rejected. So I decided that since my son wasn't allowed to make any decisions in regard to the pills, treatments, tests, or hospital stays, he wouldn't be forced to eat everything nutritious if he didn't want to. Whether this was a right or wrong decision, I don't know. I just know that I served him a lot of processed foods during those years, and he's a healthy and happy boy 10 years later. After he was finished with chemotherapy, however, we did require that he eat healthier foods.

Chapter 21

Medical and Financial Record-keeping

*Prosperity is not without many fears
and distastes; and adversity is not
without comfort and hopes.*

— Francis Bacon

KEEPING TRACK OF voluminous paper work—both medical and financial—is a trial
for every parent of a child with cancer; but keeping accurate records prevents medical errors and reduces insurance overbillings. Checking results of tests allows parents
to identify changes in lab reports that might otherwise go unnoticed and untreated.
Having easy access to medical reports and properly organizing bills can also mean less
time spent in conflicts with insurance companies and collection agencies. This chapter
suggests a few basic systems for keeping both medical and financial records.

Keeping medical records

Think of yourself as someone with two sets of books, the hospital's and yours. If the
hospital loses your child's chart or misplaces lab results, you will still have a copy. If
your child's chart becomes a foot thick, you will still have your simple system that
makes it easy to spot trends and retrieve dosage information. The following are suggested items that you should record:

- Dates and results of all lab work

- Dates of all scans and type of scan (e.g., CT, MRI)

- Dates of chemotherapy, drugs given, and doses

- All changes in dosages of medicine

- Any side effects from drugs

- Any fevers or illnesses

- Dates of all scheduled and unscheduled hospitalizations

- Dates of all medical appointments and name(s) of the doctor(s) seen

- Dates for any procedures performed (both surgical and non-surgical)

- Dates of radiation therapy, including total dose delivered and areas treated

- Dates of diagnosis, completion of therapy, and recurrences (if any)

- Your child's sleeping patterns, appetite, and emotions

Keeping daily records of your child's health for months or years is hard work. But remember that your child will be seen by pediatricians, oncologists, neurosurgeons, neurologists, residents, radiation therapists, lab technicians, nutritionists, psychologists, social workers, and physical, occupational, and speech therapists. Your records will help keep it all straight and help pull all the information together. Your records will help you remember questions to ask, prevent mistakes, and notice trends. In short, your records will help the entire team provide your child with the best possible care.

The following sections describe several record-keeping methods parents have used successfully.

Journal

Keeping a notebook works extremely well for people who like to write. Parents make entries every day about all pertinent medical information and often include personal information such as their own feelings or memorable things their child said or did. Journals are easy to carry back and forth to the clinic, and journal entries can be written while waiting for appointments. Journals have the advantage of unlimited space; but one disadvantage is that they can be misplaced.

> *Stephan's oncologist is kind of hard to communicate with. I learned early on to keep a journal of Stephan's appointments, drugs given, side effects, and blood counts. That way if I ever had to call the doctor I would have it right in front of me. I also recorded Stephan's temperature when his counts were low to keep track of infections.*

In *You Don't Have To Die*, Geralyn Gaes writes of the value of keeping a journal:

> *Some days my entries consisted of only a few words: "Good day. No problems." Other times I had so many notes and questions to jot down that my handwriting spilled over into the next day's space. I must confess that I probably went overboard, documenting every minute detail of Jason's life down to what he ate for each meal. If he gets over this disease, I thought, maybe this information will be useful for cancer research.*

I'm not so sure I was wrong. Jason went 2 years without a blood transfusion, unusual for a child receiving such aggressive chemotherapy. Studying my journal, one of his physicians remarked, "This kid eats more oatmeal than anybody I've ever seen." Which was true. Jason wolfed it down for breakfast, after school, and before bedtime. The doctor speculated, "Maybe that's why Jason's blood is so rich in iron and builds back up so fast."

Many institutions give families a notebook that contains information about their child's cancer and treatment plan. Often, these notebooks have blank pages for recording blood counts.

Record-keeping—very important! My father came to the hospital soon after diagnosis and brought a three-ring binder and a three-hole punch. I would punch lab reports, protocols, consent forms, drug information sheets, etc., and keep them in my binder. A mother at the clinic showed me her weekly calendar book, and I adopted her idea for recording blood counts and medications. Frequently the clinic's records disagreed with mine as to medications and where we were on the protocol. I was very glad that I kept good records.

Calendar

Many parents report great success with the calendar system. They buy a new calendar each year and hang it in a convenient place, such as next to the telephone. You can record counts on the calendar while talking on the phone to the nurse or lab technician and take the calendar with you to all appointments.

Each year I purchase a new calendar with large spaces on it. I write all lab results, any symptoms or side effects, colds, fevers, and anything else that happens. I bring it with me to the clinic each visit, as it helps immensely when trying to relate some events or watch trends. I also use it like a mini-journal, recording our activities and quotes from Meagan. Now that she's off treatment, I'm superstitious enough to still bring it to our monthly checkups.

· · · · ·

I wrote the counts on a calendar or on little pieces of paper that got lost. But, to be honest, I didn't keep the medical records very well. I'm upset with myself when I think of it now.

· · · · ·

For a long time I was unorganized, which is very unlike the way I usually am. I found that my usual excellent memory just wasn't working well. It all seemed to run together, and I began to forget if I had given her all of her pills. Then I began using a calendar for both counts and medications. I wrote every med on the correct days, then checked them off as I gave them.

Blood count charts

Many hospitals supply folders containing photocopied sheets for record-keeping. Typically, they have spaces for the date, white blood cell count, absolute neutrophil count, hematocrit, platelet level, chemotherapy given, and side effects.

> *My record-keeping system was given to me by the hospital on the first day. We were given a notebook with information about the illness and treatment. Also included were charts that we could use to keep all the information about my child's blood work, progress, reactions to drugs, etc. While we were at the hospital we were able to get the information off one of the computers on our floor each afternoon. My notebook holds records and notes for 3 years. Perhaps I was being compulsive with my record-keeping, but it made me feel that I was part of the team working on bringing my boy back to health.*

Tape or digital recorder

For parents who keep track of more information than a calendar can hold, and who find writing in a journal too time consuming, using a voice recording device works well. Small machines are very inexpensive and can be carried in a pocket or purse. Digital devices can be downloaded to a flash drive or computer for storage. If you want to transcribe the recordings to a written record, there are programs such as Dragon Speak® that you can train to understand your voice, and that can be used to change your spoken word into a written document.

> *I started keeping a journal in the hospital, but I was just too upset and exhausted to write in it faithfully. A good friend who was a writer by profession told me to use a tape recorder. It was a great idea and saved a lot of time. I could say everything that had happened in just a few minutes every day. I kept a separate notebook just for blood counts so I could check them at a glance.*

Computer

For the computer literate, saving all medical records on the computer hard drive is a good option. Parents can print out bar graphs of the blood counts in relation to chemotherapy and quickly spot trends. You can also keep a running narrative of your thoughts, feelings, and concerns during your child's treatment. As with all other computer records, keep a backup copy on a flash drive or external hard drive.

At our hospital, the summary of counts for a given child can be formatted to print out as a "trend review," with each date printed out on the left side of the page and the various lab values in columns down the page. The system permits printouts from the very first blood draw if that is desired. Periodically, on slow days, I'll ask if I can have a trend review. Then I can discard the associated single printouts (much less paper that way).

Keeping financial records

You will not need a calendar or journal for financial records, just a big, well-organized file cabinet. It is essential to keep track of bills and payments. Dealing with financial records is a major headache for many parents, but keeping good records can prevent financial catastrophe. Financial record-keeping is most important in countries such as the United States, where most individuals are covered by private medical insurance. In countries with standardized healthcare, such as Canada, parents never receive a bill for their child's cancer treatment. The following are ideas about how to organize financial records:

- Set up a file cabinet just for medical records.

- Have hanging files for hospital bills, doctor bills, all other medical bills, insurance explanation of benefits (EOBs), prescription receipts, tax-deductible receipts (e.g., tolls, parking, motels, meals), and correspondence.

- Whenever you open an envelope related to your child's medical care, file the contents immediately. Don't leave it on the desk or throw it in a drawer.

- Keep a notebook with a running log of all tax-deductible medical expenses, including the service, charge, bill paid, date paid, and check number.

- Don't pay a bill unless you have checked over each item listed to make sure the charge is correct.

- Start new files every year.

> *To be honest, the paper trail really gets me down. I can only deal with the stacks every few months. I open things and make sure the insurance company is doing its part, and then I try to sort through and pay our part.*
>
> • • • • •
>
> *I started out organized, and I'm glad I did because the hospital billing was confusing and full of errors. I cleared out a file cabinet and put in folders for each type of bill and insurance papers. I filed each bill chronologically so I could always find the one I needed. I made copies of all letters sent to the insurance company and hospital billing department. I wrote on the back of each EOB any phone calls I had to make*

about that bill. I wrote down the date of the call, the person's name who I spoke to, and what she said. It saved me a lot of grief.

Deductible medical expenses

It is estimated that families of children with cancer spend 25 percent or more of their income on items not covered by insurance. Examples of these expenses are gas, car repairs, motels, food away from home, health insurance deductibles, prescriptions, and dental work. Many of these items can be deducted from federal income tax. Often parents are too fatigued to go through stacks of bills at the end of the year to calculate their deductions. If a monthly total is kept in a notebook, then all that needs to be done at tax time is to add up the monthly totals.

The Internal Revenue Service (IRS) generally allows you to deduct any reasonable cost for procedures or expenses that are deemed by a doctor to be medically necessary. You may also deduct certain ancillary expenses with proper documentation; some of the costs that are currently deductible include wheelchairs, wigs, acupuncture, psychotherapy and counseling, and HMO fees, special education or tutoring costs for sick children, meals at the hospital, parking at the hospital, and transportation and lodging costs while your child is in the hospital.

To find out what can be deducted legally for the years your child is undergoing treatment, get IRS Publication 502 for the relevant tax year. You can download this publication from the IRS website at *www.irs.gov* or make a copy from a hard-copy master at your local library. You can contact an IRS representative at (800) 829-1040, Monday through Friday.

Canadian families are able to deduct many of the same medical expenses as U.S. families. To find out what can be legally deducted in Canada, visit the Revenue Canada website at *www.cra-arc.gc.ca* and type in the search term "deductible medical expenses," or call (800) 959-8281.

If you keep a calendar, an easy way to keep track of tax-deductible items is to glue an envelope to the inside cover. Whenever you incur an expense that may be tax deductible, put the receipt in the envelope and file it when you get home.

Dealing with hospital billing

Unfortunately, problems with billing are common for parents of children with cancer. Here are two typical experiences:

Insurance was an absolute nightmare. It almost gave me a nervous breakdown. After all we go through with our children, to have to deal with the messed-up hospital billing was just too much.

We would stack the bills up and try to go through them every 2 or 3 months. Our insurance was supposed to pay 100 percent, but the billing was so confusing that they refused to cover some things because it wasn't clear what they were being billed for. The hospital frequently double billed, especially for prescriptions. We just stopped getting our prescriptions there.

We would call them to try to get the mess straightened out, but the billing department was just as confused as we were. They kept sending our account to collections. We did everything in our power to get it straight, but we never did.

• • • • •

We had two distinctly different experiences at the two institutions we dealt with. The university hospital where my daughter received her radiation gave me a folder the first day. It included, among other things, a sheet from a financial counselor giving all the information needed for preventing and solving billing problems. I never needed to call her because the hospital billing was clear, prompt, and organized.

The children's hospital where my daughter was a frequent inpatient and clinic patient was another story altogether. They billed from three different departments, put charges from the same visit on different bills, frequently over-billed, continuously made errors, and constantly threatened to send the account to collections. I never spoke to the same billing clerk twice. It was a never-ending grind and a constant frustration.

It is impossible to prevent billing errors, but it is necessary to deal with them. Here are step-by-step suggestions for solving billing problems:

• Keep all records filed in an organized fashion.

• Check every bill from the hospital to make sure there are no charges for treatments not given or errors such as double billing.

• Check to see if the hospital has financial counselors. If so, make contact early in your child's hospitalization. Counselors provide services in many areas, including help with understanding the hospital's billing system, billing insurance carriers, understanding explanations of benefits, managing hospital/insurance correspondence, dealing with Medicaid, working out a payment plan, designing a ledger system for tracking insurance claims, and resolving disputes.

• If you find a billing error, call the hospital immediately. Write down the date, the name of the person you talk to, and the plan of action.

I often couldn't even get through to the billing representative; I was just put on hold forever. Then I tried to discuss the problems with the director of billing, but she was never in. After about 20 phone calls, I finally said to her secretary, "You know, I have a desperately sick child here, and I have more important things to do than call your boss every day. I've been as patient and polite as I can. What else can I do?" She said, "Honey, get irate. It works every time." I told her to put me through to somebody, anybody, and I would. She connected me to the person who mediates disputes, I got irate, and we went through all the bills line by line.

- If the error is not corrected on your next bill, call and talk to the billing supervisor. Explain the steps you have already taken and how you would like the problem fixed.

  The hospital billing was so bad, and I had to call so often, that I developed a telephone relationship with the supervisor. I always tried to be upbeat, we laughed a lot, and it worked out. She stopped investigating every problem and would just delete the erroneous charge.

- If the problem is still not corrected, write a brief letter to the billing supervisor explaining the steps you have taken and requesting immediate action. Keep a copy of each letter that you write and all written responses.

- Every time you receive an EOB from your insurance company, compare it to the hospital bill. Track down discrepancies.

- If you are inundated with a constant stream of bills and there are major discrepancies between the hospital charges and what is being paid for by your insurance, ask both the hospital billing department and your insurance company, in writing, to audit the account. Insist on a line-by-line explanation for each charge.

  Within 5 months of my daughter's diagnosis, the billing was so messed up that I despaired of ever getting it straight. When the hospital threatened to send the account to a collection agency, I took action. I wrote letters to the hospital and the insurance company demanding an audit. When both audits arrived, they were $9,000 apart. I met with our insurance representative, and she called the hospital, and we had a three-way showdown. We straightened it out that time, but every bill that I received for the duration of treatment had one or more errors, always in the hospital's favor.

- If you are too tired or overwhelmed to deal with the bills, ask a family member or friend to help. That person could come every other week, open and file all bills and insurance papers, make phone calls, write all necessary letters, and even scan your records into your computer for storage.

- Don't let billing problems accumulate. Your account may end up at a collection agency, which can quickly become a nightmare.

Our insurance was constantly months behind in paying our bills to the Children's Hospital. The hospital sent our account to collections, despite my assurances that I was doing everything I could to get the insurance to pay. We were hounded on the phone constantly by the collection people, often until we were in tears. We finally just took out a second mortgage and paid off the hospital, but now I don't know if we will be reimbursed by insurance.

Not all stories are so grim. People who are in a socialized healthcare system, some managed care systems, or on public assistance never even see bills. Many people with insurance encounter no problems throughout their child's treatment.

Our insurance paid 80 percent of everything, no questions asked, and always paid us within a month. People shouldn't have to worry about finances or their insurance program at a difficult time like this.

· · · · ·

We have a low income, so we are on the state plan. They give us coupons for each child, and we just hand over a coupon at each visit. I have never seen a bill.

· · · · ·

Although hospital billing was not ever perfect anywhere we went, we did have an absolutely great relationship with our regional HMO for 4 years. Whenever an out-of-area appointment was needed, I called the pediatrician to start their paperwork, then immediately let our insurance nurse coordinators know. We also kept in touch through phone calls and cards. Michael and Gail were interested in our son and his progress, and we will never forget their support.

Coping with insurance

Finding one's way through the insurance maze can be a difficult task. However, understanding the benefits and claims procedures can help you get the bills paid without undue stress. The following sections outline some steps to help prevent problems with insurance.

Understand your policy

As soon as possible after diagnosis, read your entire insurance manual. Make a list of any questions you have about terms or benefits.

• Learn who the "participating providers" are under the plan and what happens if you see a non-participating provider. It is possible you will be penalized financially or that your claims may be denied if you go outside the network.

- Determine whether your physician needs to document specific requirements to obtain coverage for expensive or extended services.

  With our insurance, neuropsychological tests, outpatient occupational therapy, speech therapy, and physical therapy are covered, but the phrasing must be that it is a "medical necessity" due to diagnosis and treatments.

- Find out what your insurance co-pays are for different levels of service (e.g., office visit, outpatient surgery, outpatient testing).

- Find out what your outpatient prescription drug benefits are for generic and non-generic drugs.

- Find out what your deductible is.

- Find out if there is a point at which coverage increases to 100 percent.

- Determine if there is a lifetime limit on benefits.

- Find out when a second opinion is required.

- Learn when you have to precertify a hospitalization or specialty consultation. Many insurance companies require precertification, even for emergencies.

  I had called the insurance carrier to see if they could tell me if they'd sent a precertification for our out-of-town follow-up visits on Monday, but it was Friday afternoon, and they had closed early, so I left a voice message. About 5:30, I got a call from someone from the insurance company who'd said she was the person who reviewed precertifications, and that she thought she remembered doing one for my daughter, but she wasn't sure. She said that since I had obviously made an effort to get the certification, she would give me an authorization number when I called on Monday. Then she asked some very nice questions about Mary Margaret, expressed shock and sympathy, realized we would still be out of town for doctor visits on Monday, and told me not to worry about it, that I could call on Tuesday to get the number. Then she told me she's the CEO of the company and anything they could do to help, they'd be glad to! Completely shocking. Somebody from an insurance company who is helpful and pleasant!

- Get a copy of every form you may need to submit—claim forms for inpatient care, outpatient care, or prescriptions. If your insurance provider allows it, you can cut down on paperwork by filling in all the subscriber information on one of each type of form (except date and signature) and making many copies. Then you will have a form ready to send in with each bill.

- Determine whether your policy has benefits for counseling. If so, find out how many visits are covered, the payment structure, and the level of training required.

- Find out the names of approved providers for home infusion supplies (e.g., IV medications, central venous catheter supplies, and home nutrition) and home nursing care. These are often separate companies. Determine policy coverage for these services.

> We changed to a new pediatrician, and he asked me if I thought it would be easier on my son to have visiting nurses come to our home to do the chemotherapy injections and some blood work. Since he had very low counts, it made a lot of sense not to have to go out. It also lessened his fears to be able to stay at home and have the same nurse come to do the procedures. It was a pleasant surprise to find these services covered by our insurance.

Find a contact person

As soon as possible after diagnosis, call your insurance company and ask who will be handling your claims. Explain that there will be years of bills with frequent hospitalizations, and it would be helpful to deal with the same person each time. Some insurance companies may assign your child's account to a case manager, who will review your child's plan of care in detail and make suggestions designed to make proper use of your policy benefits. Ask the case manager for answers to any questions you have about benefits. Try to develop a cooperative relationship with your case manager, because she can really make your life easier. Also, your employer may have a benefits person who can operate as a liaison with the insurer.

> My employee benefits representative was Bobbi. She was just wonderful. The hospital would send her copies of the bills at the same time they sent mine. Since I found so many errors, she would hold the bills a week until I called to tell her that they were correct before she paid them. She was very pleasant to deal with.

Negotiate

Don't be afraid to negotiate with the insurance company over benefits. Often, your case manager may be able to redefine a service your child needs to allow it to be covered.

> I did have to fight to get my HMO to cover Michael at an out-of-plan pediatric brain tumor center for surgery. I wrote a long letter, sent lots and lots of backup documentation, got help and support from the Cancer Advocacy Group, and in the end, my local, fantastic hometown neurologist called the director of the HMO, pushed hard on them and helped me out, but we got approval and Michael's medical costs were covered fully in plan for all services.

Challenging a claim

The key to obtaining the maximum benefit from your insurance policy is to keep accurate records and challenge any denied claims, sometimes more than once. Some tips for good record-keeping follow:

- Make photocopies of everything you send to your insurance company, including claims, letters, and bills.

- Pay bills by check or credit card, and keep all your canceled checks and/or credit card monthly summaries of charges.

- Keep all correspondence you receive from billing companies and insurance.

- Write down the date, name of person contacted, and content of all phone calls concerning insurance.

- Keep accurate records of all medical expenses and claims submitted.

Policy holders have the right to appeal a claim denied by their insurance company. The following are suggested steps to contest a claim:

- Keep original documents in your files and send photocopies to the insurance company with a letter outlining why the claim should be covered. Make sure to request the reply in writing and keep a copy of the letter for your records.

> We were making inquiries into hospice care, feeling it was time to explore that option. I found out that the only pediatric hospice provider in the state of Georgia was not on the preferred provider list. Our insurance company would pay for benefits, but at a reduced rate; not a good thing since the lifetime maximum for hospice care was $7,500. With these benefits, we would get 78 days of hospice care. I felt like my only options were reduced pediatric care or full benefits using adult services. I wrote a letter of appeal stating that medically and ethically, neither of these were good choices. Well, we got a better outcome than I asked for. Not only will they cover the pediatric provider, but they have waived the lifetime maximum!

- Contact your elected representative to the U.S. Congress. All Senators and members of the House of Representatives have staff members who help constituents with problems. You can also contact your state insurance board with concerns and complaints.

> When I ran into insurance company problems, I wrote a letter to the insurance company detailing the facts, the decisions the insurance company made, and a logical explanation about why the procedure needed to happen. I also noted on the letter that a copy was going to our state insurance commissioner, and I sent both letters by certified mail. Within 2 days, the insurance company all of a sudden decided to cover the procedure. I later found out that the insurance commissioner's office started an investigation against them. Letters help, especially when sent by certified mail.

- If none of the above steps resolves the dispute, take your claim to small claims court (which does not require you to hire an attorney), find an attorney who will represent you for free (called pro bono), or hire an attorney skilled in insurance matters to sue the insurance company.

It may not feel comfortable being so persistent, but sometimes it is necessary to ensure you get the support you and your child are entitled to.

> When I finally got an advocate assigned for my child within our insurance company, I fretted to her one day that every single claim was initially rejected. She replied that the agents were trained to reject all claims the first two times they were submitted as a cost-saving strategy. She said, "Very few subscribers are tenacious enough to come back three times, so we save millions of dollars each year just because they give up."

Sources of financial assistance

Sources of financial assistance vary from state to state and town to town. To begin tracking down possible sources, ask the hospital social worker for assistance. In addition, some hospitals have community outreach nurses or case workers who may point out potential sources of assistance.

Hospital policy

If you are unable to pay your hospital bills, don't sell your house or let your account go to collections. Ask the hospital social worker to set up an appointment for you with the appropriate person to discuss the hospital policy for financial assistance. Many hospitals write off a percentage of the cost of care if the patient is uninsured or underinsured. Be proactive and talk to the hospital about setting up a monthly payment plan.

> We flew to a pediatric neuro-oncology center this time around (it was Michael's second craniotomy) and they did the surgery and the resection went great. It wasn't as expensive an undertaking as you would think. We used the Corporate Angel Network to get plane tickets. No free flight they had would work for us, but we got the cheapest rate available. The hospital provided us with the flight company information and also a list of hotels in the area that provided rooms at a reduced medical rate. We stayed at a hotel for $69 a night (there were cheaper ones) and this place included free van service to take us to the clinics, the hospital, the local mall, and restaurants. While Michael was in the hospital, we ate in the cafeteria with our parent discount. Altogether, our costs were under $2,000 (there were three of us and we stayed in the area 7 days). Michael checked into the hospital the day before surgery to be started on steroids, had surgery first thing the next morning, left the hospital 3 days later, hung out at the hotel until our follow-up visit 2 days after that (at the follow-up, stitches were removed and we were cleared to head home). It was probably the best $2,000 I will spend this year. We kicked tumor butt!

Supplemental Security Income (SSI)

SSI is an entitlement program of the U.S. Government that is based on family income and administered by the Social Security Administration. Recipients must be blind or disabled and have a low family income and few assets. Children with cancer qualify as disabled for this program, making some of them eligible for monthly aid if the family income and assets are low enough. To find out whether your child qualifies for SSI, contact your nearest field office.

In addition, if you need legal help appealing a denial for SSI, there is a professional organization of attorneys and paralegals called the National Organization for Social Security Claimants' Representatives (NOSSCR). NOSSCR can refer you to a member in your geographic location. You can contact NOSSCR by phone at (800) 431-2804, or online at *www.nosscr.org*.

Medicaid

Medicaid is administered by state governments in the United States, with the federal government providing a portion of the entitlement. Rules about eligibility vary, but families with private insurance sometimes are eligible if huge hospital bills are only partially covered. Call your local or county social service department to obtain the number for the Medicaid office in your area. If they tell you your child is ineligible, ask if the state has an "Aged, Blind, Disabled, Medically Needy" program.

Medicaid sometimes also pays transportation and prescription costs. Some states cover children under the age of 21 if they are hospitalized for more than 30 days, regardless of parental income. States are supposed to have Children's Medical Services programs to pay for medical treatment of physically disabled children; these programs allow a higher income level than Medicaid. Ask for a detailed list of benefits available in your state.

Free medicine programs

Children with cancer often need expensive medications, and they sometimes cannot afford them. Most major U.S. drug companies have patient-assistance programs, and you can apply to obtain free or low-cost prescription drugs. Although each company has its own criteria for qualification, in general, you must:

- Be a U.S. citizen or legal resident
- Have a prescription for the medication you are applying to get
- Have no prescription drug coverage for the medication
- Meet income requirements

You may qualify even if you have health insurance, if it does not cover the medication prescribed to your child. For expensive medications, the income cut-off is high, so it is worth investigating whether or not you qualify. Several organizations that can help you find and apply to patient-assistance programs are listed in Appendix B, *Resource Organizations*. Because the application process takes time and includes obtaining information from your child's doctor(s), plan ahead so you do not run out of medication.

> *Our insurance does not cover the growth hormone that my daughter needs. Her physician cannot believe that our insurance company denied coverage for a survivor with a history of radiation to the brain and multiple late effects to the endocrine system, but that's our situation. The medication is incredibly expensive. We applied to a patient-assistance program and were thrilled to find out that we qualified if our adjusted gross income was less than $100,000 a year. The application process the first year was hard and took a few months, but now we just fill in a form and send in our tax return every year, and she is requalified. We get a shipment of growth hormone every 3 months and keep it in the fridge.*

Although the cost of in-hospital treatment in Canada is covered by provincial governments, families have to pay for other medications at their own expense. For those without private insurance, this usually creates an extreme financial hardship. In many instances, the Department of Social Services can help pay for medications. The qualifications vary in each province and the decision is based on financial need. Canadian parents should contact their provincial Department of Social Services for further information.

State-sponsored supplemental insurance

Most states have supplemental insurance programs for families with children who are living with chronic conditions. These programs often help cover services, prescriptions, and co-payments that your primary insurance will not. You can get more information about the specific programs in your state from your medical team or hospital social worker, or by calling your state's department that regulates insurance (e.g., State Insurance Commission).

> *In Michigan, besides my husband's insurance, we also have what is called Children's Special Health Care Services (CSHCS). It is a secondary insurance that pays for what our primary insurance doesn't: Jake's co-pays and prescriptions, trips back and forth to the hospital, doctor appointment and prescription co-pays for my husband and me, our stay at the Ronald McDonald House. Any expenses related to treatment that our primary insurance won't cover, this will. The amount you pay for this coverage is based on family income. It has been a lifesaver for us.*

Service organizations

Numerous service organizations help families in need, providing aid such as transportation, wigs, special wheelchairs, and food. Often, all a family has to do is describe its plight, and good Samaritans appear. Some organizations that may exist in your community are: American Legion; Elks Club; fraternal organizations such as the Masons, Jaycees, Kiwanis Club, Knights of Columbus, Lions, and Rotary; United Way; Veterans of Foreign Wars; and religious groups of all denominations. In addition, local philanthropic organizations exist in many communities. To locate them, call your local health department, ask to speak with a social worker, and ask for help.

Organized fund raising

Many communities rally around a child with cancer by organizing a fundraiser. Help is given in various ways, ranging from donation jars in local stores to an organized drive using all the local media. There are many pitfalls to avoid in fund raising, and great care must be exercised to protect the sick child's privacy to the fullest extent possible. Because there have been some unfortunate scams in which generous people were bilked out of contributions for sick children who did not exist, if you decide to try fundraising, it is best to obtain legal assistance and to establish a trust fund for the express purpose of paying the child's medical expenses.

If your child is on or seeking Social Security or Medicaid eligibility, funds must be held in a special needs trust and paid directly to providers. If the family receives the money, or the child's social security number is used to open the bank account, the child can lose funding from both Social Security and Medicaid.

Miscellaneous insurance issues

Loss of insurance coverage is every parent's worst nightmare. If you lose your job, change jobs, or move while your child is on treatment, speak to your employer's benefits manager promptly. You can continue insurance coverage with your previous employer through the Consolidated Omnibus Budget Reconciliation Act (COBRA) plan until you are certain your new insurance coverage is in effect or you can look for coverage under the Affordable Care Act (ACA). Although using COBRA may impose some financial strain on your family for several months, it will ensure your child's coverage without interruption.

We just switched to an ACA plan from COBRA, as did a friend of mine with cancer. I am saving $300 per month and she is saving $400. ACA covers preexisting conditions, and you can get a special tax credit that is not available with COBRA if your income level is within certain limits.

Speak to your employer about whether participation in a Section 125 Plan (sometimes called a cafeteria plan, flexible spending account, or health savings account) is an option at your place of employment. These plans generally allow you to have your employer withhold pre-tax dollars from your pay for expenses such as childcare costs and non-reimbursed medical expenses. However, you often need to fill out reimbursement forms and submit them by year's end, or the money is lost.

We had excellent insurance coverage, so we never experienced any major financial difficulties during my son's treatment. However, insurance company literature can be so complicated that I felt I almost needed an advanced degree in rocket science to decipher our coverage. Our hospital has a financial counselor available for families that need help. Given the enormous stress that parents are under, I think it's an invaluable service.

Chapter 22

End of Treatment and Beyond

The best formula for longevity:
Have a chronic disease, and cure it.

— Oliver Wendell Holmes

THE LAST DAY OF TREATMENT is a time for both celebration and fear. Most families are thrilled that the days of pills and procedures have ended, but some fear a future without treatments to keep the disease away. Concerns about relapse are an almost universal parental response at the end of treatment; but for many families, the months and years roll by without recurrence of the tumor.

However, most children and teens have lingering or permanent effects from treatment for a brain or spinal cord tumor. This chapter covers the emotional and physical aspects of ending treatment, the need for excellent medical follow-up, and employment and health insurance issues.

Emotional issues

Treatment for a brain or spinal cord tumor can span just a few weeks (for slow-growing tumors completely removed with surgery) to months or years. Regardless of the type of tumor, all children eventually reach a point in the treatment process when they move to an observation mode with no immediate plan for surgery, radiation, or chemotherapy. This period of observation may include treatments such as physical, occupational, or speech therapy, medical treatment of seizures or hormonal imbalances, and follow-up scans. It may last for months or go on indefinitely. It is during this inactive period that the family tries to return to normal life.

Parents should anticipate that, after many months or years spent watching their child go through the rigors of active treatment, they may have lost the feeling of a normal life. They may experience relapse scares and may frequently need to call the doctor to describe the symptoms and be reassured.

Sam received focal radiation to the tumor bed following surgery as a toddler for an ependymoma. When the radiation treatments were over, it was weird. Suddenly, Sam was no longer under treatment and we didn't have any reason to go to the hospital. No reason to see any doctors or nurses. I had thought that I would be thrilled, and I mostly was, but I was also scared to be on our own. I was filled with thoughts of "what if." What if he gets a fever? What if he has a headache? What if he vomits? I really missed the security of seeing a nurse every day.

Sam had his first follow-up MRI and lumbar puncture (LP) a week and a half after finishing radiation. They looked good—no signs of cancer! He was done with treatment and cancer-free! All we had to do now was go back to living normally, if that were ever possible, and come back in 2 months for his next MRI and spinal tap.

One of the ongoing issues that I still have as a parent is judging what to do in a medical situation. For a long time, I called our pediatrician for every fever or cough. Thankfully, Sam hasn't had many stomach viruses with vomiting. It's hard to go back to being normal about their health. On the one hand, I don't want to panic and make too big a deal out of anything; but on the other hand, what if it's a sign of something serious? I don't want to under-react either.

Today Sam is cancer-free and a healthy, normal 5-year-old kindergarten student. Sam having cancer is the hardest thing our family has had to deal with. I think the best way to describe it is it's like being on a roller coaster of good news/bad news. The highs and lows were more dramatic in the beginning. Even today, each MRI/LP follow-up puts us back on the ride.

With diagnosis came the awareness that life can be cruel and unpredictable. Many parents feel safe during treatment and feel that therapy is keeping the tumor from growing. The end of treatment leaves many parents and children feeling exposed and vulnerable. When treatment ends, parents must find a way to live with uncertainty—to find a balance between hope and reasonable worry.

I had a lot of anticipatory worry—it started about 6 months before ending treatment. By the last day of treatment I had been worrying for months, so it was just a relief to quit.

· · · · ·

We were thrilled when treatment ended. I knew many people who felt that celebrating would jinx them; they just didn't feel safe. Well, I felt that we had won a big battle—getting through treatment—and we were going to celebrate that. If, heaven forbid, in the future we had another battle to fight, we'd deal with it. But on the last day of treatment, we were delighted.

Last day of treatment

The last day of treatment usually includes a physical examination, blood work, an MRI scan, and a discussion with the neuro-oncologist. The doctor should review the treatment that was given, outline the schedule for MRI scans and blood tests for the future, and sensitively discuss the potential for long-term side effects. One group of parents presented the following suggestions for the last day of treatment to doctors at a major children's hospital:

• Schedule enough time to have a conversation

• Bring a sense of closure to the active phase of treatment

• Express happiness that all has gone well

• Be realistic but hopeful about the future

• Praise the child for handling a very difficult time in her life with grace (or courage, or whatever word is appropriate)

• Praise the parents for all of their hard work

• Allow time for the parents to give the doctor feedback and thanks

• Give a certificate of accomplishment to the child

• Be aware that families are relieved but fearful of the future

> The nurses at our clinic really made a big deal on the last day of treatment. They brought out a cake and balloons, and sang "Going off Chemo" to the tune of "Happy Birthday to You." They made Gina a banner and bought her a present. I sat in a corner and cried, because I was scared to death of the future. A nurse came over, hugged me, and said, "This must be so hard; we're taking away your security blanket." She was exactly right.

Catheter removal

Children and teens usually cannot wait to have the catheter removed, as it symbolizes that treatment has truly ended. Venous catheters are usually removed soon after treatment ends.

Removal of an external catheter is usually an outpatient procedure. The child is given a mild sedative, then the oncologist gently pulls the catheter out of the child's body by hand.

> Kristin's Broviac® removal wasn't too bad. They gave her fentanyl ahead of time, so she was fairly relaxed. I wish they had offered me a sedative as well! One of the

nurses had her hand on Kristin's shoulder and quietly talked to her to try to keep her focused elsewhere. I held her legs, and my wife held her hand. The doctor put one hand on her chest, and pulled on the tubing with the other. It only took about 2 seconds to come out. There was little blood; they just put a Band-Aid® on the site and sent us home.

Implanted catheters such as the PORT-A-CATH® are removed surgically in the operating room. Children are usually given general anesthesia, and the operation usually takes less than half an hour. Only one incision is made, generally just above the port at the same place as the scar from the implantation surgery. The sutures holding the port to the underlying muscle are cut, and the port with tubing is pulled out. The small incision is then stitched and bandaged. When the child begins to awaken, he is brought out to the parent(s). The family then waits until the surgeon approves their departure. Often, the wait is short, because as soon as the child is awake enough to take a small drink or eat a Popsicle®, he is released. However, if your child becomes nauseated from the anesthesia, the wait can be several hours; he won't be released until he is feeling better.

Brent had a very easy time with his port-removal surgery. We scheduled him to be the first patient early in the morning, so there was no delay getting in. Then the anesthesiologist asked him what flavor of gas he wanted, which he liked. They brought him out to us while he was still groggy, and he woke up feeling goofy and happy. We went home soon thereafter. It felt more like the ending than on the last day of treatment.

• • • • •

Our docs said that Will's port could come out after the next MRI, which was just after treatment ended. It was a short procedure under general anesthesia, and he actually woke up without thrashing or crying this time. He was so happy to have it gone. He was just barely 5. We talked a little before about the "button" and the tubing coming out, just so he understood it wasn't part of his body that was being taken out.

Ceremonies

Some families enjoy having ceremonies to celebrate the end of cancer treatment. For younger children who have spent much of their lives taking pills and having procedures, ceremonies really help them grasp that treatment is truly over. Here are ideas from many families about how to commemorate this important occasion:

• Take "last day of treatment" pictures of the hospital and staff

• Take a picture of your child taking her last pill

- Give trophies to your child and siblings
- Ask the clinic to present your child with a certificate
- Go on a trip or vacation to celebrate
- Throw a big party for friends and family

> *Erica ended treatment in December, and we threw a big party at the church. We called it a "Celebration of Life." We invited all of the families that we had become so close to through the support group. We especially wanted the families who had lost their children to cancer, and they all came. My normally even-tempered husband gave a talk about Club Goodtimes (the support group) and how it was a club that no one ever wanted to join. When he talked about the many wonderful people we met there, his voice shook with emotion. Then the preacher prayed for the children who weren't with us. We ate a huge cake, and the children were entertained by a clown. It was both moving and fun.*

- Throw a big party at school

> *When Joseph finished treatment he was in kindergarten. The kids had gone through almost an entire year with him. They had known all about his treatments and frequent hospitalizations and had talked as a group about it when we made a presentation to the class, and at other times as well. It seemed appropriate to have an "all done with treatment" celebration. We even had his two best friends who go to different schools come over to join us; and his big brother, Nate, came down from his class to share in the fun.*
>
> *It was a very joyous occasion, and we made it as much like a birthday party as we could. I made cupcakes and juice and we played games. A friend who leads the story hour at our children's bookstore came and did some songs and stories with the kids; and I even sent each classmate home with a treat bag. At the end, right before time to go home, Joseph pulled out several cans of his favorite hospital discovery, and the kids took turns blasting a shower of Silly String® on everyone else! We all clapped and cheered, and Joseph's wonderful teacher and I had a chance to have a good celebratory cry while the kids put on their things to go home. Clean-up wasn't too darn bad, and it meant a lot to all of us.*
>
> *There's still a tiny remnant of green Silly String® on one of the fluorescent light fixtures, and my big second-grader likes to go down and admire it when he visits his old kindergarten teacher.*

- If your child has been seeing a counselor, schedule a visit to talk about the accomplishment
- Have friends and family send congratulations cards

- If consistent with your beliefs, have a religious ceremony of thanksgiving

> *I preached the sermon at church after Kristin ended treatment. It was the first Sunday of Lent, and I related our experience to that. Other than that, we didn't celebrate, because it's still not over. We still have to be vigilant. Ending treatment was a big milestone, but it paled in comparison to having the line pulled. We all have so much more freedom: no more lines to flush, changing bandages, or wrapping up for baths and swimming.*

Some parents do not feel comfortable celebrating the end of treatment. One mother described her feelings this way:

> *Finishing treatment was very difficult. I thought that I would feel like celebrating and cheering—but all I felt was fear. Treatment was over, but cancer was still a part of our lives. I think we will always live with the fear of relapse. It has taken me some time to come to grips with that reality.*

As you have read so often in this book, every child, brother, sister, parent, and relative reacts differently to treatment—and to the end of treatment. The differences do not matter. What is important is that you feel free to express your feelings, whatever they may be. You may feel joyful, relieved, fearful, or terrified, but the end of treatment is emotionally charged for every member of the family.

What is normal?

After years of treatment, families grapple with the idea of returning to normal. Unfortunately, most parents no longer really know what "normal" is. Parents realize that returning to the carefree pre-tumor days is unrealistic, that life has changed. The constant interaction with medical personnel is ending, and a new phase is beginning in which routines do not revolve around caring for a sick child, giving medicines, and keeping clinic appointments. Although it is true that the blissful ignorance of the days prior to cancer are gone forever, a different life—one often enriched by friends and experiences from the cancer years—begins.

> *You can't tell from looking at James, who is 6 now, that he's had brain surgery and chemo. There are no obvious scars or deficits. When he starts to talk or tries to run, then you notice it. He's very friendly and verbal, but his speech is off for his age, his motor skills are slower, he tires easily, and he has partial seizures. He gets services at school, including speech and physical therapy, and we're working on a plan for next year to accommodate schoolwork because of seizures. We've been doing fun things all along, like trips to zoos, walking in the park, and swimming to increase his overall strength. People see us using his wagon to give him a rest when he needs it. Usually someone will look at us strange when they see a big kid using a wagon, and*

if the moment is right, I've been known to offer some insight. But when you're out having fun, you don't always want to have to explain.

• • • • •

Chemo is such a horrible thing for your child to endure, but at least you are actively fighting the beast; so when it ends you feel a bit like you're flying without a net. You get so used to this bizarre new "normal" of treatments and blood tests and doctor visits, and then suddenly you stop, but you don't get the old normal back.

I think it's probably best to approach the end of treatment as a chance to see your child get his healthy color and energy back, and an opportunity to create and explore a new "normal" for your family that is richer and more meaningful than the one you left behind. It's also really nice to finally have the chance to reconnect with your spouse (and other children) and heal all the relationships that have taken a beating during the stressful treatment period.

As for me, for perhaps a year after Joseph's treatment, I existed in a dazed mix of emotions and thoughts. I was fearful of relapse, thrilled that Joseph had survived the cancer and the treatment, concerned about what late effects lay around the corner, all tempered with a warm and thankful feeling that I knew I would never, EVER take my kids or my good life for granted anymore or sweat the small stuff the way I used to. There were days I felt like I didn't want to crawl out from under the bed, and other days I couldn't stop singing and being silly.

I think off treatment is a lot like on treatment—you just have to take it one day at a time.

"Normal" is a moving target—different for every person and family. No one can tell you what your normal will be. Normal is what keeps the family alive and planning and moving together to face their individual and collective futures.

For many people, helping others is a satisfying way to reach out or bring closure to the active phase of cancer treatment. Serving others can create something enormously meaningful out of personal challenges, which is why many parents and children like to give back to the cancer community in some way. Some examples of ways people have reached out include the following:

- I requested that the clinic and local pediatricians refer newly diagnosed families to me if the parents wanted someone to talk with. I remembered how impossible it was to go to meetings in the first few months, and how desperately I needed to talk to someone who had already traveled the same road.

- We started a Boy Scout project to keep the toy box full at the clinic.

- My children are counselors at the camp for kids with cancer.

- We organized a walk to raise funds for the Ronald McDonald House.

- We (a group of parents of children with cancer) requested and were granted a conference with the oncology staff to share our thoughts about ways to improve pain management and communication between parents and staff. It was very well received.

- We circulated a petition among parents to request increased hospital funding for psychosocial support staff. We presented it to the director of the hematology/oncology service.

- I give platelets and blood regularly.

- I took all of our leftover catheter line supplies to camp and gave them to a family who needed them.

The possibilities are endless. Parents and children can use whatever talents they have to help others—from designing head coverings to writing newsletters for families struggling with childhood cancer.

> I have administered several online support groups for parents of children with cancer over the past decade. Many of these groups have over 500 participants who live all over the world. Some of the members' children have been cancer free for years, some are newly diagnosed, and some are parents of children have died. These online communities are an important way to find comfort, support, and information. Parents who are far out from treatment remain involved in order to help those who are newly diagnosed. When my son was first diagnosed I was so reassured that people survive the ordeal. After treatment ended I wanted to be there to help others.

An equally healthy response to ending treatment is to put it behind you. Many families, after years of struggles, just want to move on. They don't want constant reminders of cancer and feel it's not good for children to be reminded of those hard times.

> I realized that it was time to put it behind us when I watched my two children playing house one day. There was only one adult and one child in the family. I asked what happened to the rest of the family and they both said, "Cancer; they died." I didn't want them to have any more cancer in their lives. They had had enough. I know people who worry all the time about the cancer returning, and it is not healthy for them or their children. I decided to get out of the cancer mode and back to being my usual upbeat self. I feel that we are finally back to normal, and it's a good place to be.

Parents and children need to talk with one another, examine their emotions, decide what course they want to chart, and work together toward creating a healthy life after cancer.

Follow-up care

Protocols for clinical trials require specific follow-up schedules. For instance, your child may require follow-up every 3 months for a period of time (usually 1–2 years), then every 4 to 6 months for a while, and then annually. Follow-up might include:

- Physical exams by primary treating doctor

- MRI scans

- Blood tests (complete blood count and hormonal tests)

- Audiograms

- Neuropsychological testing yearly or biyearly

If your child was not on a clinical trial, find out from the oncologist what the required schedule will be and where the appointments will take place. Make sure your child understands that, after treatment ends, doctor appointments, MRI scans, and blood draws will still be an occasional necessity. Follow-up care for possible late effects of treatment is a separate process.

> *Shawn is a year off treatment and I find myself letting go of the bad memories more and more. They are just fading away. What I am left with is awe, admiration, and amazement that my son handled all of the hardships of treatment and survived. He's very determined and strong-willed, and I'm so proud of him. When people say to me, "Oh, you were so strong to make it through that," I respond, "All I did was drive him to the appointments; he did the rest."*

> *This experience has really changed me and my entire family. My marriage is much better, my other sons are stronger and closer to us, and Shawn has shown us all how tough a little kid can be. We take each precious day, one at a time, and try to get the most out of it. I so appreciate life and my family.*

Possible late effects

At diagnosis, parents do not know the price their child will ultimately pay for reprieve from the brain or spinal cord tumor. Short-term effects may be discomfort, seizures, weakness in an arm and/or leg, and school absences. Long-term effects range from none to severe. These can include subtle or pronounced physical disabilities, learning disabilities, an impaired endocrine system, hearing loss, altered bone growth, infertility, and an increased risk of second cancers.

It is important to know the possible risks based on the treatment your child received. You can then store this knowledge in the back of your mind. As one mother said, "I hope for the best and I deal with the rest." For detailed information about possible late effects from childhood cancer, read *Childhood Cancer Survivors: A Practical Guide to the Future, 3rd edition,* by Nancy Keene, Wendy Hobbie, and Kathy Ruccione.

> *Our daughter was diagnosed with medulloblastoma when she was 10 months old. She had surgery and 2½ years of chemotherapy. She needed two second-look surgeries when MRIs showed a shadow. Both times they found only scar tissue, no tumor. She had minor delays in motor development that a short course of physical therapy resolved. Other than that, she has no late effects. She is a normal, happy, giggling 13-year-old girl She talks on the phone a lot and likes Backstreet Boys. She is just wonderful and we all feel blessed.*

Physical disabilities

Permanent weakness of an arm, leg, or entire side of a body can occur from the tumor itself or from swelling related to the treatment. Weakness of the muscles of the eyes and face or those involved in swallowing can also occur from the tumor and treatment. Physical, occupational, and speech therapy may be necessary for months or years. These services should be provided through the child's Individualized Education Program (IEP) at school (see Chapter 18, *School*). As the child gets older, an exercise program can be established with a physical therapist, occupational therapist, or personal trainer. Insurance companies are often reluctant to pay for long-term rehabilitation, so it is helpful for parents to request a case manager or advocate to help them obtain these services.

Educational issues

School entry and reentry for children who have spent months or years receiving treatment is difficult. Physical changes make it hard for some children who had brain or spinal cord tumors to socially fit in at school. To compound matters, side effects and late effects of the treatments used for brain or spinal cord tumors often include decline in academic functioning. A decrease in IQ is a side effect for children who received radiation treatments and sometimes for those who deal with seizures. Difficulty with memory or changes in attention span, verbal fluency, and speed of information processing can also affect children.

It is imperative that all children who received treatment for brain or spinal cord tumors receive neuropsychological testing to identify learning problems. The results of these tests can be incorporated into your child's IEP. A neuropsychologist can also use the results of these tests to help adult survivors identify strategies to cope with learning issues. For further information, refer to Chapter 18, *School*.

My son was treated for medulloblastoma when he was 5 years old, and had posterior fossa syndrome after surgery. He was paralyzed on the right side, and had to switch handedness as a result. Between that and the vincristine, he has seriously impaired fine motor skills, despite years of occupational therapy. His handwriting is illegible, he is a slow typist, and he even has trouble buttoning buttons. He has poor reading comprehension, but he is an excellent auditory learner, so he has everything read out loud to him and a scribe for tests in school. He has slowed information processing, which means that he really has trouble thinking quickly when presented with new information. He learns well when he has time to think things through, but standardized testing is a challenge for him. That said, he is a college freshman this year and with a lot of support, he is taking a full course load at a 4-year college.

Hormonal problems

Hormonal problems occur in children with pituitary and hypothalamic tumors and as a late effect of radiation to the brain. The following are types of hormonal problems that your child may develop:

- Growth hormone deficiency, resulting in short stature
- Deficiency in hormones required to develop normally in puberty
- Thyroid hormone deficiency

Long-term follow-up should include a visit to an endocrinologist with experience treating survivors of childhood cancer, who can screen for these late effects. Hormones (pills or injections) can be given to your child to help correct any deficiencies. It is essential that problems with growth and pubertal hormones be identified early, because treatment needs to begin when your child is young. Thyroid hormone replacement (a daily pill) can start at any time. If your child is fatigued or has decreased energy, make sure the doctor tests thyroid functioning.

Hearing loss

Decrease in hearing (with high-frequency hearing lost first) occurs most often in children treated with cisplatin. The hearing loss is sometimes worse if the child receives radiation therapy as well. Audiograms (hearing tests) are done at frequent intervals while the child is receiving cisplatin and should be part of the long-term follow-up upon completion of treatment. Children with hearing loss are often unable to filter out background noise. This presents a problem for children in the classroom, where background noise is common. Your child's audiologist may be able to recommend devices that will help your child. Hearing aids are sometimes needed for children with significant hearing loss.

We are lucky to have good insurance for hearing aids and have replaced them every 3 years with the best technology available. The aids Josh uses now are incredible— they operate independently and communicate with each other via WiFi. Each aid has four independent speakers that evaluate the surrounding environment and work together to modify amplification. Now also compatible with smartphones, the aids can serve as ear buds when Josh is enjoying his music or watching a video. This generation of hearing aids has made the FM system obsolete. Hearing is such an important part of development that I consider quality hearing aids to be a necessity, not a luxury. They were expensive ($6,000), but in my mind were worth every penny.

Survivorship

An essential aspect of survivorship is making healthy choices. Good health habits and regular medical care help protect survivors' health and lessen the likelihood of late effects from cancer treatment. A sizable number of adult cancers are linked to life-style choices. Eating a healthy diet, staying physically active, using sunscreen, avoiding excessive alcohol consumption, maintaining a healthy weight, and not smoking all help keep survivors healthy and cancer-free. To protect survivors from injury, it is also important to wear bike or motorcycle helmets, use seat belts, and call a cab if the person driving has had too much to drink. Survivors have little or no control over their genetic make-up or the environment in which they live. But making healthy choices about how to live the rest of their lives gives them control over some of their future.

Immunizations

If your child was diagnosed before she received all her immunizations, ask the neuro-oncologist when she should resume the regular schedule for immunizations. If your child had one or more peripheral stem cell transplants, then all immunizations may need to be repeated. Your child's neuro-oncologist will order blood tests to determine which immunizations need to be repeated.

My doctor said to wait a year before beginning to catch up on shots. It was nice for her to get a long break before any more pokes.

Risks of smoking

Teens need continuing counseling about problems associated with smoking cigarettes or engaging in other high-risk behaviors. The combination of effects from treatment and smoking increases the chance of heart disease; heart attack; congestive heart failure; stroke; cancer of the mouth, throat, and lungs; and death from sudden cardiac failure. An article about survivors and smoking in a youth newsletter ends with these words:

If you've had cancer and your friends haven't, they don't face the same risks from smoking that you do. You've fought hard for your life. Don't put it out in an ashtray.

Safe sex

Every teen and young adult who has survived cancer should be counseled about safe sexual practices. Despite the prevalence of sexual messages in our culture, most teens and young adults are woefully underinformed about the facts. Even though the administration of many chemotherapueutic drugs may cause infertility, many babies have been born to long-term survivors of brain and spinal cord tumors. Survivors should not assume that they are infertile.

In addition, sexually transmitted diseases are of concern for anyone engaging in sexual activity. All sorts of diseases, some potentially fatal (e.g., hepatitis C, HIV/AIDS) and some not (e.g., genital herpes, genital warts, gonorrhea), can be transmitted through sexual intercourse. One nurse practitioner at a large follow-up clinic stated:

> I tell every teenager who comes through the door, regardless of their medical background, that I think he or she is too young to have sex, and I explain why. But then I say, in the event that you do choose to become sexually active, you always need to use a condom, and not just any condom. I tell them to only use a latex condom with a spermicide, which is the most barrier-protective. I explain that no sex is the only guarantee to avoid the many diseases out there, but a latex condom with spermicide offers the next best protection. And I really stress that this should be done whoever the partner is, and for whatever type of sex. So many teenagers think that diseases only happen to other kinds of kids.

Treatment summaries

Once treatment and follow-up for recurrence of disease are completed, many children and young adults will no longer be cared for by pediatric neuro-oncologists who are familiar with their history. A transition back to their local doctor often occurs. Moreover, many primary care doctors—pediatricians, family practice doctors, internists, gynecologists—are not fully aware of all the different treatments used for the multitude of childhood cancers, or of the late effects they can cause.

Additionally, when treatment ends, patients and parents are not always given adequate information about the risks of developing late effects in the months, years, or decades after treatment ends. The risks of delayed effects are real, and it is imperative that survivors become informed advocates for their own health care. They need to be educated, in a supportive and responsible way, about the risk of future physical adversities; then if a problem does arise, it will be recognized early and receive prompt attention. Young adults who have survived childhood brain or spinal cord tumors need to be fully informed of their unique medical history and be able to share this information with all doctors who care for them in the future.

A few months before the end of treatment, ask the oncologist to fill out the treatment record, *Cancer Survivor's Treatment Record* at the back of this book. Make several copies of the completed form, because this health history will become an indispensable part of your child's medical records for the rest of her life. It should be kept in a safe place, and a copy should be given to each medical caregiver. When your child leaves home to begin her adult life, this treatment summary should go with her and a copy should be kept in a safe place.

If you do not have a copy of the health history booklet, write down the following important information, which should be in your child's treatment summary:

- Name of disease

- Date of diagnosis and relapse, if any

- Place(s) of treatment

- Dates of treatment

- Names of attending oncologist and primary nurse

- Name and number of clinical trial (if your child was treated on one)

- Names and total dosages of chemotherapeutic agents used

- Type and amount of radiation used and areas treated

- Name of radiation center

- Date(s) when radiation was received

- Dates and types of surgeries

- Date and type of stem cell transplant, if any

- Any major treatment complications

- Any persistent side effects of treatment

- Recommended medical follow-up for late effects

- Contact numbers for treating institutions

Because many survivors of brain and spinal cord tumors face complex medical, psychological, and social effects from their years of treatment, some institutions have established comprehensive follow-up clinics to provide a multidisciplinary team to monitor and support survivors. The nucleus of the team is usually a nursing coordinator, pediatric oncologist, pediatric nurse practitioner, social worker, and psychologist. The team also includes specialists such as endocrinologists and cardiologists.

Yearly appointments with follow-up programs usually include a review of treatments received, counseling about potential health risks (or lack thereof), and case-specific diagnostic tests (e.g., hormonal studies or testing for learning disabilities). Follow-up clinics not only provide comprehensive care for long-term survivors, they also participate in research projects that track the effectiveness of and side effects from various clinical trials. In addition, the follow-up clinics act as advocates for survivors with schools, insurance companies, and employers. If your institution does not provide comprehensive, long-term, follow-up care, you can find a list of survivor programs at *www.acor.org/ped-onc/treatment/surclinics.html*. Many survivors travel to comprehensive programs for their yearly follow-up visits.

Employment

The population of adults who have survived childhood cancer is growing at a rapid rate. It is estimated that there are 350,000 survivors of childhood cancer in the United States. Thousands of survivors are staying well, growing up, and successfully entering the workforce.

Despite their numbers, some survivors still face job discrimination. Under federal law and many state laws, an employer cannot treat a survivor differently from other employees because of a history of cancer. The Americans with Disabilities Act of 1990 (ADA) prohibits many types of job discrimination by employers, employment agencies, state and local governments, and labor unions. In addition, most states have laws that prohibit discrimination based on disabilities, although what these laws cover varies widely.

The ADA prohibits discrimination based on actual disability, perceived disability, or history of a disability. Any employer with 15 or more workers is covered by the ADA. The ADA requires the following:

- Employers cannot make medical inquiries of an applicant, unless the applicant has a visible disability (e.g., uses a wheelchair), or the applicant has voluntarily disclosed her cancer history. Such questions must be limited to asking the applicant to describe or demonstrate how she would perform essential job functions. Medical inquiries are allowed after a job offer has been made or during a pre-employment medical exam.

- Employers must provide reasonable accommodations unless it causes undue hardship.

- Employers may not discriminate because of family illness.

The U.S. Equal Employment Opportunity Commission (EEOC) enforces Title 1 (employment) for the ADA. Visit *www.eeoc.gov* or call (800) 669-4000 (voice) or (800) 669-6820 (TTY) for enforcement publications. Other sections are enforced or have their enforcement coordinated by the U.S. Department of Justice (Civil Rights Division, Public Access Section), which can be contacted online at *www.ada.gov* or by calling (800) 514-0301.

The Job Accommodation Network (JAN) is a service provided by the U.S. Department of Labor's Office of Disability Employment Policy (ODEP). The service supports the employment, including self-employment and small business ownership, of people with disabilities. JAN can be reached at *www.askjan.org* or by calling (800) 526-7234 (voice) or (877) 781-9403 (TTY).

In Canada, the Canadian Human Rights Act provides essentially the same rights as the ADA. The Act is administered by the Canadian Human Rights Commission. You can get more information by visiting the national office's website at *www.chrc-ccdp.ca*.

Health insurance

Job discrimination can spell economic catastrophe for cancer survivors because most health insurance is obtained through one's place of employment. As survivors mature, seek employment, and move away from home, many encounter barriers to obtaining health insurance, such as rejection of application based on cancer history, policy reductions, policy cancellation, preexisting condition exclusions, increased premiums, or extended waiting periods.

The Patient Protection and Affordable Care Act (ACA) of 2010 and its companion amendments allow access to healthcare for survivors, who in the past could often not get healthcare due to preexisting conditions. You can find up-to-date information about the law at *www.healthcare.gov*.

The ACA offers the following provisions that are relevant to childhood cancer survivors:

- Young adults are allowed to stay on their parents' insurance plan until they turn 26 years old, whether or not they are in college.

- Certain preventive services are covered, including services that are important aspects of survivorship care.

- If a survivor is unemployed or has a limited income— up to about $15,000 per year for a single person—he may be eligible for health coverage through Medicaid.

- If an employer doesn't provide health insurance, survivors can buy it through the Health Insurance Marketplace (sometimes called an "exchange"), which offers a choice of health plans. To learn about the options in your state, visit *https://www. healthcare.gov/what-is-the-health-insurance-marketplace*.

- You may get tax credits to help pay for insurance if your income is less than about $43,000 for a single individual and your job doesn't offer affordable coverage.

- Health plans can no longer limit or deny coverage to anyone with a pre-existing condition.

Following are some legal remedies for insurance discrimination.

- **COBRA.** The Comprehensive Omnibus Budget Reconciliation Act (COBRA) is a federal law that requires public and private companies employing more than 20 workers to provide continuation of group coverage to employees if they quit, are fired, or work reduced hours. Coverage must extend to surviving, divorced, or separated spouses, and to dependent children. You must pay for your continued coverage, but it must not exceed by more than 2 percent the rate set for the company's full-time employees. By being allowed to purchase continued coverage, you have time to seek other long-term coverage. The U.S. Department of Labor provides a COBRA fact sheet at *www.dol.gov/ ebsa/faqs/faq_consumer_cobra.html*.

- **ERISA.** The Employee Retirement and Income Security Act (ERISA) is a federal law that protects workers from being fired because of the cancer history of the employee or beneficiaries (spouse and children). ERISA also prohibits employers from encouraging a person with a cancer history to retire as a "disabled" employee. ERISA does not apply to job discrimination (denial of new job due to cancer history), discrimination that does not affect benefits, or to employees whose compensation does not include benefits.

- **Health Insurance Portability and Accountability Act of 1996 (HIPAA).** This law allows individuals to change employers without losing coverage, if they have been insured for at least 12 months. It prevents group health plans from denying coverage based on medical history, genetic information, or claims history, although insurers can still exclude those with specific diseases or conditions. It also increases portability if you change from a group to an individual plan. For additional information, a HIPAA fact sheet with frequently asked questions is available by visiting *www.dol.gov/ebsa/ faqs/faq_consumer_hipaa.html*.

Appendix B, *Resource Organizations*, lists organizations that can help if you or your child faces job discrimination or problems with insurance due to treatment for cancer.

Well, we finally did it. We took a deep breath, a heavy sigh, and we packed up the medical supplies. While this step may seem insignificant for some, those who have dealt with a chronic/life-threatening illness in their family know that the disposal of your arsenal of medical supplies is a symbolic rite of passage. It can only mean two

things: your loved one has passed on, or you simply don't need them anymore. We thank God every day that we ended up with the latter reason.

Katy's medical "tower" was stored in our hallway, and included various bins and drawers full of central line supplies, a mini IV pump, masks and gloves, hypodermics, and sharps containers. It was very conspicuous. You simply couldn't miss it if you walked through the house. It was our constant reminder that we had a sick child, and at times, for me, a crutch. I think I felt that as long as the tower was there and properly stocked and arranged, I was somehow in control of Katy's illness. I feared disposing of, or putting anything away, thinking that if I did, she would most assuredly relapse and I'd need it again. No, of course that's not rational, but rationality has never been one of my strong points.

However, as the months passed, the tower gathered its dust, and soon, I couldn't remember the last time we'd even used any of the supplies. A few more months passed, and I began to realize what an eyesore this bunch of junk was! So, after my husband brought some big boxes home from work, it was time. We did it together. Into the boxes went the tubing and syringes, the masks and dressing change kits for the kids' oncology camp. Into the garbage went all the expired meds, heparin, and saline. It was so liberating! I can't imagine why we kept that stuff around for so long. It felt like the end of an era. And in a way it was.

Chapter 23

Recurrence

Hold fast to dreams
For if dreams die
Life is a broken winged bird
That cannot fly.

— Langston Hughes

CHILDHOOD BRAIN AND SPINAL CORD TUMORS are different than other childhood cancers because periods of active treatment often alternate with observation in an attempt to "do no harm." Sometimes tumors never regrow. But if they do regrow, there are either new treatments to try or perhaps already-existing treatments that couldn't be given earlier (such as radiation, if the child is now older than age 3). The terms the doctor might use are *recurrence* (reappearance of a tumor that previously disappeared with treatment) or *progression* (an increase in the size of an existing tumor).

Parents frequently describe the recurrence or progression of their child's tumor as more devastating than the original diagnosis. They sometimes feel betrayed, guilty, and/or angry. They worry that if the previous treatments didn't work, what will? Mostly, they are afraid. And their often unspoken but most crushing fear is: What if my child dies?

If your child's tumor has returned or grown, it is worth remembering that you now have several strengths you didn't have before. You have already done this. You know the language, and you have a relationship with the medical team. You probably have friendships with other parents of children with brain or spinal cord tumors and you know they will be there for you. You can also hope that during the time your child's tumor was in remission researchers were able to develop newer and more effective treatments. You know that something that seems insurmountable can be endured, one day at a time.

This chapter describes signs and symptoms of recurrence or progression, what emotional responses you can expect, and how to set goals and decide on a treatment plan. In addition, several parents and patients share their stories about how they managed to cope.

Signs and symptoms

Recurrence or progression can happen at any time during treatment or after therapy is completed. Occasionally the child has no symptoms of tumor growth (or regrowth) but the MRI scan shows an increase in tumor size. More frequently, however, the signs and symptoms include many or all of the indicators that were present at diagnosis. For a brain tumor these include:

- Headaches (often with early morning vomiting)
- Fatigue
- Dizziness
- Seizures (convulsions)
- Staring spells
- Visual changes: loss of peripheral vision, double vision, jiggling of an eyeball, inability to look up, an eye turning inward or outward
- Weakness in hands on one or both sides of the body
- Unsteady gait
- Word-finding problems
- Drowsiness
- Facial drooping
- Nausea and vomiting
- Hormonal or growth problems
- Hearing loss
- Changes in appetite or thirst
- Behavioral changes
- Changes in school performance

For a spinal cord tumor the symptoms may be:

- Back or neck pain that awakens your child from sleep
- Scoliosis (curvature of the spine resulting in leaning of shoulders to one side or a hump noticeable in the back)
- Torticollis (tilting of the head and upper spine to one side)
- Weakness or sensory changes in arms or legs
- Changes in bowel and bladder control

I think our respite is ending. Jen had a scan on Monday and we knew when we looked at them it would probably not be good news and that was confirmed today when we met with her oncologist. I don't have the radiology report yet but the scans will be discussed at tumor board Friday. It seems the original area of tumor continues to look stable and maybe even a little better, but there appears to be an area of new growth definitely crossing the midline now to the right side of her brain. Instead of starting what would have been her seventh round of Temodar® she is on hold until Friday. Two possibilities mentioned were CPT-11 and high dose Tamoxifen®.

This has been a hard day. I have already made some phone calls as I know from our discussion with the doctor he doesn't think there's much lag time before she needs to be on something. The last 4 weeks of Procrit® shots have moved her blood count from anemic to normal and she is physically active and still feeling good with the exception of some fatigue. She has been having some slight difficulty with her right hand grasping and holding but I am more concerned with her description of losing awareness of what it does. She's having more memory problems and the beginning of some incontinence. The 29th of this month will be the end of 12 years she has been dealing with this. Enough! But it doesn't look like that is meant to be.

The majority of brain and spinal cord tumors regrow or progress at the original tumor site. However, occasionally, the tumor spreads to another area of the brain or spinal cord.

Morgan was 4 years old when she relapsed. The tumor was found on a routine scan almost exactly 2 years from the day of first diagnosis. The tumor was again a medulloblastoma and it was small in size, but that didn't matter; the only thing I could think of was that we did the strongest chemotherapy out there and it didn't work, now what? Doctors presented us with options, and none seemed all that promising. We talked to the top doctors in the country and many of them told us that Morgan had such a small chance of survival at this point that it might be better to stop treatment all together. Those that did offer treatment told us about traditional photon beam radiation therapy whose long-term side effects could leave Morgan seriously mentally disabled. Our options seemed dismal. Then we heard about a doctor who had just started working with a new kind of radiation (proton). We got on a plane with Morgan's scans in hand and went to Boston where we were told that the new treatment might not only cure Morgan but possibly also spare her some cognitive late effects. This was the first doctor who had given us hope. Literally the next day, Chris and I packed up our home as well as Morgan and her two younger sisters (aged 2 and 10 months) and drove to Boston. Morgan is now 18 and doing great. [To read the rest of Morgan's story, see Chapter 25, Looking Forward].

Emotional responses

Parents who have children with a brain or spinal cord tumor in remission think or speak of regrowth of the tumor with an almost palpable dread. Just the thought can cause an eruption of the same emotions that surged in them at diagnosis. Parents, their child, and the siblings may feel a wide array of emotions at relapse: numbness, guilt, dread, anger, fear, confusion, denial, and grief. For parents whose child has had many years of stable MRI scans with no tumor growth, the scan that confirms their worst nightmare feels overwhelming.

> I found that relapse was far worse than the original diagnosis. At diagnosis, after a certain period of adjustment, you think that treatment has a beginning, a middle, and an end. But relapse creates a bigger burden to accept. You begin to feel that maybe the disease is more powerful than the medicine. I found that for a while I just stopped functioning and thinking rationally. I felt like I was on a runaway freight train, hurtling toward an end that didn't look so good anymore.

Parents often experience physical symptoms such as dizziness, nausea, fainting, and shortness of breath. They wonder how they can ask their child to endure treatment again. They wonder how they will survive it themselves. They may oscillate between optimism and panic.

> My first relapse was the worst emotionally. Neither my parents nor I ever thought that after 5 years it would be back. I also had been so young when I was first treated that I didn't understand that I could die from it. But at 13, I remembered clearly what I had been through, and all I could think was that it hadn't worked. I told my parents that I wouldn't do it again. My father sat me down and gave me a reality check. He explained that I would die if I didn't get treatment. He said, "If you don't do it for yourself, please do it for me and your mom." The next morning I went into the clinic and started all over again.

Goal setting and treatment planning

A difficult but necessary step in making plans is discussing and deciding on your and your child's goals. Health Canada's publication, *This Battle Which I Must Fight: Cancer in Canada's Children and Teenagers,* states:

> This [relapse] is a time of crisis and ambivalence. The decision to be made is whether to continue to try to achieve a remission or to replace this hope with the hope for comfort for the child and a special time together. Each parent, and the child who is old enough to understand, requires differing amounts of time to reach a decision about how to proceed. Careful and frequent discussions with the medical team,

as well as with trusted friends and relatives, may help clarify issues and bring some peace of mind.

In a newsletter for parents of children with cancer, Arthur Ablin, MD, (Director Emeritus of Pediatric Clinical Oncology at the University of California, San Francisco), wrote of the importance of goal setting in the decision-making process after relapse:

> *Before determining which treatment is to be chosen, a decision must be made to determine the goal of treatment—in other words, what is it that we are trying to achieve. This crucial first step is the basis upon which any decision concerning treatment must be made. But it is too often omitted from consideration and/or discussion, even by the most experienced. The frustrations accompanying the previous failure of treatment, the fear of the loss of the hope for cure, the pressure of urgency to find solutions, the new awareness of the possibility or probability of death, lead us all to want to consider treatments first rather than these more difficult considerations involved in establishing goals. These also force us to deal with reality earlier, which could mean the almost intolerable confrontation with the death of a very-much-loved child, a tragedy to be avoided at all costs.*

If after discussion of goals your family decides to pursue aggressive treatment, there may be more than one option available. Therefore, it is important to understand the treatment avenues that are open to you. Treatment plans for a first recurrence may be specified in the standard treatment or clinical trial protocol document, or your child's doctor may suggest a different approach. Suggestions for treatment may include surgery, radiation, stem cell transplantion, more intensive chemotherapy, a clinical trial, or a combination of several treatments.

> *Twenty-five days after surgery for medulloblastoma, Ayla (32 months) started chemo. Six chemo treatments were planned, but we only got through the first three, consisting of vincristine, etoposide (VP-16), cisplatin, and cyclophosphamide. They also collected stem cells for a stem cell transplant, which was never done. During this time, the MRIs showed that there was additional spread in 10 spots in the midbrain. Chemo was stopped and the last three treatments (thiotepa and carboplatin) weren't used. Exactly 1 day after Ayla's third birthday, she started radiation, and got the maximum doses for cranial and spinal radiation. Ayla sailed through radiation. She didn't get that sleepy period, although she did add an extra couple hours of nap every day. She had her radiation treatments early in the morning for 6 weeks. The whole thing took half an hour, and just a few minutes for the actual procedure. The radiation tech would give her the sedative, her special "milkshake" medicine, through her Hickman®. Afterwards, we'd go out for the day and play. Most, if not all, of the spots that they were watching are gone now and her original tumor site is showing scar tissue.*

Do not rush into treatment if you or your family feel uncomfortable about the plan. There is always time to obtain answers to all of your questions and to get a second opinion. Doctors make recommendations based on knowledge, experience, and consultations with other experts in the field. Do not hesitate to ask your child's doctor why she has suggested a certain treatment approach to your child's relapse. Ask the doctor about treatment goals, methods, and possible side effects. Also ask if she has consulted with others in the decision-making process, and if so, with whom. Be certain older children and teens are involved in decisions regarding their care and treatment choices.

> Our 18-year-old daughter was diagnosed with medulloblastoma in the cerebellum when she was 2 years old. She was treated with high-dose chemotherapy followed by stem cell transplant. At her 2 year off treatment MRI, the tumor was back—tiny and at the same site. It was again totally resected and this time we knew she needed radiation. The question was: what kind?

Making a decision about treatment

Treatment for children with brain and spinal cord tumors is evolving. The information gleaned from second opinions or your own research may reinforce what your doctor recommended, or it might provide you with additional treatment options. Either way, the information may increase your comfort level during the treatment planning process. You might want to ask your child's treatment team the following questions about the suggested treatment plan:

• Why do you think this treatment is the best option? What are the other choices, and why are you recommending this one?

• Have you consulted with other doctors? If so, with whom? Did you all agree on this treatment or were several choices suggested?

• Is there a standard treatment for this type of recurrence or progression? If so, what is it?

• Are any clinical trials are available?

• What are the potential benefits and possible side effects of the suggested treatment?

• How long is the proposed treatment?

• If transplant is recommended, what is the timing strategy for the transplant?

• If radiation is to be included, what type and dose are you recommending?

• What are the known or potential risks of the treatment?

• Is any neurocognitive testing done prior to treatment/transplant and what kind of follow-up is there post-treatment/transplant?

- How often will my child need to be hospitalized?

- If the treatment is investigational, is there scientific evidence that it works for brain and spinal cord tumors?

- Does insurance cover this type of treatment?

- What supportive services are available? How do we contact the people responsible for these services? (Contacts might include a hospital school coordinator, social worker, psychologist, and physical therapist.)

- What is the goal of this treatment? Remission? Comfort?

When older children and parents disagree about how to proceed, you can ask the primary nurse practitioner, social worker, or psychologist to help your family talk about the options. These discussions will help clarify each family member's thoughts and feelings and will allow the child's emotional and physical well-being to be part of the equation.

After you have set goals, received answers to all of your questions, obtained a second opinion if desired, and decided on a treatment plan, it is time to proceed. Your knowledge and experience may prove to be a double-edged sword. You have no illusions about the difficulties ahead because you've done it before, but you also will be strengthened by your ties to the cancer community, your comfort with your doctors and hospital routines, and your ability to work with the system to get what your child needs. Many parents shared how their child took the lead with relapse treatment. While the parents agonized, their child simply said, "Let's just do it." And they did.

Evan, who had his first surgery shortly after his ninth birthday, wrote the following essay about his journey. In addition to having a brain tumor, Evan has a diagnosis of high-functioning autism.

> I was 9 when I found out I needed brain surgery. I was nervous then, but I would be scared out of my mind if I was put in that situation now. When I came out of surgery, I couldn't walk, I couldn't even swallow very well or talk much. My first memory after surgery, I was in intensive care. It was bright. I was sound-sensitive, and my head was throbbing. I found out the type of tumor I had, a pilocytic astrocytoma, is the least malignant, but it was in the brainstem. That meant it was still very serious.
>
> After that surgery, I lost weight. I looked like a Holocaust survivor. I couldn't even stand on the scale, so someone had to hold me. They did a test that I had to swallow food with some chemical thing in it, and then they found out that I had cranial nerve damage so it was hard for me to swallow.

I went to rehab to learn to walk and for physical and occupational therapy. In rehab I could wear regular clothes, and they had a school, too. They had something like periods. At certain times, I'd go to therapy, and then I'd be in school, and so on. Some things were fun, and some things were not.

Some things I enjoyed were seeing movies and playing Uno®. Things I did not enjoy were blood tests and the physical therapy, or PT. Finally after 6 weeks, I got to go home. When they sent me home, I could walk and talk, but I had to wear a helmet. That's it for the first time around.

A year later, I started to get worse again. I had an MRI, and the tumor had grown, so it was time for another surgery. I was afraid, but I had more of an idea what to expect. After surgery, I didn't lose as much weight, but I had crossed eyes and high blood pressure. It felt like a '57 Chevy on my head, as I described the pain then. It was around Halloween, so I didn't go trick-or-treating. I was also eager to get to rehab, because it made me feel so much better the last time.

Chapter 24

Death and Bereavement

*The loss of my son has illuminated for me the true definition of love:
the giving of oneself, body and spirit, to another. His death, like that
of any child, is a story of withered hopes and unfulfilled dreams.
In this book I have tried to capture a few remembered strains of the
brief, glad music of his life. These are all I have of him now,
and they comfort me even as they break my heart.*

— Gordon Livingstone, MD
Only Spring

THE DEATH OF A CHILD causes almost unendurable pain and anguish for the loved ones left behind. Death from a brain or spinal cord tumor comes after months or years of debilitating treatment, emotional swings, and financial crises. The family begins the years of grief already exhausted from the years of fighting the tumor. It is truly every parent's worst nightmare.

In this chapter, many parents share their innermost thoughts and feelings about their decisions to transition from active treatment, to involve hospice, to choose death at home or in the hospital, and experiencing grief. It made no difference whether parents had recently lost a child or whether it happened decades before—tears flowed when talking about their family's experience. Because family members and friends can be strong sources of support, or casualties of the grieving process, parents describe words and actions that help, and they offer suggestions about what words and actions to avoid. Grief has as many facets as there are grieving parents; what follows are the experiences of a few.

Transitioning from active treatment

For children or teenagers whose disease is progressing, medical caregivers and parents at some point need to decide when to end active treatment and begin to work toward making the child comfortable for his remaining days. This is an intensely personal decision. Some families want to try every available treatment and exhaust all possible remedies. Others reach a point where they feel they have done all they can and want to transition to a time of sharing memories, expressing love, and preparing for death.

This has been a very difficult weekend with many tears. We have had so many wonderful years beyond what we ever thought was possible with such a good quality of life for Jen and us. In spite of everything, we have no regrets. We selfishly want every moment we can have, but we have come to the crossroad where we are asking at what cost to Jen. While we have not made the commitment to hospice yet, we are all feeling that we are not far from that place unless there is a dramatic change in Jen soon. She has really fought hard. She made this damn brain tumor work really hard to slow her down. She is very, very tired and while my head understands this, my heart is breaking.

Dr. Arthur Ablin, Director Emeritus of Pediatric Clinical Oncology at the University of California, San Francisco, wrote about the difficulties of deciding to end active treatment:

All too often, the decision to abandon the goal for cure and, reluctantly, accept the reality of inevitable death of a child is too painful and, therefore, never made. This paralyzing pain occurs with equal frequency, perhaps, for the family and the doctor. We of the medical profession have no equal in our ability to prolong dying. We have a powerful array of mechanical, electronic, pharmaceutical, and biotechnical interventions at our command. We can keep people dying for months and even years. Applying or withholding this armamentarium is an awesome responsibility, and it requires infinite wisdom to know how to manage wisely and correctly. We can do great good by applying these tools correctly, but can also do incalculable harm through over-utilization. Physicians and families alike must work together to avoid the possible pitfalls. When cure is beyond all of us, then the challenge is to make the rest of life as worthwhile and rich as possible. There is much to do for the terminally and critically ill child and his or her family. They have that right, we have the privilege, to be of service.

One of the more difficult tasks a parent will face is sharing the news with their child that treatments have stopped working. Older children and teenagers need to be an integral part of the subsequent discussions with the healthcare team. Their thoughts and feelings are crucial during the decision-making process. Honest, thorough communication between the ill child or teen, family members, and involved professionals helps everyone work together.

My niece was diagnosed right after her third birthday and died 2½ months short of her fifth birthday. We told her about the "tumor in her head" and she knew that was what was causing all the symptoms she was experiencing. She knew she was sick and wasn't getting better, but we never told her specifically that she would die until after we had stopped all treatment and the outcome was inevitable, probably a month or so before she died.

When we told her, we sat down with her and her 2½ year old brother and told them. She acted exactly as though she had already known what was going to happen to her, that we were telling her nothing new.

About 2 months before we told her, the movie "Little Women" came out on video. We had previously taken her to see it in the theatre. We got the video right away, and she watched it probably three times a week or more. She would always tell me, when I watched it with her, that her favorite part was the part where Jo died. It wasn't like she got any pleasure out of that part, but it was like she knew what would happen to her and she could identify very closely with Jo.

In retrospect, I think she had known for some time, long before we told her, but she did not speak of it because she had already come to terms with it, and she was not fearful. I think she desperately wanted to live and be cured, but she somehow knew that if a cure could not be found, she would die.

Sometimes, children take the lead in making the decision to stop treatment.

When my 6-year-old son Greg was in the hospital in intensive relapse treatment, he would repeat over and over again, "I want to go home." When he was finally well enough to come home for awhile, he kept saying, "I want to go home." In frustration, I said, "Greg, you are home, why do you keep saying that?" He looked up and quietly said, "I want to go to my heavenly home. I want to go to God." I said, "Honey, please don't say that," and, knowing how much we loved him, he replied, "Okay, Mom, I'll fight, I won't go." And he did fight hard for several more months. But he was way ahead of us in acceptance, he was at peace, and he knew it was time to let go.

When it is clear that death is inevitable, parents struggle with the thought of how to discuss it with the ill child and siblings. All too often in our culture, children are perceived as having to be protected from death, as if this somehow makes their last days better. On the contrary, children, often as young as age 4, know they are dying. If the parents are trying to spare the child from knowing, an unhealthy situation develops. The child might pretend that everything is okay to please the parents, and the parents might try to mask their deep grief with false smiles. Everyone loses.

Aidan was diagnosed at 4 ½ and at the time didn't know what the word cancer meant. We kept it that way. A little while later we told him about bad cells, in relation to having radiotherapy. I think this was easier for all of us than with an older child with a better understanding of death. Even so, Aidan now talks about that initial time in the hospital as "when you were very worried about me." I think he has some idea about how close he came that week. More recently, now 6, Aidan faced a recurrence from the medulloblastoma. When he was having a lumbar puncture I told him the doctor would put a needle in his back. He asked why and I answered that he needed to see if there were any bad cells there.

After a bit of thinking he asked, "What happens if there are?" I put on my brave face and said we hoped there weren't but we just have to wait and see. Then he said, "They'll go everywhere won't they?" My brave face was certainly tested then and so was his, he was very quiet that afternoon.

Denial sometimes prevents children and parents from finishing up business—distributing belongings, telling each other how much they love one another, and saying good-bye. It also strips parents of their ability to prepare their child for the journey from life to death. Children need to know what to expect about dying. They need to know that they will be surrounded by people they love and that their parents will be holding them as they pass on. They also need to know the family's beliefs about what happens after death.

> Jennifer contracted a respiratory fungal infection that resulted in her being hospitalized on a ventilator. She was given lots of morphine so that she wouldn't feel air hungry. She was alert off and on for a few days. We read to her and played tapes. After 1 week on the respirator, she took a turn for the worse. She didn't respond to me after that. Her kidneys were ceasing to function, and she started to get puffy. Her liver was deteriorating, and her painful pancreatitis had come back. After 10 days on the respirator, I couldn't bear it any longer. I lay down in her bed, took her in my arms, and kissed her at least 200 times. I talked to her for a long time, and told her that we would take care of her cats, and that I was sorry that she had to suffer so much, and how beautiful Heaven is. I told her to go be with Jesus, her Grandpa, and her dog. I also told her how much we all loved her and how proud we were of her. I got off the bed to change positions, and the nurse rushed in. Her heart had suddenly stopped the second I got up. I believe she heard me and just needed to know it was okay to go. She didn't want to leave until she knew her mommy was ready.

> Jennifer had told me that she wasn't afraid to die, and this has been a great source of comfort to us. I believe that she was preparing for her death, even as we hoped for her remission. Before she went to the hospital, she spent all her money, gave away some of her possessions to her sisters, and said a final good-bye to her home, cats, teachers, and friends.

One father shares how his family faced his daughter's terminal prognosis:

> When Stacia was diagnosed with glioblastoma, the prognosis was given as 9 to 12 months. With experimental treatments, I guessed that I might be able to extend her life another year. But the bottom line was that our child, our beautiful Stacia, was going to die. The recognition of this truth is a paralyzing event. Simply said, it breaks your heart in half, and leaves you weeping uncontrollably. When the crying subsided, the questions came flooding. Whatever in the world am I going to do? Two ideas came to mind. The first was absolutely normal: I will scour the world for treatments and try to save my child's life. This thought occurs to every parent in this situation. Understandably, most parents become completely absorbed by this single idea.

> My second thought was: How can I give Stacia the best possible life in the time that she (and we) have left? The concept I came up with was LIVING BIG. And live big we did. I set about with my wife Linda, our children, Jodi and David, Stacia's extended family, and all of her good friends, to create a network of love and support that would always be there to help her live life to the fullest, no matter what happened. In practical terms,

what this meant was creating a schedule of "living" to complement her schedule of "treatments."

We did not play it safe. We took Stacia everywhere: Canada, Yosemite, Shasta Lake, Tahoe, Pinecrest, Cayucos, San Francisco, even Mexico. That was one of the greatest weeks of our lives. Pure fun, pure memories. You see, Stacia was the life of the party. All we had to do was treat her that way.

There is another element of living big, other than just taking big trips. That's the intimate part. Setting aside a night, when you take your child out for dinner—just you and her. I asked Stacia if it would be okay to make Thursday nights our father-daughter night. She readily agreed. We went to our favorite pizza parlor, every Thursday, even if she did not eat. At the beginning, she could walk in on her own. Later she used a cane, still later we did a Texas two-step, where we walked in hand in hand, still later a 4-point walker, and still later her wheelchair. We never missed a night. And she often did not eat or drink much. She didn't really care. Because we were together. We made small talk, most of the time. Other times, we spoke about life and death. Mostly about life.

The rest of the family set about making their own special days or weekends with Stacia. We threw parties and had her friends over. Her friends threw parties, and we brought her over, even when I had to carry her inside, in my arms. We never left her out.

We tried to enjoy life to the fullest, even when we knew the situation was terminal. We packed a lifetime of living into 2 years. Stacia lived 26 months from her initial diagnosis. Cut down in her prime by a disease that the medical community doesn't understand all that well. An orphan disease that could have made orphans of my whole family, except that we did not let it.

We miss Stacia terribly, and our hearts are still broken over losing her. But our spirits are not broken, because we lived big, with the life of the party. God bless you, Stacia Jennifer.

Supportive care

In the United States, there are very active and effective hospice home care services for children. Hospice organizations ease the transition from hospital to home and provide support for the entire family. Hospice personnel ensure adequate pain control, allow children to control their last days or weeks of life, and provide active bereavement support to the family after the child's death.

If the family wishes for the child to die at home, a smooth transition usually occurs from the oncology ward to home hospice care. Unfortunately, sometimes pediatric patients are not referred to hospice, and the parents are left to deal with their child's last days at home with no experienced help and no clear idea of what is to come. Your nurse practitioner, case manager, or hospital social worker can refer you to, or help you find, a pediatric hospice organization in your area. Before you leave the hospital, it is wise to find out the name of a contact person at the agency who will be taking over the home care of your child.

> *Yesterday we got a visit from the hospice nurse. We had been putting it off but felt that we should have it in place for when we really need it for Ryan. Everyone keeps telling me what a great thing it is, and maybe that's how they feel, but personally, birthday parties are great, Disneyland® is great, even Chuck E. Cheese® is great. Hospice is not great.*

· · · · ·

> *When our children were babies and learning, I always used the principle of reinforcing things I wanted them to learn or understand with all their senses: hearing, seeing, touch, smell, and taste. During Jen's last days, we kept her room filled with light the way she liked it, and even a soft low light at night so whenever her eyes opened so she knew one of us was right there. We played her favorite music continuously, more upbeat during the day and softer choices at night, and we talked with her and then to her when she could no longer respond with her voice, although the squeeze of her hand and her big blue eyes spoke volumes.*
>
> *We touched her constantly, sometimes just sitting next to her holding her hand and not moving, other times stroking her head, rubbing "udder" cream on her elbows and heels so she didn't get bedsores. She had lost quite a bit of her sense of smell, but we kept everything very fresh and all the flowers that came to the house were all around her because she visually could remember their wonderful scent. We learned to use the great swabs that hospice provided with very cool water and a bit of mint Listerine so her mouth felt clean and fresh, especially as she became less able to take care of herself and even more so when she was no longer able to take in water and then food. One of the nurses told us to take ice chips and put them in a very worn piece of cloth and make it tiny so she wouldn't gag and let in rest in her mouth for a few minutes at a time so she had some moisture, and when that became impossible because she could hardly open her mouth, we swabbed her lips and the gums outside of her closed teeth. All this was meant to convey the message you are loved and cared for and we will be right here for you every step of the way.*

Hospice not only provides assistance in physically caring for your child, it can also provide emotional support for your child, you and your spouse, and any other children in your home. If you have questions about hospice or what support is available, you can contact Children's Hospice International online at *www.chionline.org* or by phone at (800) 242-4453 (800-24-CHILD).

> *We were very fortunate in our hospice experience, which lasted a mere 8 days. On the first day, a nurse arrived to meet all of us. She came in with a big smile and introduced herself. The nurse began by taking a very complete medical history, and*

I remember being surprised by the depth of information she wanted. It was like she wanted to fully understand the entire brain tumor journey and what he had been through, while I suppose I had expected her to laugh off with disinterest everything that had happened before "the end," as if it wouldn't matter anymore. She listened intently, reacted appropriately at incidents that had been a bit unusual, and wrote down a great deal. Then she did a brief exam, just blood pressure, pulse, and general appearance, and assured him that she wouldn't bother him anymore. He relaxed when he realized that she wouldn't be poking him as so many others had already done. We had been apprehensive before her arrival, but afterward, it felt like the night crew had arrived after a very long day shift.

Dying in the hospital

Some children die in the hospital suddenly, while others slowly decline for weeks or months. If your child is slowly dying, you may have choices about where he will spend his last days. There are no right or wrong choices. Much depends on the number of people available to provide care at home and how comfortable they are doing so. Many parents ask their child where she would prefers to be. Some children and teens want to be with the nurses in a hospital environment, but others want to stay at home with brothers, sisters, friends, and pets.

Parents, children, and staff should talk honestly to decide on the appropriate place for the child and then obtain the support (e.g., hospice care, private nurses in the hospital, family members) needed to make the choice a comfortable reality. Remain flexible so that as the situation changes, options remain open. If the choice is made to die in the hospital, most hospitals have a palliative care team that can help families make choices that emphasize comfort.

Although we had been advised that it didn't look good for Greg, we were trying one last time to get him to transplant. He was sleeping quietly in his hospital bed. He had been complaining of severe head pain, and was on a low morphine drip. The afternoon nurse woke him to take vitals, and he chatted with her. He told me, "Mom, I'm going to go back to sleep, I love you." Two hours later the night nurse tried to wake him up to give him some medicine, and she couldn't wake him. They called the doctor in from his home, and he ordered a CT scan. When the film came up to the floor, the doctor took me out in the hall and said, "He's not going to live through the night." He held up the film showing a massive cerebral infarction; Greg was bleeding into the brain. He quietly died less than an hour later. Family and staff were in total shock. Nobody expected it. But, looking back, Greg had decided he had had enough; he was ready to go. I am grateful that he didn't die on a transplant floor in a strange city. We were able to call in friends and family, and we were surrounded and supported by the wonderful nurses whom we knew so intimately. I couldn't leave him until three nurses promised to stay with him and escort him to the morgue. They are still dear friends.

Parents of children who died in the hospital stressed the importance of clear communication. Parents need to be strong advocates for adequate pain control, and they need to clearly tell the staff their wishes for their child's end of life. For example, in most hospitals, if a patient's heart stops or if he stops breathing, the staff immediately begins cardiopulmonary resuscitation (CPR) and electric shocks to the heart—this is called a "code." If the parents have decided they are ready to let their child die naturally, they need to discuss their wishes with the oncologist and ensure that an order of "NO CODE" is put in the chart and on the child's door. A No Code order is also called a DNR, or "Do Not Resuscitate" order. Family members should understand that a DNR does not mean "Do not care for my child." On the contrary, it allows the medical team to provide comfort measures, such as:

- Allowing the child to sleep during the night without interruptions for temperature and blood pressure

- Providing adequate pain medication

- Allowing family and friends open visitation without restrictions as to length and time of stay and the number of people allowed in the room

- A private room

> *Alannah was medicated at any indication of discomfort, and after a week of semi-consciousness followed by a week of coma, we finally got up the guts to have her taken off the respirator, to let her go. She opened her mouth a couple of times, as if trying to breathe, and that was it. With her mother and I holding her, the staff just left us alone. Fifteen minutes later, the attending doc came back and declared time of death. She left very peacefully. We were told to expect that she might seem to be struggling or gasping, and that it would just be reflex, that she wouldn't really be struggling. It didn't happen.*

Parents also should discuss whether they want nurses or doctors present when their child dies. Many families feel very close to the hospital staff and feel supported by their presence, while others prefer to have only family and close friends at the child's bedside. Advance planning helps to ensure that, as death approaches, the family's wishes are understood and respected.

Dying at home

A child's death at home and the time just before can be a peaceful experience, depending on the extent of preparation and the quality of support available to the family. Unlike other childhood cancers, pain and its control are rarely associated with brain and spinal cord tumors, although families should keep their doctor or hospice team apprised if their child is experiencing any discomfort. For this reason, many families of children with brain and spinal cord tumors choose for their children to die at home.

Four weeks before Stacia died, she called us into her room. One by one, she proclaimed her love for each of us, and thanked us for being the best family a girl could ever have. She told us not to worry, that she was going to be all right, and that one day, we would all be together again. On Memorial Day, Stacia died in her mother Linda's arms, with all of us at her side.

· · · · ·

Just before Thanksgiving, 10 days before Jay's 15th birthday, my worst fear was realized—the tumor was back, an anaplastic ependymoma, and this time, in the brainstem. Because of location, surgery was not possible. And this time, radiation wasn't possible either. We faced the decision of attempting an aggressive and not usually very successful chemotherapy or calling it quits and letting him go. Choosing hospice was the hardest decision of our lives.

Jay wanted to die at home, it was important to him. Toward the end, we sat near Jay's bed talking softly. A few minutes later, I leaned over to check on our son. He seemed to be slipping away.

"Squeeze my finger if you can hear me," I pleaded. Jay gave my finger a light squeeze, so weightless I could barely feel it. He slept in a classic fetal position, knees beneath his chest, occupying as small a space as possible. A few minutes later, I spoke to him again, this time no response. Gently, I grasped his wrist with my thumb and forefinger and counted a pulse. We called hospice and they offered to send a nurse over, but we refused, preferring to receive their support by telephone.

We sat at Jay's bedside. At 9:00, our daughter Vanessa came home. She spoke to her brother, his eyebrows arched, but he didn't respond in any other way. We felt positive he could hear her. At first, I thought I must have given my son too much morphine. Gary called the doctor and the doctor insisted that I hadn't. Deep down I knew I hadn't done anything wrong. There wasn't anything I could have done differently to help my son become fully alert again.

Throughout the night, we all stayed with Jay. We folded ourselves onto the bed with him, surrounding him. In the center, Jay lay between the three of us, small, quiet, immobile, with his dog at his side. All night, his breathing stopped and then started again.

"Maybe we need to tell him that it's okay to die," Vanessa offered. "Jay, I love you," she said. "Don't worry, I'll do your chores and help Mom. Time is different in heaven; we'll be there with you before you know it," she cooed.

I kissed Jay on his forehead. "It's okay," I whispered. "Don't wait for anything, it's time for you to go." At that moment, Jay smiled the sweetest smile, and a peaceful feeling as wide as the sky settled over us, something warm and cozy fell across my heart, and then he was gone.

Involving siblings

Whether your child is dying at home or in the hospital, any siblings should be included in the family response. Being part of things and having jobs to do help brothers and sisters remain involved, contributing members of the family. Young children can answer the door, go on errands, or make tapes or CDs to play for the sibling. Older children can help with meals, stay with the ill child to give parents a break, answer the phone, or help make funeral arrangements. These jobs should not be "make-work"—children should truly be helping. This not only allows them to clarify their role in the family, it helps them to prepare for the death, as well as have an opportunity to say good-bye.

> We gave our children free rein to pick out the clothes that Jesse would be buried in. They made very thoughtful choices: her favorite, very comfortable pajamas with little tea cups on them, and her teddy bear.

The Compassionate Friends (see Appendix B, *Resource Organizations*) has dozens of resources to help all members of the family.

The funeral

Funerals and related rituals (e.g., memorial services, wakes, burial, shiva) are important not only as a time to say good-bye and to begin to accept the reality of death, but also to provide an opportunity to recognize the relationships and impact that the child or teen had on others. Funerals allow friends and family to gather together to share memories and show support for the remaining family members. A funeral is a tangible demonstration of love.

> As the car drove us to Guildford Cathedral, the rain started to come down in torrents, even the angels were crying. It got darker and darker and I felt lower and lower.

> As we walked around the corner into the Nave, we were absolutely amazed. There were 700 people in the Cathedral. 700. I could not believe my eyes. Michael obviously touched a lot of hearts.

> When the service started, the singing was just out of this world. And right next to me our son Christopher shut his eyes and sang along with his friends from St. George's who had come along to bolster the Guildford Choir. And that was quite something, to see the boys from the two choirs sitting side by side in the choir stalls, together with the men of two choirs. Michael had always wanted to sing with his brother when he was still a chorister. He finally got the two Choral Foundations together.

> The tribute from his godfather was perfect: funny, witty, poignant, and included a wonderful tribute to Christopher as well. The sermon from Canon Maureen told everyone what a strong faith Michael had and how he was so sanguine in living and in dying. "Here was someone who was alive from top to toe!" she said. And he WAS.

The anthem was moving, the prayers touching, and then the undertakers moved in to pick up the coffin, and Graham, Christopher, and I moved behind it to take that long, long walk down the Nave. By now I was in tears—and walking past 700 people, most of whom were also in tears, was not easy. As we got to the Great West Door, the pallbearers turned round so that Michael was facing the altar, and everything was so quiet you could hear a pin drop. Suddenly, over the speakers, came the sound of Michael singing, "In the morning when I rise …"

Christopher and I stood with our arms round each other and tears pouring down our cheeks. As it finished, the organ swung into action and Michael's body was turned around and carried out for the last time of his beloved Cathedral, just as the sun came out.

Children of all ages should be allowed to attend the funeral if they wish, but only after they have been prepared for what to expect. They need an explanation of what the event is for, where they will be going, and what will happen. They need to know what death is, what type of room they are going to, whether the casket will be there, whether it will be open, whether there will be flowers, who will be there, how the mourners will behave, who will stay with them, what they will be expected to say or do, how long they will be there, and what will happen after the service (e.g., burial, reception). All questions should be answered honestly and the children's feelings respected. Many siblings benefit from giving one last gift to the departed, such as writing a private note and dropping it in the casket, or bringing some of their sister's favorite flowers to put in her hands.

We celebrated our 3-year-old son's Kevin's life today. The past week has been a whirlwind. All of Kevin's favorite women worked nonstop for 48 hours leading up to last night. The funeral home was beautiful. There were pictures everywhere—on pedestals, in photo albums, collages, and frames.

There were children's books throughout the funeral home as well as red balloons, Kev's favorite color. We had patchwork squares out to create a memorial quilt for his younger sisters, Courtney and Katie. People wrote special messages and drawings on them to capture their feelings: "Kevin, Sending you love and kisses and one BIG scoop of mashed potatoes!"

We also had sheets of paper to write stories and memories of Kevin to make a memorial book for the girls. Kevin's favorite things were on a memorial table: his green blankie with the hole in it, his books, his Buzz Lightyear, his green bike, his catcher's mitt, his baseball and yellow bat, golf clubs, and more.

We rented a 6' projector screen and a big screen TV to display a 20-minute video in both rooms at the funeral home. It showed Kevin's life over the past year. And it was a pretty good life too: putting candles on Grammy's cake with Matthew, gymnastics with Grampie, wrestling with Courtney, reading with Daddy, playing football with Nana, kissing Auntie JoJo and Auntie Karin, playing golf in the yard, laying on the floor laughing, telling knock knock jokes, riding bikes in the house, at the beach at the Cape.

What does a mom do? She loves, cherishes, teaches, protects, and lets go. For one brief, shining moment, we had Kevin. For happily ever after we have our memories of him.

For families that are involved in a spiritual community, their clergy have a unique opportunity to provide support, love, and comfort to the grieving family and friends. They usually know the family well and can evoke poignant memories of the deceased child or teen during the service. Members of the clergy often have excellent counseling skills and can visit the family after the funeral to provide ongoing help during mourning.

The role of family and friends

Family members and friends can be a wellspring of deep comfort and solace during grieving. Some people seem to know just when a hug is needed or when silence is most welcome. Unfortunately, in our society there are few guidelines for handling the social aspects of grief. Sometimes well-meaning people voice opinions concerning the time it is taking to "get over it" or question the parents' decision to not give away their child's clothing or other belongings. Others do not know what to say, so they are silent, pretending that life's greatest catastrophe did not occur. Many friends never again mention the deceased child's name, not knowing that this silence, as if the cherished child never existed, only adds to parents' pain. Holidays can become uncomfortable, because they bring sadness as well as joy.

In an attempt to alleviate these difficulties, bereaved parents helped compile the following lists of what helps and what does not, in the hope that it may guide those family members and friends who deeply care, but just don't know how to help. Parents or family members can copy these lists to share with people who want to help.

These suggestions are offered with the understanding that what works for one family may not work for another. Family members and friends should use their knowledge of the bereaved family to choose options that they think will be most helpful. If in doubt, they should ask the parents. As Mother Teresa said, "Kind words can be short and easy to say, but their echoes are truly endless."

Things that help

The long lists of things that help from Chapter 16, *Family and Friends* (e.g., keeping the household running, feeding the family, and helping with bills), are still appropriate here. The following lists are specific suggestions for support with grieving.

Helpful things to say:

- I am so sorry.
- I cannot imagine the pain you are feeling, but I am thinking about you.
- I really care about you.
- You and your family are in our thoughts and prayers.
- We would like to hold a memorial service at the school for your child if you think that it would be appropriate.
- I will never forget John's sunny smile.
- I will never forget Jane's gentle way with children and animals.

Parents also offer a list of helpful things to do:

- Go to the funeral or memorial service.

  We were overwhelmed and touched by all of the people who came to the funeral. Even people that I had not seen in years—like some of my college professors— attended. Her oncologist and nurse drove 100 miles to be there.

- Show genuine concern and caring by listening.

  What has helped me the most is for people to just listen. Finding time to remember and reminisce is sometimes very difficult and painful, yet other times I feel much pride and happiness. Friends whose children also have cancer have been the greatest help to me during my daughter's illness and after her death.

- Help the siblings.

  We had friends just call and say, "We will pick up Nick on Saturday and take him to Water World, then to our house for dinner. We were hoping he could spend the night. Will that be all right?" They did this many times, and it not only was fun for him, but gave us a chance to be alone with each other and our grief.

- Write the parents a note instead of sending a preprinted sympathy card with your signature. Include special things you remember about their child or your feelings about their child. Letters, poems, or drawings from classmates and friends allow children to share their feelings with the family of the deceased, as well as provide poignant testimonials that the family will cherish.

- Talk about the child who has died. Parents forever carry cherished memories of their child and enjoy hearing others' favorite recollections.

Months after the funeral, we gathered family members and some close friends to share memories on tape. We did a lot of laughing as well as shed a few tears. But I will always cherish those tapes.

. . . . .

I think most of all parents want their child to be remembered. It really comforts me to go to Greg's grave and find flowers, notes, or toys left by others.

- When parents express guilt over what they did or did not do, reassure them that they did everything they could. Remind them that they provided their child with the best medicine had to offer.

- Remember anniversaries. Call or send a card or flowers on the anniversary of the child's death.

- Respect the family's method of grieving.

- Give donations in the child's name to a favorite charity of the child or parents, for example, the child's school library, the local children's camp, or U.S. Children's Hospice International.

  Every year we still get a card saying that Caitlin's occupational therapist donated money to Camp Goodtimes. It makes me feel good that she is remembered so fondly and that the money will help other kids with cancer and their brothers and sisters.

- Commemorate the child's life in some tangible way. Examples of this are planting trees, shrubs, or flowers; erecting a memorial or plaque; or displaying a picture of the child.

  The spring after Matthew's death, his school contacted me and said they wanted to do something special in his honor. They planted a little leaf linden tree in front of the building and built a wonderful seat around its base. They picked this particular tree because of its wonderful fragrance, and because the leaves were shaped like little hearts. A plaque beside the tree proclaims that this is Matthew's Friendship Tree. In addition to his name and the date of his birth and death, it reads: "When you remember me, please have a smile and cherish the good times we shared. And in these memories I will live with you forever."

- Be patient. Acute grief from the loss of a child lasts a long, long time. Expectations of a rapid recovery are unrealistic and hurtful to parents.

- Encourage follow-up from medical personnel.

  Caitlin had a very kind, very gentle radiation oncologist. I went back to see her after Caitlin died; she said, "We were so happy when we saw the progress that Caitlin made, from a stretcher to sitting to talking and walking again; and then our hearts broke when she relapsed. I wept." It was so human and so wonderful for her to let me know that she cared.

What not to say

Please do not say the following to grieving parents:

- I know exactly how you feel.
- It's a blessing her suffering has ended.
- Thank goodness you are young enough to have another child.
- At least you have your other children.
- Be brave.
- Time will heal.
- God doesn't give anyone more than they can bear.
- It was God's will.
- He's in a better place now.

> *Every time someone approached me at the funeral home with the words, "He's gone to a better place," I felt as if I would scream. Matthew's place was with me, his mother. Seven-year-old boys need their mother. It also really angered me when people repeatedly said, "Oh, with all he suffered, you wouldn't wish him back if you could." Well, yes, I would wish my child back! I would wish him back healthy and well. To this very day I would wish my child back, even if I could hold him for just a moment or hear the sound of his laughter one more time.*

- God must have needed another angel.
- It's lucky this happened to someone as strong as you.
- Don't worry, in time you'll get over it.
- Why did you decide to cremate him?
- How is your marriage holding up?
- You need to be strong for your other children.

Please do not say to the siblings:

- You need to be strong for your mom and dad.
- Don't cry, it upsets your parents.
- You're the man of the house now.
- How does it feel to be the big sister now?

Even if bereaved parents have deep religious faith, it is often tested by their child's death. Parents are not comforted by well-meaning friends who assume faith is making the grief bearable; indeed, many parents find it to be infuriating. It's better to just say "I'm sorry."

In the months and years following the child's death, any of the following are unlikely to be appreciated and may, in fact, be hurtful:

- Don't you think it's time to get over it?

- It's been 6 months; it's time to put the past behind you.

- Life goes on.

- You need to get on with your life.

- You shouldn't be feeling that way.

- Don't you think you should give away all her clothes?

- Don't cry.

- Doesn't it bother you to have his pictures around?

- Please don't talk about Johnnie, it just stirs up all those memories.

- It's not good to just sit around, you need to get out and have some fun.

Don't let your own sense of helplessness keep you from reaching out, even if you are unsure about what to say or do. It hurts the grieving family members when others stay away or pretend nothing is wrong or avoid (or refuse) to talk about the child who has died.

What not to do

The following are suggestions from parents about what not to do:

- Don't remove anything that belonged to the child who died, unless specifically asked to by the parents.

    One family member took my son's toothbrush out of the bathroom and threw it away. I missed it immediately. She probably felt that she was doing me a favor, but it made me so angry. I needed to keep things. I have his hair from the second time it fell out, because he wanted to save it, and I've kept his teeth which had to be pulled during treatment. I just need to have those things, and I resent people who insist you must clear out a child's things. Parents should be able to keep things or get rid of them— whichever is comfortable—regardless of others' opinions.

- Don't offer advice.

    Christie's room is still her room. We still refer to it as Christie's room. People just don't have the right to say you shouldn't leave that room empty: it's not empty, it's full of her life. I know that they are not trying to hurt us. It just bothers them to see that room. Sometimes it is just a reminder of death; yet, there are times when being in there and surrounded by all her things brings us closer to her and her time with us.

- Don't say anything that in any way suggests that the child's medical care was inadequate.

    I can't tell you how many people said things like "If only you had gone to a different treatment facility," or "If only you had used this or that treatment." What people need most is support for what they are doing or did do.

- Don't look on the bright side or find silver linings.

    I became unexpectedly pregnant the month after my daughter died. I can't tell you how many people said things like "The circle of life is complete," or "God is taking one and giving you another," or "God is replacing her." She can never be replaced. It was horrible to hear those things, and I felt it was unfair to both the unborn baby and to my daughter who died.

- Don't make comments about the parents' strength.

    People would say things to me like "You're so strong," or "I just couldn't live through what you have." It makes me want to scream. Do they mean I loved my child less than they love theirs because I have physically survived?

Sibling grief

Siblings are sometimes called the "forgotten grievers" because attention is typically focused on the parents. Children and teens sometimes hesitate to express their own strong feelings in an attempt to prevent causing their parents additional distress. Indeed, adult family members and friends may advise the brothers and sisters to "be strong" for their parents or to "help your parents by being good." These requests place a terribly unfair burden on children who have already endured months or years of stress and family disruption. Siblings need continual reinforcement that each of them is an irreplaceable member of the family and that the entire family has suffered a loss. They have the right, and need, to mourn openly and in their own way.

The family requires such reorganization after a child's death, and there is nowhere to look for an example. Each person in the family constellation has different feelings and different ways of grieving; there is just no way to reconcile all of this when the supposed leaders of the group are totally out of it. Not to mention the fact that both my husband and I wanted more understanding and compassion from each other than we were possibly able to give.

Children express grief in many ways. Some children develop physical manifestations, such as stomach aches, a loss of appetite or voracious eating, or changes in sleeping or toileting habits. Many younger children regress; they may revert to diapers or baby talk, stop walking, or stop talking. Fears and phobias, such as a fear of the dark or of being alone, are common responses to loss. Children may develop unpredictable or disruptive behaviors, such as tantrums, crying, sadness, anxiety, withdrawal, or depression. Older children and teens may appear nonchalant, angry, withdrawn, or engage in risky behaviors, such as sexual promiscuity, alcohol abuse, and drug use.

Parents need to engage siblings of different ages at their appropriate developmental levels. Private time together, or individual outings with the parents, can be very helpful for siblings.

Families can pull apart when individuals within the family have incompatible ways of expressing grief. Men and women tend to express grief in profoundly different ways, which may seem intolerable or inexplicable to one another. In these situations, family therapy or some other form of counseling can help.

Some parents worry that if they start talking about their feelings, they will "break down" in front of the children. But the children know their parents are grieving and it hurts them to feel excluded. They are grieving, too, and if they see their parents pulling away from them, they are likely to feel that their parents do not love them as much as they loved the child they lost. Here are suggestions from families about ways to pull together while mourning:

- Let the siblings go to the funeral. They have suffered a loss and they need to say good-bye. They need support for their grief just as much as adults.

- Children and teens experience the same feelings as adults. By sharing your own feelings, you can encourage them to identify their own. (For example, "I'm really feeling sad today. How do you feel?")

- Some families establish a regular meeting time to talk about their feelings. Both tears and laughter erupt when family members talk about funny or touching memories of the departed child.

- Jointly discuss how holidays and anniversaries should be observed. Each family devises different ways to handle holidays, the child's birthday, and the anniversary of her death.

> Last year we marked our first Christmas since Matthew's death. It was so incredibly hard for me to open the boxes of decorations knowing that inside I would find treasures he had made for me over the years with his own two little hands. I cried when I found his stocking, because I didn't know what to do with it. Somehow it didn't seem right to not hang it as usual.

I decided that I would continue to place Matthew's stocking beside David's and Kristina's. Instead of Santa filling it with treats, I asked my family to fill it for me. A few weeks before Christmas, I ask members of my family to write a memory of Matthew on a piece of paper. The only stipulation is that it must be a happy memory. On Christmas morning I look forward most of all to the gifts my children have made for me in school, and the memories that fill Matthew's stocking. Matthew will always be included in our Christmas. That's because he will always be an important member of our family.

Parental grief

Losing a child is one of life's most horrific and painful events. There is no "right way" to grieve. There is no timetable, no appropriate progression from one stage to the next, and no specific time when parents should "be over it." The death of a child shatters the very order of the universe—children are not supposed to die before their parents; it seems unnatural and incomprehensible. Losing a child, especially after such a long and grueling battle to save them, feels cruel and unjust. When a child dies, parents mourn not only the child, but all of the hopes, dreams, wishes, and needs relating to their child. When you lose a child, you lose part of yourself and an important part of your future. Below, parents themselves share their thoughts about grief.

I truly think that it is the worst thing in the entire world. Nothing worse can happen than losing your child. There is no reprieve. None.

• • • • •

I was having a very hard time grieving when a wonderful therapist that I was seeing said to me, "You are beating yourself up about grieving. Think about it. When you enter marriage, what are you called? A wife. When your spouse dies, what are you called? A widow. When you don't have a home and you are living on the street, what is the name for that? A homeless person. When you lose a child, what's it called, what's the name?" I said, "I don't know." She said, "Exactly. There is not even a word in our vocabulary. That's how terrible it is. It doesn't even have a name."

• • • • •

Every day when I walk out of my house I tell myself to grab the mask. I feel like I walk different than everybody and talk different than everybody and look different than everybody. It's the worst part of bereavement, the isolation caused by people who just don't know how to talk to you, when really all they need to do is listen and remember with you.

• • • • •

I found myself getting busier and busier, thinking that I could outrun the pain. I realized that I couldn't avoid the hurt; I just had to grit my teeth, cry, and live through it.

I felt like our sick daughter was the center of our universe for so long, that now I need to start feeling some responsibility for my other kids whom I've been away from for so long, both physically and emotionally. I told my husband the other night that I didn't even know if I loved the three kids anymore. I cannot feel a thing. Pinch me, I don't feel it. Hug me, I don't feel it. I'm numb.

• • • • •

It's hard to admit, but there was an element of relief when my daughter died. Not relief for myself, but for her. I was almost glad that she wouldn't face a life full of disabilities, that she wouldn't face the numerous surgeries that would have been required to repair the damage from treatment, that she wouldn't face the pain of not having children of her own. I just felt relief that she would no longer feel any pain.

• • • • •

At first we didn't feel like a family anymore. Now it's better, but it's still not the family that I was used to, that I want. I still feel like the mother of four children, not three. I find it very hard to answer when someone asks me how many children I have. I also can't sign cards like I used to, with all of our names, so now I just write "from the gang." I guess that's not fair to the boys, but I just can't bear to leave her name off.

• • • • •

I had always heard that time heals all things. I was afraid of healing, because I didn't want to feel any farther away than I felt when he died. It's been 7 years, and he still feels really close—a presence. But I still ache to touch his body so, that little back and fat tummy.

• • • • •

Birthdays are hard for us. Greg's birthday was June 10, and his brother's is June 9. So it's pretty hard to ignore. On Greg's birthday and the anniversary of his death, we blow up balloons, one for every year he would have been alive, write messages on them with markers, and release them at his grave.

• • • • •

It seems like just about every holiday has some difficult memory attached to it now. He was diagnosed on Easter, and then relapsed the next year on Valentine's Day. I hate them both now. Christmas is always hard. And Halloween is tough because he so loved to dress up. I see all those little ones in their costumes and I'm just flooded with pain.

• • • • •

This evening my heart was so saddened. I paced up and down in front of the mantel pausing to look at each picture of my daughter. Something that I cannot describe catches in my chest, and I can't breathe right. I look at her face and try to will it to life for a kiss and a touch, for softly spoken endearments at night. How we love all of our children, yet one missing leaves such a stabbing pain.

• • • • •

The past few weeks have been tough. Everything is a reminder of Kevin, a spoon with his name on it, toys throughout the house, syringes in the drawer, the dozens of books on the shelf. I can hear his 3-year-old singsong voice with the things he used to say at least a thousand times, "Momma, you shut the TV off?" "Momma, where are ya?" "Momma, I want my blankie" "Momma, how come Courtney's not cooperating" "Momma, you read me a book" "Momma, you lay down and scratch my back" "Momma, you sing hush baby."

The "firsts" are going to be the hardest, going to the park, going food shopping, going to the Maine house, going to Target®, driving by the library and not popping in to pick up a book for Kev. I find that I don't want to spend time with anyone who didn't know Kevin. I'm not sure if it's because they won't know of how big the loss is or because I need to have people around who can talk about him and the things he used to say and do. So when people say, "How are you doing," I say, "We're doing." We're doing a lot of thinking, a lot of laughing, and a lot of crying.

• • • • •

It's hard when people I have just met ask, "How many children do you have?" In the beginning I always felt that I had to explain that I had two but one died. Now, I just say one. I don't want their sympathy, I don't want their pity, but most of all I just don't want to have to explain. After 2 years or so, I started to feel uncomfortable giving out my life history and then having to deal with other people's discomfort. So now I just say one, and yet it still feels like I'm betraying him every time I do it.

• • • • •

That 1-year rule, when you are supposed to start feeling better, I've found to be true. Not that any of the pain is lessened, but I realized I had managed to live through a year of holidays and anniversaries. I knew it was possible to do it a second, then a third time. One year isn't magic, but it does prove to you that you can survive.

• • • • •

On the anniversary of my son's death we all went to the cemetery, and his girlfriend's parents planted a cherry tree at the foot of his grave. That was on a Sunday. I woke up on Monday feeling just as bad as I did the day before. All I could think was, "Oh hell, I have to go through that whole cycle again." The first year did not bring me any peace.

• • • • •

This morning was the 4-year anniversary of my daughter's death. While I was at church I wanted to write in the intentions book, "I want my daughter back," but then

I didn't because nobody would understand. I guess I'm pretty unreal in my thoughts a lot of the time.

• • • • •

From the minute I turn the calendar over to August, I'm on a knife edge. The twentieth of August just pulses on the calendar. I become depressed, spacey; I'm just in a very bad mood. I get sick a lot those first 3 weeks of August. But when it's over, I begin to relax and look forward to fall.

• • • • •

At church, we always sit with the same group of close friends who helped us through Jesse's illness and are helping us grieve her death. If they begin to sing a hymn that reminds one of us of Jesse, we all start to cry, and someone produces a box of tissues, which gets passed down the aisles. People must wonder at the group that sobs through services. But it has helped me so much to have a community of grievers, it's been a very cleansing thing. It has spread out the tears.

• • • • •

I think parents need to know that it hurts like hell and they will feel crazy. But it is a normal craziness. If they talk to other bereaved parents, they will know that pain, guilt, rage, and craziness are how normal human beings feel when their child dies.

Bereaved parents are frequently reassured that "time will ease the pain." Most find that this is not the case. Time helps them understand the pain; the passage of time reassures them that they can adjust and they will survive. The acute pain becomes more quiescent, but it still erupts when parents go to what would have been their child's graduation, hear their child's favorite song, or just go to the grocery store. Grief is a long, difficult journey, with many ups and downs. But, with time, parents report that laughter and joy do return. They acknowledge that life will never be the same, but that it can be good again.

I just wish that I had armfuls of time.

— Four year old with cancer
Armfuls of Time

Chapter 25

Looking Forward

Behind the curtain's mystic fold,
The glowing future lies unrolled.

— Bret Harte

IT'S HARD TO BELIEVE that when the first astronaut walked on the moon, the technology available to diagnose and treat children with brain and spinal cord tumors was primitive, at best. Many children were placed on medication for seizure disorders without ever knowing that the cause of the seizures was a tumor. When diagnosed, most children died from their tumor.

Treatments have come a long way in the past 4 decades. New techniques and technologies are now available to successfully diagnose, treat, and cure many children with brain and spinal cord tumors. Diagnostic tools, especially the MRI, allow for earlier diagnosis and treatment. The MRI helps neurosurgeons plan delicate surgeries and is also used to give them a three-dimensional picture of the tumor during surgery. MRI is also used to plan radiation treatments and allows the newer radiation therapy machines to deliver more focused doses of radiation, thus sparing nearby healthy brain cells. Chemotherapy has been shown to penetrate the blood/brain barrier, and many drugs have been found to be effective in destroying brain and spinal cord tumor cells.

The enrollment and participation in national clinical trials has fueled great success in understanding and treating these tumors. Many children with fast-growing tumors have enrolled in clinical trials over the last few decades, which has enabled researchers to learn about the many different subgroups of tumors and how each should be treated. Research has also shown that:

- Children diagnosed with the same type of tumor have incredibly variable responses to treatment. Therefore, some children with grim prognoses are cured, while others with a tumor considered to be very treatable are not.

- Children with tumors that are totally removed with surgery have a much better prognosis than those whose tumors cannot be totally removed.

- Slow-growing tumors may be observed and remain dormant for months or years without any treatment.

- Some slow-growing tumors shrink over time.

- New surgical instruments and improved intraoperative monitoring provide valuable information to pediatric neurosurgeons during operations.

- Chemotherapy, whether used alone or in conjunction with radiation therapy, is effective in treating some brain and spinal cord tumors.

- Radiation therapy, which used to be the gold standard, is now not used for some tumors until other treatment methods have been tried.

When you have an aggressive malignant tumor growing in your child's brain, the choice to wait for newer, superior treatments to come along may not be an option. In the case of our daughter Morgan, who was first diagnosed with a malignant medulloblastoma a few days before her second birthday, the decision to wait on having her undergo radiation therapy was a hard and complicated one. After a successful resection of her tumor, Morgan went on to receive six rounds of intense chemotherapy followed by a stem cell transplant. Afterward, her doctors requested that we follow her therapy with radiation treatments. Because of her age, not yet 3, we opted to not expose her to the powerful tool of radiation, which may have increased her chance of long-term survival but at the same time may have left her cognitive abilities severely handicapped. Our decision was not a hasty one. We also had well-respected doctors telling us not to do any other therapy, including radiation, because Morgan's chemo treatment was the most powerful of its day and some kids were actually achieving long-term survival without radiation.

Morgan stayed cancer free for 2 years. It was at Morgan's 2-year MRI scan that a small tumor was found—she had relapsed at the original tumor site. Now we had no choice but to treat Morgan with radiation therapy. What we immediately realized was that by waiting, we bought Morgan some time. Now almost 5, Morgan's cognitive development would fare better after radiation than if she were 3. What we didn't know was that technology in radiotherapy had improved greatly with the introduction of a sophisticated treatment called proton beam radiation. Different from the traditional method, proton beam causes less damage to the good brain cells and delivers a more direct hit to the tumor bed. The result, many doctors believe, is less damage to the good brain tissue (sparing cognitive impairment) and similar results for long-term survival as traditional radiation treatments.

Morgan received proton beam radiation for 6 weeks to her head and spine. Today she is 18 years old, a senior in high school, and is currently looking at colleges. Does she have learning disabilities? Yes. Are they stopping her from pursuing her dreams? No. She has continued to stay mainstream throughout her high school academic career with some support. She has been able to join the cross country team and run all 4 years of high school. She has a fun group of friends who she goes to movies with and hangs out with. She drives, has a job, and stresses about the clothes she is going to wear. She is a typical teenager who just happens to have had a brain tumor.

There is good reason to believe that the technological advances on the horizon will result in a more positive outlook for children and teens diagnosed in the future. These advances, combined with continued enrollment of children with brain and spinal cord tumors in national clinical trials, will expedite the identification of effective treatments.

The increased number of long-term survivors has raised awareness of late effects of the disease and treatments. The expansion of rehabilitative medicine has allowed for physical, occupational, and speech therapy to be available at home, at school, and in the community. Special education and the mandate for individualized educational programs provide appropriate education for children who have cognitive problems from the tumor or its treatment. Such programs have expanded to include career and college counseling.

As researchers, doctors, and nurses forge ahead in the fight to improve diagnosing and treating children with brain and spinal cord tumors, they share the same dreams of the patients and their families.

During the 30 years that I have spent as a nurse and a nurse practitioner, I have worked only with children with cancer. Twenty five of those years were spent working with children who have brain and spinal cord tumors. I have witnessed countless families coping with the diagnosis and treatment of their children. In the early days, there were no MRI scans, no venous catheters, and most children who had brain tumors died. As clinicians, we would sigh to ourselves with each new diagnosis thinking in the back of our minds, "How many months or years will this child live?"

Technological advances and laboratory research have completely changed the pessimism associated with brain and spinal cord tumors. We now know that many tumors can be cured or controlled with surgery. Chemotherapy and radiation can cure or control those that grow back or can't be removed with surgery. We have learned that to do nothing but watching often buys us time for a newer treatment that may come along. Aggressive research continues with the support of many groups organized by families of children with brain and spinal cord tumors to find a cure for each and every type of tumor.

In the bigger picture, it isn't the diseases or the treatments that I remember, it is the children:

- *Kristen who had four surgeries and 2 years of chemotherapy for her medulloblastoma, which was diagnosed when she was 9 months of age. She is now 25, a college graduate.*

- *Ryan had a brainstem and spinal cord tumor diagnosed at age 2 and underwent several surgeries and radiation. He couldn't move a muscle, was dependent on a respirator, and had a feeding tube because he could not swallow. I cried 4 years later when I got a holiday card with a picture of Ryan riding a bicycle. He is now 26.*

- *Brian, diagnosed at 15, underwent surgery, chemotherapy, and radiation. Ten years later, I went to his wedding. Three years ago, I got a birth announcement. He is the proud father of a daughter.*

- *Charlie was operated on at ages 4 and 8 for a brain stem tumor. He invited me to his bar mitzvah at 13, graduated from college, and emailed me recently that he is working in finance and applying to law school.*

- *Colette was diagnosed with a frontal lobe, low-grade astrocytoma after a seizure in 8th grade. It was surgically removed, and eventually she was taken off seizure medications and the seizures did not return. She wrote an excellent college essay based on her story and she is now a junior in college.*

There is reason to hope.

Appendix A

Blood Tests and What They Mean

KEEPING TRACK OF THEIR CHILD'S BLOOD counts becomes a way of life for parents of children with brain or spinal cord tumors. Unfortunately, misunderstandings about the implications of certain changes in blood values can cause unnecessary worry and fear. To help prevent these concerns, and to better enable parents to spot trends in the blood values of their child, this appendix explains the blood counts of healthy children, the blood counts of children being treated for brain or spinal cord tumors, and what each blood count value means.

Values for healthy children

Each laboratory and lab handbook has slightly different reference values for each type of blood test. There is also variation in values for children of different ages. For instance, in children ranging in age from newborn to 4 years, granulocytes are lower and lymphocytes are higher than the numbers listed below. The following table lists blood tests and blood count values for healthy children.

Blood Test Type	Values for Healthy Children
Hemoglobin (Hgb)	11.5 to 13.5 g/100 mL
Hematocrit (HCT)	34 to 40%
Red blood cells (RBCs)	3.9 to 5.3 million/cm^3 or 3.9 to 5.3 x 10^{12}/L
Platelets	160,000 to 380,000/mm^3
White blood cells (WBCs)	5,000 to 15,000/mm^3 or 5 to 15 K/uL
WBC differential:	
Segmented neutrophils	40 to 70%
Band neutrophils	1.5 to 8%
Basophils	<0.3%
Eosinophils	<0.5%
Lymphocytes	20 to 50%

Blood Test Type	Values for Healthy Children
Monocytes	2 to 10%
Liver function tests	
ALT (sometimes called SGPT)	0 to 48 IU/L
AST (sometimes called SGOT)	0 to 36 IU/L
Bilirubin (total)	0.3 to 1.3 mg/dL
Direct (conjugated)	0.1 to 0.4 mg/dL
Indirect (unconjugated)	0.2 to 1.88 mg/dL
Kidney function tests	
Blood urea nitrogen (BUN)	6 to 20 mg/dL
Creatinine	0.5 to 1.5 mg/dL
Electrolytes	
Carbon dioxide (CO2)	24 to 30 mEq/L
Chloride	98 to 108 mEq/
Glucose	70 to 115 mEq/L
Potassium	3.5 to 5.0 mEq/L
Sodium	135 to 145 mEq/L
Minerals	
Calcium	8.5 to 10.5 mg/dL
Magnesium	1.5 to 2.9 mg/dL

Values for children on chemotherapy

Blood test results of children being treated for brain and spinal cord tumors often fluctuate wildly. WBCs can go down to zero or be above normal. RBCs may go down periodically during treatment, necessitating transfusions of packed red cells. Platelet levels may also decrease, sometimes requiring platelet transfusions. Absolute neutrophil counts (ANC) are closely watched, as they give the doctor an idea of the child's ability to fight infections; ANCs vary from zero to in the thousands.

Neuro-oncologists consider all of the blood test results to get the total picture of a child's reaction to illness, chemotherapy, radiation, or infection. Trends are more important than any single value. For instance, if the values were 5.0, 4.7, and 4.9, then the second result (4.7) was insignificant. If, on the other hand, the values were 5.0, 4.7, and 4.3, then the trend would indicate a decrease in the cell line.

Children with brain and spinal cord tumors who are on medications for seizures or chemotherapy can have changes in kidney and liver function, along with changes in electrolytes and mineral levels in the blood. The section below describes the most common blood tests given to children with brain or spinal cord tumors. If you have any questions about your child's blood test results, ask the doctor for a clear explanation.

Common blood tests

The following sections explain each blood test listed in the table in section "Values for healthy children."

Hemoglobin (Hgb)

Red cells contain Hgb, the molecules that carry oxygen and carbon dioxide in the blood. Measuring Hgb gives doctors an exact picture of the ability of the child's blood to carry oxygen. Children may have low Hgb levels at diagnosis and during the intensive parts of treatment; this is because both cancer and chemotherapy decrease the bone marrow's ability to produce new red cells. Signs and symptoms of anemia—paleness, shortness of breath, fatigue—may occur if the Hgb gets very low.

Hematocrit (HCT)

The HCT is sometimes called the packed cell volume. The purpose of the HCT test is to determine the ratio of plasma (the clear liquid part of blood) to red cells in the blood. For this test, blood is drawn from a vein, a finger prick, or central catheter and is spun in a centrifuge to separate the red cells from the plasma. The HCT is the percentage of red cells in the blood. For example, if the child has a HCT of 30 percent, it means that 30 percent of the amount of blood drawn was red cells and the rest was plasma.

When a child is on chemotherapy, the bone marrow does not make many red cells and the HCT goes down. When the HCT is low, less oxygen is carried in the blood, so your child will have less energy. Your child may be given a transfusion of packed red cells if the HCT goes below 18 or 19 percent.

Red blood cell count (RBC)

Red blood cells are produced by the bone marrow continuously in healthy children and adults. These cells contain hemoglobin, which carries oxygen throughout the body. To determine the RBC, an automated electronic device is used to count the number of red cells in a blood sample.

White blood cell count (WBC)

The total WBC determines the body's ability to fight infection. Some treatments for brain and spinal cord tumor tumors kill healthy white cells or decrease the ability of the bone marrow to make new white cells. To determine the WBC, an automated electronic device counts the number of white cells in a blood sample.

White blood cell differential

When a child has blood drawn for a complete blood count (CBC), one section of the lab report will state the total WBC and a "differential," meaning that each type of white blood cell will be listed as a percentage of the total. For example, if the total WBC count is 1,500 mm³, the differential might appear as in the following table:

White Blood Cell Type	Percentage of Total WBC
Segmented neutrophils (also called polys or segs)	49%
Band neutrophils (also called bands)	1%
Basophils (also called basos)	1%
Eosinophils (also called eos)	1%
Lymphocytes (also called lymphs)	38%
Monocytes (also called monos)	10%

The differential is obtained by microscopic analysis of a blood sample on a slide.

Absolute neutrophil count (ANC)

The ANC (also called the absolute granulocyte count or AGC) is a measure of the body's ability to withstand infection. Generally, an ANC above 1,000 means the child's infection-fighting ability is near normal.

To calculate the ANC, add the percentages of neutrophils (both segmented and band) and multiply by the total WBC. Using the example above, the ANC is 49 percent + 1 percent = 50 percent, and 50 percent of 1,500 (.50 x 1,500) = 750, so the ANC is 750.

Platelet count

Platelets are needed to repair the body and stop bleeding by forming clots. Because platelets are produced by bone marrow, platelet counts decrease when a child is on chemotherapy. Signs of low platelet counts are bruises and bleeding from the gums or nose. When their platelets are low, children with a brain or spinal cord tumor should be watched carefully for symptoms of bleeding in the brain (such as sudden headache, seizures, or any other changes in level of consciousness). Platelet transfusions are sometimes given when the count is lower than 20,000 or when there is bleeding. Platelets are counted by passing a blood sample through an electronic device.

Alanine aminotransferase (ALT)

ALT is also called serum glutamic pyruvic transaminase (SGPT). When doctors talk about *liver functions,* they are usually referring to blood sample tests that measure liver damage. If chemotherapy is causing liver damage, the liver cells release an enzyme called ALT into the blood serum. ALT levels can go up into the hundreds, or even thousands, in some children on chemotherapy. Each institution and protocol has different points at which chemotherapy drug dosages are decreased or stopped to allow the child's liver to recover.

Aspartate aminotransferase (AST)

AST is also called serum glutamic oxaloacetic transaminase (SGOT). AST is an enzyme present in high concentrations in tissues with high metabolic activity, such as the liver. Severely damaged or killed cells release AST into the blood. The amount of AST in the blood is directly related to the amount of tissue damage. Therefore, if your child's liver is being damaged by chemotherapy, the AST count can rise into the thousands. Viral infections or reactions to an anesthetic can also cause an elevated AST.

Bilirubin

The liver converts hemoglobin released from damaged red cells into bilirubin. The liver then removes bilirubin from the blood and excretes it into bile, which is a fluid released into the small intestine to aid digestion. If too much bilirubin is present in the body, it causes a yellow color in the skin and whites of the eyes that is called jaundice.

The two types of bilirubin are indirect (also called unconjugated) and direct (also called conjugated). An increase in indirect bilirubin is seen when destruction of red cells has occurred, and an increase of direct bilirubin is seen when there is a dysfunction or blockage of the liver.

Blood urea nitrogen (BUN)

The BUN blood test is used to assess kidney function. It is also used to detect liver disease, dehydration, congestive heart failure, gastrointestinal bleeding, or shock. The test measures the amount of an end product of protein metabolism, called urea nitrogen, in the blood. For children with kidney or liver damage, BUN is often at abnormal levels.

Creatinine

Creatinine is a breakdown product of protein metabolism found in the urine and the blood. In children with brain or spinal cord tumors, creatinine is measured to assess kidney function. An elevated blood creatinine level is often seen in children with kidney insufficiency or failure.

Carbon dioxide (CO2)

The CO2 test measures the acidity of the blood. Low CO2 levels can be caused by chronic excessive breathing (hyperventilation). High CO2 levels in children with brain or spinal cord tumors indicate dysfunction in the brainstem, which controls breathing.

Chloride

Chloride helps the body maintain its normal balance of fluids. The most common chloride abnormality seen in children with brain or spinal cord tumors is a low chloride level caused by excessive sweating or fast breathing.

Glucose

The amount of glucose (sugar) in blood changes throughout the day, depending on when, what, and how much people eat, and whether or not they have exercised. A normal fasting (no food for 8 hours) blood glucose level is between 70 and 99 mg/dL. A normal blood sugar level 2 hours after eating is less than 140 mg/dL. Elevated glucose levels can occur in children with brain and spinal cord tumors who are taking steroids.

Potassium

Potassium is important for the proper functioning of the nerves and muscles, particularly the heartbeat. Too much or too little potassium increases the chance of irregular heartbeats. Potassium levels can be altered by chemotherapy or other treatments for children with brain or spinal cord tumors.

Sodium

The amount of sodium (salt) in the body is regulated by the brain, kidneys, and adrenal glands. Tumors in the pituitary, hypothalamus, or brainstem can cause high or low sodium levels. In addition to frequent blood tests for sodium levels, a careful record of urine output is necessary for children with abnormalities in sodium regulation. High blood sodium is associated with excessive urination, and low sodium levels result in low urine output.

Calcium and magnesium

Calcium and magnesium are minerals that can be compared to the spark plugs in your car—they spark the chemical reactions in your body needed to make it function properly. Calcium and magnesium also help to develop and maintain the strength of bones. In addition, magnesium is necessary for the development of muscle and for nerve conduction throughout the body. Many chemotherapy drugs given to children with brain or spinal cord tumors decrease the calcium and magnesium levels in the blood.

Your child's pattern

Each child develops a unique pattern of blood counts during treatment, and some parents like to track the changes. You can put lab sheets in a binder or enter blood test results in a computer program that shows trends over time. Doctors consider all of the laboratory results before deciding on a course of action. They should be willing to explain their plan so you can better understand what is happening and worry less.

If your child is participating in a clinical trial and you have obtained the entire clinical trial protocol (discussed in Chapter 5, *Choosing a Treatment*), it will contain a section that clearly outlines the actions that should be taken by the neuro-oncologist if certain changes in blood counts occur. For example, most protocols list each drug and when the dosage should be modified. The following is an example from a protocol for the drug vincristine.

Vincristine
  1.5 mg/m^2 (2 mg maximum) IV push weekly x 4 doses days 0, 7, 14, 21.

Seizures
  Hold one dose, then reinstitute.

Severe foot drop, paresis, or ilius
  Hold dose(s): when symptoms abate, resume at 1.0 mg/m^2; escalate to full dose as tolerated.

Jaw pain
  Treat with analgesics; do not modify vincristine dose.

Bilirubin
  Withhold if total bilirubin is >1.9 mg/dL.
  Administer 1/2 dose if total bilirubin is 1.5–1.9 mg/ dL.

Resource
Organizations

THE RESOURCE ORGANIZATIONS LISTED in this appendix are starting points for finding the information or help you need. The organizations are listed in the following order:

Pediatric neurosurgeons

The American Society of Pediatric Neurosurgeons
www.aspn.org/member-directory/active-members

Maintains an updated list of pediatric neurosurgeons and where they practice.

Brain tumor organizations (United States)

American Brain Tumor Association
(800) 886-2282
www.abta.org

Provides publications about brain tumors, holds patient conferences, offers support by telephone, publishes newsletters, and funds research.

Brain Tumor Foundation for Children, Inc.
(404) 252-4107
www.braintumorkids.org

Provides educational information, scholarships, and some financial assistance to families at specific institutions.

Children's Brain Tumor Foundation
(866) 228-4673
www.cbtf.org

Provides support for families and children, resource guides, funds for research, toll-free phone support by neuro-oncology social workers, and a peer mentoring program for parents.

Making Headway Foundation, Inc.
(914) 238-8384
www.makingheadway.org

Offers a variety of supportive services for families in the New York/New Jersey area, including in-hospital programs, educational programs, scholarships, and counseling with trained specialists.

National Brain Tumor Society
(617) 924-9997
www.braintumor.org

Provides information and advocacy opportunities, funds research, and promotes public policy initiatives.

Pediatric Brain Tumor Foundation of the United States
(800) 253-6530
www.curethekids.org

Funds childhood brain tumor research, development of educational materials, college scholarships for survivors, and Ride4Kids motorcycle charity events.

We Can, Pediatric Brain Tumor Network
(310) 739-3433
www.wecan.cc

Offers information and emotional support to all members of the family via educational programs, social events, and family camps. Services offered in Spanish.

Brain tumor organization (Canada)

Brain Tumour Foundation of Canada
(800) 265-5106
www.braintumour.ca

Supplies a free handbook, information line, support groups, chat groups, and educational conferences.

Brain tumor organization (Australia)

Brain Tumour Alliance Australia
(800) 857-221
www.btaa.org.au

Provides information, toll-free number for support, and representatives for advisory bodies.

Other service organizations (United States)

American Childhood Cancer Organization
(855) 858-2226
www.acco.org

ACCO (formerly Candlelighters Childhood Cancer Foundation) provides a toll-free information hotline, various handbooks to help families of children with cancer, and national advocacy.

American Speech-Language-Hearing Association (ASHA)
(800) 638-8255
www.asha.org

Provides referrals to local speech/language/hearing specialists.

Cancer Care
(800) 813-HOPE / (800) 813-4673
www.cancercare.org

Provides referrals, one-on-one counseling, specialized support groups, and educational programs.

Chai Lifeline/Camp Simcha
(877) CHAI-LIFE / (877) 242-4543 or (212) 465-1300
www.chailifeline.org

Provides support service programs to Jewish children and their families, including medical referrals, support groups, visits to hospitalized and housebound children, financial aid, transportation, and a camp for kids with cancer.

Epilepsy Foundation of America
(800) 332-1000
www.epilepsy.com

Provides support nationally and locally for seizure management at home and school, sponsors self-help groups and summer camps, provides information about laws and legal rights, and hosts forums for discussion.

Flashes of Hope
(440) 442-9700
www.flashesofhope.org

Creates powerful, uplifting photographic portraits of children fighting cancer and other life-threatening illnesses.

Hydrocephalus Association
(888) 598-3789
www.hydroassoc.org

Provides support, education, and advocacy through conferences, newsletters, and informational pamphlets. Materials available in Spanish.

National Association for Parents of Children with Visual Impairments
(800) 562-6265
www.spedex.com/napvi
www.familyconnect.org

Maintains a national support network via telephone and mail correspondence; provides publications, information, referrals, conferences, outreach programs; and publishes a quarterly newsletter.

National Center for Complementary and Alternative Medicine
(888) 644-6226
http://nccam.nih.gov

Dedicated to exploring complementary and alternative healing practices in the context of rigorous science; training researchers; and disseminating authoritative information.

National Hydrocephalus Foundation
(888) 857-3434
www.nhfonline.org

Membership entitles families to quarterly newsletters, publications, access to a reference library, and peer mentors.

Physician Data Query (PDQ)
(800) 4-CANCER / (800) 422-6237
www.cancer.gov/cancertopics/pdq

PDQ is the National Cancer Institutes' computerized listing of accurate and up-to-date information for patients and health professionals about cancer treatments, research studies, and clinical trials.

Ronald McDonald House Charities
(630) 623-7048
http://rmhc.org

Committed to helping families of seriously ill children by providing Ronald McDonald Houses, the Ronald McDonald Learning Program, and Ronald McDonald Family Rooms within hospitals.

Songs of Love Foundation
(800) 960-SONG / (800) 960-7664
www.songsoflove.org

Volunteer group of more than 200 artists who produce personalized musical portraits for children with chronic or life-threatening diseases.

Other service organization (Canada)

Childhood Cancer Canada Foundation
(800) 363-1062
www.childhoodcancer.ca

Invests in collaborative cancer research and provides support programs for families, such as a teen connector website, scholarships for survivors, and financial assistance.

Other service organizations (Australia)

CanTeen, The Australian Organization for Young People Living with Cancer
National Office
www.canteen.org.au

Provides support services for young people aged 12 to 24. Programs include face-to-face counseling, phone support, peer mentors, and printed resources.

Challenge Foundation
www.challenge.org.au

Offers services for families who have children with cancer. Programs include camps, hospital support, respite and holiday accommodations, parent support, and family activity days

Childhood Cancer Association
www.childhoodcancer.asn.au/services

South Australia organization dedicated to providing emotional, practical, and financial support to families. Programs include peer, family, and sibling support; accommodations for families from rural areas; respite support; educational assistance; and bereavement services.

Childhood Cancer Support
www.ccs.org.au

Provides counseling, financial assistance, recreational therapy activities, and most importantly, love and support.

Humour Foundation
www.humourfoundation.com.au

The Humour Foundation's core project is Clown Doctors, which touches the lives of more than 100,000 people every year. The focus is children's hospitals, and Clown Doctors are now part of hospital life in all major children's hospitals around Australia.

Ronald McDonald Children's Charities
www.rmhc.org.au

Committed to helping families of seriously ill children by providing Ronald McDonald Houses, the Ronald McDonald Learning Program, Ronald McDonald Family Rooms within hospitals, and the Ronald McDonald Family Retreat (free holiday accommodations).

Country Care Link
www.sistersofcharityoutreach.com.au

Provides support and hospitality to country people visiting Sydney for medical purposes; has been assisting rural families since 1992.

Camps

For a comprehensive list of camps for children with cancer, visit *www.acor.org/ped-onc/cfissues/camps.html*.

Camp Simcha
(877) CHAI-LIFE / (877) 242-4543 or (212) 465-1300
www.chailifeline.org

A camp run by the national, nonprofit Jewish organization Chai Lifeline.

Children's Oncology Camping Association International
(404) 661-5723
www.cocai.org

Umbrella organization of groups that provide camps for children with cancer.

Camp Quality (Australia)
www.campquality.org.au

Provides fun therapy for children and families of children with cancer, including camps for ill children and their siblings, family camps, fun days, pamper days for moms and daughters, and fishing weekends for fathers and sons.

Clinical trials

American Brain Tumor Association's TrialConnect™
(877) 769-4833
www.abtatrialconnect.org

The American Brain Tumor Association's clinical trial matching service.

Educational and legal support

The Disability Rights Education and Defense Fund
(800) 348-4232
www.dredf.org

Trains and educates people with disabilities and parents of children with disabilities about their rights under state and federal disability rights laws; educates lawyers, service providers, government officials, and others about disability civil rights laws and policies.

Federation for Children with Special Needs
(617) 236-7210
www.fcsn.org

Federally funded organization with representation in every state that provides information about special education rights and laws, conferences, referrals for services, parent training workshops, publications, and advocacy information.

Job Accommodation Network (JAN)
(800) 526-7234
www.jan.wvu.edu

Facilitates the employment and retention of workers with disabilities by providing employers, employment providers, people with disabilities, their family members, and other interested parties with information about job accommodations, entrepreneurship, and related subjects.

Learning Disabilities Association of America
(412) 341-1515
www.ldanatl.org

Serves parents, professionals, and individuals with learning disabilities; has local chapters and provides educational materials.

National Center for Learning Disabilities
(888) 575-7373
www.ncld.org

Offers extensive resources, referral services, and educational programs about learning disabilities. Promotes public awareness and advocates for effective legislation to help people with learning disabilities.

U.S. Department of Justice ADA Information Line
(800) 514-0301
TTY: (800) 514-0383
www.ada.gov

Answers questions about the Americans with Disabilities Act (ADA), explains how to file a complaint, and provides dispute resolution.

Financial help

First Hand Foundation
(816) 201-1569
www.firsthandfoundation.org

Assists children who have health-related needs when insurance and other sources of financial resources have been exhausted.

Friends4Michael Foundation
(845) 774-4809
www.friends4michael.org

Provides financial assistance to families of children being treated for a brain tumor. Requests must be submitted by a social worker.

National Children's Cancer Society
(800) 532-6459
www.nationalchildrenscancersociety.org

Serves as a financial, emotional, and educational resource for families that can't make ends meet when their child is diagnosed with cancer. Since inception, has provided more than $57 million in direct financial assistance to more than 33,000 children nationwide.

Free air services (United States)

Air Charity Network
(877) 621-7177
http://aircharitynetwork.org

Made up of independent member organizations identified by specific geographical service areas. These organizations are groups of volunteer pilots or groups that coordinate free airline tickets or reduced-price ambulatory services.

Air Care Alliance
(888) 260-9707
www.aircarealliance.org

Nationwide association of humanitarian flying organizations that provides flights for medical treatment.

Angel Flight America
(800) 296-3797
www.angelflightmidatlantic.org

Provides free transportation to medical treatment for people who cannot afford public transportation or who cannot tolerate it for health reasons. (A member of Air Charity Network.)

Miles For Kids In Need (American Airlines)
www.aa.com/kids

Provides free travel for ill children and their families. A third party, such as a charitable organization, hospital, or other tax-exempt organization, must submit travel requests.

Corporate Angel Network, Inc.
(866) 328-1313
www.corpangelnetwork.org

Gives patients with cancer available seats on corporate aircraft to get to and from recognized cancer treatment centers. Patients must be able to walk and travel without life-support systems or medical attention. A child may be accompanied by up to two adults. There is no cost or financial-need requirements.

Mercy Medical Airlift
(800) 296-1217
http://mercymedical.org

Dedicated to serving people in situations of compelling human need through the provision of charitable air transportation. (A member of Air Charity Network.)

Miracle Flights for Kids
(800) FLY-1711 / (800) 359-1711 or (702) 261-0494
www.miracleflights.org

Purchases commercial airline tickets, uses private aircrafts, and combines resources from individual donors to provide free transportation to medical treatment centers all across America.

PatientTravel.org
24-hour hot line: (800) 296-1217
www.patienttravel.org

Refers callers to the most appropriate, cost-effective charitable or commercial services, including volunteer pilot organizations and special airline transport programs. (A member of Air Charity Network.)

Free air service (Canada)

Hope Air
(877) 346-HOPE / (877) 346-4673
www.hopeair.org

Provides free air transport to Canadians in financial need who must travel from their communities to recognized facilities for medical care.

Free air service (Australia)

Angel Flight Australia
www.angelflight.org.au

Coordinates free, non-emergency flights to help people dealing with bad health, poor finances, and daunting distances.

Insurance

Patient Advocate Foundation (PAF)
(800) 532-5274
www.patientadvocate.org

Offers a legal resource network of attorneys who provide pro bono (free) advice; helps mediate disputes with insurance companies by acting as a liaison; and provides publications about managed care and health insurance appeals.

Medications (low-cost or free)

Partnership for Prescription Assistance
(888) 477-2669
www.pparx.org

Helps find companies and agencies that provide prescription medicines free of charge to physicians whose patients might not otherwise have access to necessary medicines.

RxHope
(877) 267-0517
www.rxhope.com

Lists patient-assistance programs that are offered by federal, state, and charitable organizations.

PatientAssistance.com, Inc.
www.patientassistance.com

Helps uninsured patients get free medication.

NeedyMeds, Inc.
www.needymeds.org

Helps people who cannot afford medicine or healthcare costs. The information at NeedyMeds is available anonymously and free of charge.

Sports organizations

PATH International
Professional Association of Therapeutic Horsemanship International
(800) 369-RIDE / (800) 369-7433
www.pathintl.org

Lists accredited therapeutic riding programs all over the world, offers educational resources, and hosts conferences about equine-assisted activities and therapies.

Special Olympics, Inc.
www.specialolympics.org

International program of year-round sports training and athletic competition for more than 1 million children and adults with cognitive challenges.

Stem cell transplantation

BMT InfoNet (blood and marrow transplant information network)
(888) 597-7674
www.bmtinfonet.org

Provides transplant patients and their loved ones with emotional support and high quality, easy-to-understand information about bone marrow, peripheral blood stem cell, and cord blood transplants.

Children's Organ Transplant Association (COTA)
(800) 366-2682
www.cota.org

Provides fundraising help for families with children who need transplants (including stem cell transplants).

HelpHopeLive
(800) 642-8399
www.helphopelive.org

Provides fundraising assistance and donor awareness materials to transplant and catastrophic injury patients nationwide.

Wish-fulfillment organizations (United States)

In addition to the large organizations listed below, there are many smaller and local organizations that grant wishes to seriously ill children. A comprehensive list of wish fulfillment organizations can be found online at *www.acor.org/ped-onc/cfissues/maw.html*.

Children's Wish Foundation International
(800) 323-WISH / (800) 323-9474
www.childrenswish.org

Fulfills the wishes of children with life-threatening illnesses in the United States and Europe.

Clayton Dabney Foundation for Kids with Cancer
(214) 361-2600
http://claytondabney.org

Provides last wishes and financial assistance to families of terminally ill children.

The Dream Factory, Inc.
(800) 456-7556
www.dreamfactoryinc.com

Grants the wishes of children ages 3 to 18 who are critically or chronically ill (has chapters in 30 states).

Make-a-Wish Foundation of America
(800) 722-WISH / (800) 722-9474
www.wish.org

Grants wishes to children under the age of 18 with life-threatening illnesses (has U.S. and international chapters and affiliates).

Sunshine Foundation
(215) 396-4770
www.sunshinefoundation.org

Grants wishes to chronically or terminally ill children ages 3 to 18 (no geographic boundaries).

Wish-fulfillment organization (Canada)

The Children's Wish Foundation of Canada
(905) 427-5353
www.childrenswish.ca

Provides a once-in-a-lifetime experience for children ages 3 to 18 with high-risk, life-threatening diseases (has chapters throughout Canada).

Wish-fulfillment organizations (Australia)

Make-A-Wish Foundation of Australia National Office
www.makeawish.org.au

Grants seriously ill children in Australia their most-cherished wish.

Starlight Children's Foundation Australia
www.starlight.org.au

Brightens the lives of seriously ill and hospitalized children and their families throughout Australia by granting wishes, providing vans that travel to remote hospitals to cheer children's lives, and offering activities, entertainment, and social engagement in hospital Starlight Rooms.

Hospice and bereavement (United States)

Children's Hospice International

(703) 684-0330

www.chionline.org

Provides resources and referrals for children and families of children with life-threatening conditions.

The Compassionate Friends National Office

(877) 969-0010 or (630) 990-0010

www.compassionatefriends.org

Offers understanding and friendship to bereaved families through support meetings at local chapters and telephone support (they match people with similar losses). Publishes a newsletter for parents and one for siblings.

Hospice and bereavement (Canada)

Canadian Network of Pediatric Hospices

http://cnph.ca

Fosters collaboration and sharing among pediatric residential hospices in Canada.

Hospice and bereavement (Australia)

Bear Cottage

www.bearcottage.chw.edu.au

New South Wales's only children's hospice, located on the grounds of St Patrick's Estate, near Sydney. It offers both respite and palliative care to children and young people with life-limiting illnesses and their families.

The Compassionate Friends New South Wales

www.tcfnsw.org.au

Assists families in the positive resolution of grief following the death of a child and provides information to help others be supportive.

Palliative Care Australia

www.palliativecare.org.au

Represents the interests and aspirations of all who share the ideal of quality care at the end of life for all.

Books and Websites

A WEALTH OF INFORMATION about childhood brain and spinal cord tumors is available through libraries and computers. This appendix briefly describes how to get the most from these resources and lists specific books and websites that you might find helpful when conducting research on your child's medical condition or treatment.

You might find there are some print books you wish to own. If they are not in stock at your local or online bookstore, ask if they can be special-ordered for you—most bookstores are happy to do this for customers. Copies of out-of-print books can often be located on the Internet through used bookstores or private sellers on sites such as Amazon.com. Ebooks are available in many different formats and from many online booksellers (e.g., *www.amazon.com, www.barnesandnoble.com*) or from local libraries.

How to get information from your library or computer

Libraries have a computerized database of all materials available in their various branches, although some libraries may still use a manual card catalog system. If you need help learning how to use these book-locating systems, ask a librarian. You can also learn how to request a book from another branch and how to put a book on hold if it is currently checked out.

If a book is not in your library's collection, ask a reference librarian if it can be obtained from another library via interlibrary loan. This is common practice, and you might be able to get medical texts from university or medical school libraries. Some local libraries also have online databases that list all publications available at regional libraries; this way, you can look up a book on the Internet, find out which library has it, and request that it be sent to your local library for pick up.

If you want to read medical journal articles, you can access them through your local library. The librarian can show you how to use the database to search for articles and where to find the periodicals. Public libraries often subscribe to only the most popular medical journals, such as the *New England Journal of Medicine* and *Journal of the American Medical Association*. If you are able to visit a university or medical school library, you will find many more print medical journals available. If you do not live close to one of these libraries, ask your local librarian to help you obtain copies of the articles you want.

An astonishing amount of information is available through the Internet. Libraries from all over the world can be accessed, and you can download information in minutes from huge databases such as MedLine or Cancerlit. Obtaining information from large medical databases, established journals, or large libraries is exceedingly helpful for parents at home with sick children. However, the huge numbers of people using the Internet has spawned websites, chat rooms, and social media sites that may or may not contain accurate information. You may want to read information from only reliable sources and adopt the motto: "Let the buyer beware."

If you do not have a home computer, many libraries provide Internet access. Ask the librarian to help you connect to MedLine, Physician's Data Query (PDQ), or other databases you wish to search.

Books

Below are some print books (many are also available as ebooks) that parents of children with brain and spinal cord tumors have found helpful.

Treatment journals

Alex's Lemonade Stand Treatment Journal. The Alex's Lemonade Stand Foundation provides a free treatment journal to help parents of children with cancer keep track of important information. Parents can request a hard copy of the journal or can create their own online journal at *www.alexslemonade.org/childhood-cancer-treatment-journal*.

Lazar, Linda; Crawford, Bonnie. *In My World.* (1999). Available by calling (866) 218-0101 or visiting *www.centering.org*. Journal for teens coping with life-threatening illnesses. Includes chapters called "Things Accomplished in My Life," "I've Been Thinking," and "Questions I'd Like Answered."

Technical reading

Bleyer, Archie; Barr, Ronald. *Cancer in Adolescents and Young Adults.* (2007). Medical textbook.

Institute of Medicine. *Childhood Cancer Survivorship, Improving Care and Quality of Life.* (2003). Comprehensive coverage of survivorship issues, including late effects of treatment and how to obtain survivorship care. Available as full text online or as a paperback ($29.70) through the National Academies Press website at *www.nap.edu*.

Keating, Robert; Goodrich, James; Packer, Robert. *Tumors of the Pediatric Central Nervous System, 2nd ed.* (2013). Medical textbook.

Physicians' Desk Reference. (2013). Reference book, published yearly, which contains accurate information about all Food and Drug Administration approved drugs. Technical language. Available at the reference desk in most libraries.

Pizzo, Philip A. and Poplack, David, eds. *Principles and Practice of Pediatric Oncology, 6th ed.* (2010). Medical textbook.

Memoirs

Fesler, Rene. *Alicia's Updates: A Mother's Memoir of Pediatric Cancer.* (2009). This book chronicles a family's journey through Alicia's treatment for a spinal cord tumor and the impact it had on their family and those around them. Honest and friendly, this book helps parents of a child with cancer feel less alone.

Strumpf, Katie. *I Never Signed Up for This! An Upfront Guide to Dealing with Cancer at a Young Age.* (2006). Written by a 25-year-old survivor with an upbeat attitude, this book covers returning to school, dealing with parents and doctors, losing your hair, and dealing with the fear of death.

MacLellan, Scott. *Amanda's Gift.* (1998). A review of the emotional and financial impact of a child's 7-year fight with cancer and other illnesses, including a liver transplant. It covers the complexities of insurance coverage and all areas of life as a caregiver, including the impact on faith and marriage.

Domozych, Patrice Mary; Buggee, Heather; Condra, Stephanie. *Hope Is Here To Stay.* (2009). A 35-page illustrated story about Lauren, her family, and her treatment for a pediatric brain tumor.

General reading (for adults)

American Brain Tumor Association (ABTA). *About Brain Tumors: A Primer for Patients and Caregivers.* (2012). Available free online at *www.abta.org/secure/about-brain-tumors-a-primer.pdf.* The ABTA also publishes many informational pamphlets about specific types of brain and spinal cord tumors and individual treatments, including *Chemotherapy; Ependymoma; Glioblastoma and Malignant Astrocytoma; Medulloblastoma; Conventional Radiation Therapy; Stereotactic Radiosurgery;* and many others.

Bracken, Jean Munn. *Children with Cancer: A Comprehensive Reference Guide for Parents.* (2010). Comprehensive coverage of childhood cancers, written by a librarian who is the parent of a survivor of a rare cancer.

Cochran, Lizzie. *Singing Away: Stories of Faith, Hope & Love in the Fight Against Childhood Cancer.* (2013). True stories written by families of children with cancer.

Jampolsky, Gerald G. *Advice to Doctors and Other Big People from Kids*. (1991). Book full of stories from children with catastrophic illnesses that offers suggestions and expresses their feelings about healthcare workers. Wise and poignant, it reminds us how perceptive and aware children of all ages are, and how necessary it is to involve them in medical decisions.

Kushner, Harold. *When Bad Things Happen to Good People, revised ed.* (2004). Rabbi Kushner wrote this comforting book about how people of faith deal with catastrophic events.

National Cancer Institute. *21st Century Pediatric Cancer Sourcebook: Brain and Spinal Cord Tumors*. (2011). Starting with the basics, and advancing to detailed patient-oriented and physician-quality information, this comprehensive ebook gives families, caregivers, nurses, and doctors information about the diagnosis and treatment of these diseases.

National Cancer Institute. *Young People with Cancer: A Handbook for Parents*. This booklet describes the different types of childhood cancer, medical procedures, dealing with the diagnosis, family issues, and sources of information. To obtain a free copy, call (800-4-CANCER) / (800) 422-6237, or read it at *www.cancer.gov/cancertopics/youngpeople*.

Sourkes, Barbara M. *Armfuls of Time: The Psychological Experience of the Child with a Life-Threatening Illness*. (1996). Written by a psychologist, this eloquent book features the voices and artwork of children with cancer. It clearly describes the psychological effects of cancer on children and explains the power of the therapeutic process.

Woznick, Leigh; Goodheart, Carol. *Living With Childhood Cancer: A Practical Guide to Help Families Cope*. (2001). Written by a mother–daughter team, this book draws on the authors' experiences with cancer, as well as their professional expertise and stories from others to help families address the psychological impact of childhood cancer.

Zeltzer, Paul. *Brain Tumors: Leaving the Garden of Eden—A Survival Guide to Diagnosis, Learning the Basics, Getting Organized, and Finding Your Medical Team*. (2004). This book includes chapters about all major types of brain tumors, medications, using the Internet to search for information, and getting a second opinion.

General reading (for children)

Bourgeois, Paulette. *Franklin Goes to the Hospital*. (2000). Franklin the turtle goes to the hospital for an operation to repair his broken shell, and everyone thinks he's being very brave. But Franklin is only pretending to be fearless. He's worried that his x-rays will show just how frightened he is inside. For young children.

Crary, Elizabeth. *Dealing with Feelings. I'm Frustrated; I'm Mad; I'm Sad Series*. (1992). Fun, game-like books to teach young children how to handle feelings and solve problems.

Gaynor, Kate. *The Famous Hat: A Storybook.* (2008). This book helps children with cancer prepare for hospitalization, chemotherapy, and hair loss.

Keene, Nancy; Romain, Trevor. *Chemo, Craziness & Comfort: My Book About Childhood Cancer.* (2002). A 200-page resource that provides practical information for children diagnosed with cancer between 6 and 12 years of age. Warm and funny illustrations and easy-to-read text help the child (and parents) make sense of cancer and its treatment. Available free from *www.acco.org/Information/Resources/Books.aspx.*

Krisher, Trudy. *Kathy's Hats: A Story of Hope.* (1992). A charming book, for children ages 5 to 10, about a girl whose love of hats comes in handy when chemotherapy makes her hair fall out.

Richmond, Christina. *Chemo Girl: Saving the World One Treatment at a Time.* (1996). Written by a 12-year-old girl with rhabdomyosarcoma, this book describes a superhero who shares hope and encouragement.

Rogers, Fred. *Going to the Hospital.* (1997). With pictures and words, TV's beloved Mr. Rogers helps children ages 3 to 8 learn about hospitals.

General reading (for teens)

Dorfman, Elena. *The C-Word: Teenagers and Their Families Living with Cancer.* (1998). Contains photos and the stories of five teenagers with cancer.

Gravelle, Karen. *Teenagers Face to Face With Cancer.* (2000). Sixteen teenagers talk openly about their experiences with cancer—from the physical difficulties of coping with treatment to the emotional trauma, which can be as painful as the illness itself. A heartfelt, honest book that demonstrates clearly how having cancer changes young people and how strength can emerge from struggles.

General reading (for siblings)

American Cancer Society. *When Your Brother or Sister Has Cancer.* To obtain a free copy, call (800) 227-2345. This 16-page booklet describes the emotions felt by siblings of a child with cancer.

O'Toole, Donna. *Aarvy Aardvark Finds Hope: A Read Aloud Story for People of All Ages About Loving and Losing, Friendship and Hope.* (1988). Aarvy Aardvark and his friend Ralphie Rabbit show how a family member or friend can help another in distress.

Dodd, Mike. *Oliver's Story.* (2004). A 40-page illustrated book for 3- to 8-year old siblings of children diagnosed with cancer. Order a free copy from *www.acco.org/Information/Resources/Books.aspx.*

Peterkin, Allan. *What About Me? When Brothers and Sisters Get Sick.* (1992). Describes the feelings of siblings whose brother or sister is hospitalized.

Diffuse intrinsic pontine gilioma (DIPG)

Hoffman, Ruth (editor). *Understanding the Journey, A Parent's Guide to DIPG.* (2012). A comprehensive resource with chapters written by pediatric neuro-oncology experts that covers all aspects of treating a child with DIPG. Order a free copy from *www. acco.org/Information/Resources/Books.aspx.*

Hydrocepahalus

About Hydrocephalus: A Guide for Patients and Families. Free booklet from the Hydrocephalus Association available at *www.hydroassoc.org.*

Mohanty, Aaron. *100 Questions & Answers About Hydrocephalus.* (2011). Provides authoritative, straightforward answers to the most common questions asked by children with hydrocephalus and their parents.

Radiation

National Cancer Institute. *Radiation Therapy and You: Support for People With Cancer.* (2007). A 52-page booklet that explains conventional radiation, what to expect, possible side effects, and follow-up care. Available online at *www.cancer.gov/ cancertopics/coping/radiation-therapy-and-you.*

School

Hoffman, Ruth (editor). *Educating the Child With Cancer: A Guide for Parents and Teachers, 2nd ed.* (2011). An book written by top researchers in the field that includes parents' personal experiences. Order a free copy from *www.acco.org/Information/Resources/ Books.aspx.*

Leukemia and Lymphoma Society. *Living and Learning with Cancer.* Booklet about returning to school and obtaining accommodations (appropriate for children with any type of cancer). Available at *www.lls.org/content/nationalcontent/resourcecenter/ freeeducationmaterials/childhoodbloodcancer/pdf/learninglivingwithcancer.pdf.*

Princeton Review. *K&W Guide to College Programs and Services for Students with Learning Disabilities or Attention Deficit/Hyperactivity Disorder, 11th ed.* (2011). Excellent reference that is available at most large libraries.

Silver, Larry. *The Misunderstood Child: Understanding and Coping with Your Child's Learning Disabilities, 4th ed.* (2006). Comprehensive discussion about positive treatment strategies that can be implemented at home and in school to help children with learning disabilities.

Siblings

Faber, Adele; Mazlish, Elaine. *Siblings Without Rivalry: How to Help Your Children Live Together So You Can Live Too, revised edition.* (2012). Offers dozens of simple and effective methods to reduce conflict and foster a cooperative spirit. Helpful information for all stressed parents.

Murray, Gloria; Jamplosky, Gerald (editors). *Straight from the Siblings: Another Look at the Rainbow.* (1995). Written by 16 children who have brothers and sisters with a life-threatening illness who met at the Center for Attitudinal Healing. A must-read for both parents and siblings.

Stem cell transplantation

Stewart, Susan. *Bone Marrow and Blood Stem Cell Transplants: A Book of Basics for Patients.* Available by calling (888) 597-7674 or visiting *www.bmtinfonet.org.* A 228-page book that clearly explains the medical aspects of bone marrow and blood stem cell transplantation, the different types of transplants, emotional and psychological considerations, pediatric transplants, complications, and insurance issues. Technically accurate, yet easy to read.

Stewart, Susan. *Autologous Stem Cell Transplants: A Handbook for Patients.* (2000). Order by calling (888) 597-7674 or visiting *www.bmtinfonet.org.*

Survivorship

Keene, Nancy; Hobbie, Wendy; Ruccione, Kathy. *Childhood Cancer Survivors: A Practical Guide to Your Future, 3rd ed.* (2012). A user-friendly, comprehensive guide about late effects of treatment for childhood cancer. Full of stories from survivors of all types of childhood cancer. Also covers emotional issues, insurance, jobs, relationships, and ways to stay healthy.

Terminal illness and bereavement

Callanan, Maggie; Kelley, Patricia. *Final Gifts: Understanding the Special Awareness, Needs, and Communications of the Dying.* (2012). Written by two hospice nurses with decades of experience, this book helps families understand and communicate with terminally ill patients. Compassionate, comforting, and insightful, *this book* movingly teaches how to listen to and comfort the dying.

Orloff, Stacy; Huff, Susan (editors). *Home Care for the Seriously Ill Child: A Manual for Parents.* (2003). Available from Children's Hospice International by calling (800) 242-4453 or online at *http://75.103.82.45/publications-hospice-care-programs-and-support.* Helps parents explore the possibility of home care for the dying child. Contains practical information about what to expect, methods of pain relief, and management of medical problems.

Price, Mary Kathleen. *Dance When the Brain Says No.* (2009). A mother's memoir about her vivacious and strong-willed daughter who was diagnosed with medulloblastoma when she was 19 and died 2½ years later.

Bereavement: A Magazine of Hope and Healing. For a free copy or to subscribe, call (888) 604-4673 or go online at *www.bereavementmag.com.*

Bernstein, Judith R. *When the Bough Breaks: Forever After the Death of a Son or Daughter.* (1998). A serious and sensitive book about how to cope with the loss of a child.

Kubler-Ross, Elisabeth. *On Children and Death: How Children and Their Parents Can and Do Cope With Death.* (1997). In this comforting book, Dr. Kubler-Ross offers practical help for living through the terminal period of a child's life with love and understanding. Discusses children's knowledge about death, visualization, letting go, funerals, help from friends, and spirituality.

Wild, Laynee. *I Remember You: A Grief Journal, 2nd ed.* (2000). A journal for recording written and photographic memories during the first year of mourning. Beautiful book filled with quotes and comfort.

Sibling grief (adult reading)

Grollman, Earl. *Talking About Death: A Dialogue Between Parent and Child, 4th ed.* (2011). One of the best books for helping children cope with grief. Contains a children's read-along section to explain and explore children's feelings. In very comforting language, the book teaches parents how to explain death, understand children's emotions, understand how children react to specific types of death, and know when to seek professional help.

Schaefer, Dan; Lyons, Christine. *How Do We Tell the Children? A Step-by-Step Guide for Helping Children and Teens Cope When Someone Dies, 4th ed.* (2010). If your terminally ill child has siblings, read this book. In straightforward, uncomplicated language, the authors describe how to explain the facts of death to children and teens and show how to include the children in the family support network, laying the foundation for the healing process to begin. Also includes a crisis section for quick references about what to do in a variety of situations.

White, P. Gill. *Sibling Grief: Healing After the Death of a Sister or Brother.* (2008). Endorsed by the Bereaved Parents of the USA, this book validates the emotional significance of sibling loss, drawing on clinical experience, research, and wisdom from hundreds of bereaved siblings to explain the five healing tasks specific to sibling grief.

Sibling grief (young child)

Buscaglia, Leo. *The Fall of Freddy the Leaf: A Story of Life for All Ages.* (1982). This wise yet simple story about a leaf named Freddy explains death as a necessary part of the cycle of life.

Hickman, Martha. *Last Week My Brother Anthony Died.* (1984). A touching story of a preschooler's feelings when her infant brother dies. The family's minister (a bereaved parent himself) comforts her by comparing feelings to clouds—always there but ever changing.

Mellonie, Bryan; Ingpen, Robert. *Lifetimes: The Beautiful Way to Explain Death to Children.* (1983). Beautiful paintings and simple text explain that dying is as much a part of life as being born.

Sibling grief (school-aged children)

Romain, Trevor. *What on Earth Do You Do When Someone Dies?* (1999). Warm, honest words and beautiful illustrations help children understand and cope with grief.

Temes, Roberta. *The Empty Place: A Child's Guide Through Grief.* (1992). Explains and describes feelings after the death of a sibling, such as the empty place in the house, at the table, and in a sibling's heart.

Sibling grief (teenagers)

Gravelle, Karen; Haskins, Charles. *Teenagers Face to Face with Bereavement.* (2000). The perspectives and experiences of 17 teenagers comprise the heart of this book, which focuses on teens coping with grief.

Grollman, Earl. *Straight Talk About Death for Teenagers: How to Cope with Losing Someone You Love.* (1993). Wonderful book that talks to teens, not at them. Discusses denial, pain, anger, sadness, physical symptoms, and depression. Charts methods to help teens work through their feelings at their own pace.

Websites

This section lists websites that are not listed in Appendix B, *Resources,* but that many parents find helpful. As with any resource, check with your child's treatment team about the accuracy of any information found on websites.

Dictionary

National Cancer Institute Dictionary of Cancer Terms
www.cancer.gov/dictionary

Education

Wrightslaw
www.wrightslaw.com

Accurate, up-to-date information about special educational law for parents, advocates, and attorneys.

General online medical resources

Clinical Trials and Noteworthy Treatments for Brain Tumors
Musella Foundation for Brain Tumor Research and Information
www.virtualtrials.com

Descriptions of and discussions about clinical trials and noteworthy treatments for brain tumors. Website features a brain tumor guide, survivor stories, a video library, links, and support group information.

Medline Plus
www.nlm.nih.gov/medlineplus/druginformation.html

A service of the National Institutes of Health, this site provides accurate information about drugs, including precautions and side effects.

National Cancer Institute
www.cancer.gov

A huge, reliable site that provides accurate information about cancer, treatments, and clinical trials.

Pediatric Oncology Resource Center
www.acor.org/ped-onc

Excellent source of information about pediatric cancers created and managed by a mother of a long-term survivor. Contains detailed and accurate material about diseases, treatment, family issues, activism, bereavement, and survivorship. Also provides links to other helpful cancer sites.

PubMed
www.ncbi.nlm.nih.gov/PubMed

The National Library of Medicine's free search service provides access to more than 23 million citations in MEDLINE and PREMEDLINE (with links to participating online journals) and other related databases.

Quackwatch
www.quackwatch.com

International network of people who post information about health-related frauds, myths, fads, fallacies, and misconduct.

Rx List—The Internet Drug Index
www.rxlist.com

Accurate information about prescription medications. Also contains a medical dictionary.

Squirreltales
www.squirreltales.com

An uplifting and practical website that encourages and empowers parents of children with cancer when they are feeling discouraged and powerless.

Online support groups

Be sure to check the accuracy of any information obtained from an online support group with members of your child's treatment team.

ACOR, The Association of Cancer Online Resources, Inc.
www.acor.org

ACOR is a unique collection of 142 online cancer communities and is designed to provide timely and accurate information in a supportive environment. It hosts several pediatric cancer discussion groups, including PED-ONC (a general pediatric cancer discussion group), Medulloblastoma and PNET, and PED-ONC-SURVIVORS (for parents of survivors).

The Healing Exchange Brain Trust
www.braintrust.org

Host to a number of online support groups, including the large Braintmr list, craniopharyngioma list, and ependymoma parents' list.

Jenna's Corner
www.jennasrainbow.org/jennas_corner.html

Online community sponsored by Jenna's Rainbow and the Children's Brain Tumor Foundation to help family members of children with brain or spinal cord tumors gain practical information, support, and guidance from professionals and each other.

Yahoo Groups

Brainstem Tumors
www.yahoogroups.com/group/brainstem

Cerebellar Mutism
www.yahoogroups.com/group/cerebellarmutism

DIPG (diffuse intrinsic pontine glioma)
www.yahoogroups.com/group/DIPG

CNS Germ Cell
www.yahoogroups.com/group/germcell

Low Grade Glioma Kids
www.yahoogroups.com/group/LGGliomaKids

Optic Glioma
www.yahoogroups.com/group/optic-glioma

Pediatric Brain Tumors
www.yahoogroups.com/group/pediatricbraintumors

JPA and Adult Pilocytic Astrocytoma
www.yahoogroups.com/group/pilocyticastrocytoma

Astrocytoma Brain or Spinal Tumor
http://health.groups.yahoo.com/group/pilomyxoid

Tectal Glioma
www.yahoogroups.com/group/tectalglioma

Stem cell transplantation

BMT InfoNet
www.bmtinfonet.org

Provides accurate and medically reviewed publications and website content for patients and family members.

Survivorship resources online

Ped-Onc Resource Center Survivor Issues
www.ped-onc.org/survivors

Collection of information for families of survivors, including resources, technical and nontechnical articles, accurate information about late effects, sources of scholarships for survivors, list of survivorship clinics, and much more.

Children's Oncology Group Long-term Follow-up Guidelines
www.survivorshipguidelines.org

Downloadable document that details current knowledge about the late effects of childhood cancer. The late effects are listed by treatment (chemotherapy drug or radiation dose/site) and guidelines for diagnostic tests are provided. Includes individual "Health Links" with information about dozens of specific late effects.

Index

Antinausea drugs,
    with chemotherapy, 211
    diarrhea from, 231
    list of, 212
Apheresis, 270
Appetite changes, 387–388
    increased appetite, 388
    as side effect, 264
    stem cell transplants, 279
    as symptom, 2
Armfuls of Time: the Psychological Experience of the Child with a Life-Threatening Illness (Sourkes), 470, 502
Aromatherapy, 126, 223
    for nausea, 243
Arrhythmia, 185
Aseptic meningitis, 171
Aseptic necrosis, 185
Aspirin
    blood clotting, 225, 240
    interactions with, 194, 200
AST (aspartate aminotransferase), 479
Astrocytomas, 33–35
    brainstem gliomas, 35
    posterior fossa syndrome, 36
    radiation therapy for, 255
Ataxia, 19
Ativan, 212
Atropine with irinotecan, 198
Attention deficits, 357
Atypical teratoid/rhabdoid tumor (ATRT), 34, 40
Audiograms, 431, 433
Auditing hospital accounts, 412
Autonomic nervous system, 27
Avastin, 184

B

Back pain
    spinal cord tumors, 2
    with chemotherapy, 187
Bactrim, 200, 210, 246
Bag Balm, 232
Balanced diet, 390
Baldness. *See* Hair loss
Balloons, 126
Bathing/showering with catheter, 142
Bed wetting, 227–228
Behavioral changes
    of children, 327–334
    of parents, 334–339

    in siblings, 351, 285–291
    as symptom, 442
Benadryl, 101, 212
BCNU, 184, 246
Benign tumors, 33
Bereavement, 458–470
Bevacizumab, 184, 187
BCNU. *See* Carmustine
BiCNU, 184
Biofeedback, 78, 223
Biologic modifiers, 42, 45
Biopsy, 157
    bone marrow aspiration/biopsy, 83
    needle aspiration biopsy, 92
Bladder control
    chemotherapy, 192, 196
    postoperative complications, 170
    spinal cord tumors, 2
    symptom of recurrence, 442
Blended families, 308
Blenoxane. *See* Bleomycin
Bleomycin, 184, 187
    lung infections, 246
Blindness. *See* Vision
Blood chemistries, 82
Blood counts. *See also* Low blood counts
    complete blood cell counts (CBC), 238
    red blood cell count (RBC), 477
    white blood cell count (WBC), 478
Blood cultures, 82,
Blood draws, 82–83
Blood patch, 94
Blood transfusions, 100, 132, 166,
Blood urea nitrogen (BUN), 476, 479
BMT InfoNet, 273, 495, 510
Board certified doctors, 57, 108, 111
Body surface area (BSA), 181
Bone growth test, 83
Bone marrow aspiration/biopsy, 83
Bowel control
    postoperative complications, 170
    spinal cord tumors, 2
    symptom of recurrence, 442
Bowel perforation, 185
Bowel movements. *See also* Constipation; Diarrhea
    pain with, 2
Brachytherapy, 254
Brain, 13
    basic anatomy diagram, 19
    cerebrum, 15
    diencephalon, 21

Growth hormone injections, 267
Growth problems, 267
    bone growth x-rays, 83
Guilt
    on death of child, 462
    of parents, 338, 378
    of siblings, 287

H

Hair loss, 51, 185, 235–236
    as radiation side effect, 264
Hand washing, 238
Headaches
    from spinal taps, 94
    hydrocephalus, 163
    intracranial pressure and, 26
    radiation therapy and, 265
    symptom, 1
    symptom of recurrence, 442
Head nurses, 109
Health history, keeping, 436
Health Insurance Portability and Accountability Act
    of 1996 (HIPPA), 439
Hearing/hearing loss
    audiogram, 82
    cranial nerves controlling, 20
    eligibility for special education, 359
    late effect, 433
    stem cell transplants, 282
    symptom of recurrence, 442
Hematocrit (HCT), 475, 477
Hematuria, 185
Hemoglobin (Hgb), 477
Hemorrhagic cystitis, 185, 279
Heparin, 139, 141, 145, 146
Hepatitis
    adolescent survivors and, 435
    chicken pox complication, 247
    from transfusions, 101–102
Herpes simplex, 280
Herpes zoster, 247
Hexadrol, 184
Hickman lines, 137, 142
High blood pressure, 186
High-grade anaplastic astrocytomas, 34
Hippocampus, 16
HIV virus
    adolescent survivors and, 435
    from transfusions, 101

Hobbie, Wendy, 266, 432
Home infusion supplies, 415
Home nursing care, 139, 415
Honesty with children, 47, 326
Hormones. *See also* Growth problems
    chemotherapy, 180
    diencephalon tumors, 21
    germ cell tumors, 37
    late effects, 433
    radiation therapy and, 266
Hospice care, 453–454
Hospitals/hospitalizations
    advocating for child, 131
    chaplains, support from, 377
    choosing, 112
    doctors at, 107
    dying in, 455
    errors, checking for, 70, 132–133
    financial assistance policies, 417
    food, 128
    nurses, 109
    parent-to-parent programs, 375
    parking issues, 128
    sleeping in child's room, 131
    staff, working with, 130
    training hospitals, 107
    tumor board, 110
    waiting and, 129
Hospital social workers, 121, 156, 369
Household rules, 336
Hycamptin, 184
Hydrocephalus
    choroid plexus tumors with, 36
    development of, 26
    fourth ventricle tumors, 24
    medulloblastoma causing, 38
    postoperative complication, 170
    surgical treatment of, 163
Hydrocortisone, 248
Hydromorphone, 216, 218
Hypafix, 153
Hyperalimentation, 165, 402
Hyperfractionation, 252
Hyperglycemia, 185
Hyperpigmentation, 186
Hyperproteinuria, 186
Hyperventilation, 87, 480
Hypnosis, 76, 223
Hypocalcemia, 274
Hypoglycemia, 185

Propofol, 79
    for bone marrow aspiration/biopsy, 83
    during radiation, 259
Protein inhibitors, 180
Protocols, 70–71
Proton beam radiation, 253
Psittacosis, 250
Psychiatrists, 370, 379, 380
Psychologists, 358. *See also* Neuropsychological
   testing
    conflict mediation with, 370
    referrals to services, 379, 380
Puberty
    after stem cell transplants, 283
    late effects and, 433
    radiation therapy and, 265–267
Pulmonary edema, 282
Pulmonary function tests, 93

Q

Questions to ask
    before anesthesia, 168
    before chemotherapy, 182
    before procedures, 81
    before surgery, 166
    before radiation, 256
    before stem cell transplants, 270–271

R

Radiation oncologists, 252
Radiation recall, 200
Radiation therapy, 43, 251–268
    cognitive problems, 266
    endocrine function and, 266
    external, 252, 261
    facilities giving, 257
    growth process and, 267
    hyperfractionation, 252
    immobilization devices, 258
    intensity modulated radiation therapy (IMRT),
      252
    internal, 254, 262
    long-term side effects, 265–268
    masks, use of, 258
    personnel administering, 257
    photon beam radiation, 252
    proton beam radiation, 253
    questions about, 256

    sedation during, 259
    short-term side effects, 263–265
    simulation, 261
    stereotactic radiosurgery, 253
    tooth development and, 268
Radioimmunotherapy, 255
Radiolabeled antibodies, 255
Radiosurgery, 253
Randomization, 63, 69
Recordkeeping. *See* Financial records; Medical records
Recreation therapy rooms, 133
Rectal temperatures, 99, 239
Recurrence, 441–448
Red blood cell count (RBC), 475–477
Regression, 53, 227, 331
Rehabilitation Act. *See* 504 plans
Rehabilitation services
    occupational therapy, 175
    physical therapy, 174
    school services, 175
    speech therapy, 175
Reiki, 78, 223
Relief Band, 244
Religious community, 377
Research. *See* Clinical trials
Residents, 108
Respiratory problems. *See* Breathing problems
RNA, 180
RNs (registered nurses), 109
Roxanol. *See* Morphine
Roxicet. *See* Oxycodone
Roxilox. *See* Oxycodone
Roxycodone. *See* Oxycodone
Ruccione, Kathy, 266, 432

S

Saliva, radiation and, 230, 265
School, 347–368
    Individual Education Program (IEP), 356
    changes in performance, 357
    communicable diseases, avoiding, 354
    communicating with, 348
    early intervention services, 364
    504 plans, 355
    Individualized Family Service Plan (IFSP), 365
    preparing to return to, 348
    preventing problems on return to, 348
    rehabilitative services, 358
    returning to, 351

pulmonary edema, 282
questions to ask, 270–271
second cancers after, 283
thyroid function and, 283
tooth development and, 283
veno-occlusive disease (VOD), 282
Sterapred, 184
Stereotactic biopsy, 157
Stereotactic radiosurgery, 253
Steroids
appetite changes, 388
lung infections, 246
side effects, 248
taste of, 98
Stomatitis, 186
Stool softeners, 240
Streptokinase
for external catheter clots, 140
for subcutaneous ports, 147
Stressed children, checklist for parenting, 345
Stroke, postoperative, 170
Subarachnoid space, 24, 164
Subcutaneous injections, 181
Subcutaneous ports, 143–147
accessing, 143
care for, 145
costs of, 152
insertion of, 143
risks of, 146
Subdural grid EEGs, 87
Substance abuse by parents, 339
Sulci, 13
Sulfamethoxazole, 210, 246, 280
Summer camps, 383, 489
for siblings, 384
Sunscreen, 194, 200, 204, 239, 247, 434
Supplements
calcium supplements, 389
nutritional supplements, 401
vitamin supplements, 396
Support groups
for children, 374
online support, 373
for parents, 371
parent-to-parent programs, 375
for siblings, 375
Suppositories, 230, 239
Suprasellar area, 37, 41
Supratentorial region, 15

Surgery, 42, 155–178
biopsies, 157
complications from, 170–173
computer-guided surgery, 161
debulking, 158
discharge, 177
for hydrocephalus, 163
intraoperative monitoring, 160
palliation, 165
presurgical evaluation, 165
questions to ask, 166
resection, 158
types of, 157
Wada test before, 104
Survivorship, 431–438
employment issues, 437
follow-up care, 431
insurance for survivors, 438
late effects, 431–435
treatment summary, 435
Swallowing,
brainstem tumors, 20
gastrostomy, for, 90
posterior fossa tumors, 19
as postoperative complication, 171
tests, 97
Swimming
with external catheters, 142
pool therapy, 176
with subcutaneous ports, 146

T

Tandem transplants, 35, 44, 270
Taste, 389
chemotherapy and, 197, 229
distortion of, 190, 229
pentamidine, 210
prednisone, 98
radiation and, 265
stem cell transplant, 276
Tax deductions, 409–410
Teachers
communicating with, 300
communicable diseases, 246
help from, 317
Individual Education Program (IEP) and, 360
notifying about diagnosis, 55
siblings, communication about, 351
of terminally ill children, 367

Cancer Survivor's Treatment Record

Taking Care of Yourself for Life

This booklet helps you keep track of your medical history with:

- A summary of your cancer treatment.
- Guidelines for health monitoring that may reduce your chances of medical problems in the future.
- Suggestions for additional resources for information and assistance.

_____

Name

_____

Clinical trial name/# (if enrolled)

_____

Clinical trial name/# (if enrolled)

_____

Medical record number

General Health History Information

1. Name of disease you had: _____

2. Date of diagnosis (month/year): _____

3. Date all treatment was completed (month/year): _____

4. Date(s) of any relapses: _____

   _____

   _____

   _____

5. Place of treatment:

   Institution _____

   Address _____

   _____

   Telephone number _____

6. The doctor and/or nurse practitioner most responsible for your care:

   Name(s) _____

   _____

   _____

   _____

   Telephone number _____

Treatment Information

Chemotherapy

Drug Name	Total Dose	How Given: IV, by Mouth, Intrathecally

Surgery

Date	Type of Surgery	Surgeon's Name

Radiation Therapy

Date	Area Treated	Total Dose
_____	_____	_____
_____	_____	_____
_____	_____	_____
_____	_____	_____
_____	_____	_____

Place of treatment:

Institution _____

Address _____

_____

Telephone number _____

Your radiation therapy was supervised by:

Dr. _____

Stem Cell Transplantation

Date and Types of Transplant(s):

Month/Year/Type _____

Month/Year/Type _____

Month/Year/Type _____

Transplant Chemotherapy

Drug Name	Total Dose	How Given: IV, by Mouth, Intrathecally
_____	_____	_____
_____	_____	_____
_____	_____	_____

Transplant Radiation Therapy

Date	Area Treated	Total Dose
_____	_____	_____
_____	_____	_____
_____	_____	_____
_____	_____	_____
_____	_____	_____

Place of treatment:

Institution _____

Address _____

_____

Telephone number _____

Doctor responsible for your transplant was:

Dr. _____

Transfusions

Date Received	Type (e.g., blood, platelets)
_____	_____
_____	_____
_____	_____
_____	_____
_____	_____

Complications During Treatment

These problems were complications you had during treatment (other than fever and low blood counts):

Date	Complication
_____	_____
_____	_____
_____	_____
_____	_____
_____	_____
_____	_____

Your Medical Follow-up

These are special instructions for monitoring your health in the future, based on the treatment you received:

Treatment	Organs at Risk	Medical Tests
_____	_____	_____
_____	_____	_____
_____	_____	_____
_____	_____	_____
_____	_____	_____
_____	_____	_____
_____	_____	_____
_____	_____	_____
_____	_____	_____

Complications After Treatment

These problems were complications you had after treatment:

Date	Complication
_____	_____
_____	_____
_____	_____
_____	_____
_____	_____
_____	_____

Things To Do For Your Health

Today more people are cured of cancer than ever before. You can help yourself and anyone who gives you medical care by:

- Knowing about your disease and its treatment.

- Having checkups once a year, with a physical examination, blood count, urinalysis, and recommended tests.

- Learning the 10 steps to a healthier life and a reduced adult cancer risk suggested by the American Cancer Society.

- Making use of available resources for information and support.

- Keeping a copy of all your test results (MRI scan, echocardiogram, etc.) so they are available if needed for comparison.

Resources

Children's Oncology Group Follow-up Guidelines
www.survivorshipguidelines.org

Childhood Cancer Survivors: A Practical Guide to Your Future,
3rd edition (2012) by Keene, Hobbie, and Ruccione

Pediatric Oncology Center: Survivor Issues
www.ped-onc.org/survivors

Other Resources in Your Area

_____

_____

_____

_____

_____

_____

This Summary of Your Disease and Treatment was Prepared by:

Name _____

Date _____

Keep this copy for your records. Make copies as needed for your doctors or nurses. Contact the following person where you were treated whenever your medical condition or address changes, or if you have questions about your follow-up:

Name _____

Telephone number _____

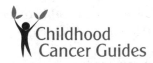

Childhood
Cancer Guides

About the Authors

Tania Shiminski-Maher received her BSN and MS in pediatric primary care from Columbia University and holds an academic appointment to the faculty of Columbia University School of Nursing. She is certified as a pediatric nurse practitioner and has held past certification as clinical neuroscience registered nurse and pediatric oncology nurse. For the past 30 years, she has worked as a pediatric nurse practitioner in pediatric neurosurgery and pediatric neuro-oncology and has published extensively in the areas of pediatric brain tumors, hydrocephalus, and multidisciplinary team communication. She has been a member of the Children's Cancer Group (CCG) and Children's Oncology Group (COG)—consortiums of researchers from more than 300 institutions that treat children with cancer—for the past 25 years.

Catherine Woodman received her BA in biology and her MD from Brown University, and she completed her residency at the University of California, San Francisco. She has been on the faculty at the University of Iowa in the departments of psychiatry and family medicine for more than 20 years. She has served as a member of COG for 10 years and is on its Patient Advocacy Committee, Ethics Steering Committee, and Central Nervous System Tumors Steering Committee. In addition, Dr. Woodman is currently a member of the Phase I/Phase II Data Safety Monitoring Committee, and she served on the National Cancer Institute's Pediatric Central Institutional Review Board for 6 years. She has published numerous papers related to ethics of pediatric research and late effects of treatment for childhood cancer. Her 19-year-old son is a survivor of medulloblastoma.

Nancy Keene, a well-known writer and advocate for children with cancer, is the parent of a 22-year survivor of high-risk acute lymphoblastic leukemia. She is one of the founders of the nonprofit Childhood Cancer Guides, and she has written many books for families of children with cancer, including *Childhood Leukemia; Your Child in the Hospital;* and *Chemo, Craziness, and Comfort.* She co-authored *Childhood Cancer: A Parent's Guide to Solid Tumor Cancers* and *Childhood Cancer Survivors: A Practical Guide to Your Future* and edited *Educating the Child with Cancer.* She served as chair of the Patient Advocacy Committees of both CCG and COG. Ms. Keene has been interviewed on National Public Radio about childhood cancer survivorship, frequently speaks to professional and parent groups, and has participated in online pediatric cancer support groups (*www.acor.org*) since they began in 1996.

Childhood Cancer Guides™

Questions Answered
Experiences Shared

When your life is turned upside down, your need for information is great. You have to make critical medical decisions, often with what seems like little to go on. Plus, you have to break the news to family, quiet your own fears, help your ill child and your other children, figure out how you are going to pay the bills, and sometimes get to work or put dinner on the table.

Childhood Cancer Guides provide authoritative information for the families and friends of children with cancer or survivors of childhood cancer. Our books cover all aspects of how these illnesses affect family life. In each book, there's a mix of:

- **Medical information**
  Dozens of experts on childhood cancer and survivorship contributed to these books to provide state-of-the-art information to help you weigh treatment options. Modern medicine has much to offer. When there are treatment controversies, we present differing points of view.

- **Practical information**
  After making treatment decisions, life focuses on coping with treatment and any late effects that develop. We cover day-to-day practicalities, such as those you'd hear from a helpful nurse or a knowledgeable support group.

- **Emotional support**
  It's normal to have strong reactions to a condition that threatens your child's life. It's normal that the whole family is affected. We cover issues such as the shock of diagnosis, living with uncertainty, and communicating with loved ones.

Each book contains stories from parents, children, and siblings who share, in their own words, the lessons they have learned and what truly helped them cope.

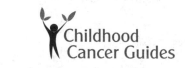

www.childhoodcancerguides.org

Other Books for Families

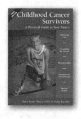

Childhood Cancer Survivors
A Practical Guide to Your Future, 3rd Edition

By Nancy Keene, Wendy Hobbie & Kathy Ruccione
ISBN 9781941089101, Paperback, 6" x 9", $29.95, 452 pages

"An extraordinary resource for survivors of childhood cancer, as well as for their families, caregivers, and friends."

— Barbara Hoffman, JD
Editor, *A Cancer Survivor's Almanac:*
Charting Your Journey

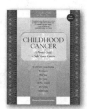

Childhood Cancer
A Parent's Guide to Solid Tumor Cancers, 2nd Edition

By Honna Janes-Hodder & Nancy Keene
ISBN 9781941089156, Paperback, 7" x 9", $29.95, 537 pages

"I recommend [this book] most highly for those in need of high-level, helpful knowledge that will empower and help parents and caregivers to cope."

— Mark Greenberg, MD
Professor of Pediatrics, University of Toronto

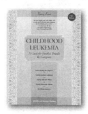

Childhood Leukemia
A Guide for Families, Friends & Caregivers, 4th Edition

By Nancy Keene
ISBN 9781941089057, Paperback, 7" x 9", $29.95, 503 pages

"What's so compelling about Childhood Leukemia is the amount of useful medical information and practical advice it contains. Keene avoids jargon and lays out what's needed to deal with the medical system."

—The Washington Post

Our helpful guides are available at
an online bookseller or a bookstore near you.